The Challenges of Integrating Religion and Spirituality into Psychotherapy

This book examines personal and professional understandings of religion in psychotherapy and advocates for integrity, competency, and cultural pluralism in clinical practice.

A major feature of this book is that it confirms the massive proliferation of religion-oriented approaches to counseling and therapy in recent years. It attributes this rise to opportunism and exaggerated individualism among therapists and to the frequent failures of professional associations, clinical preparation programs, and other influences. In response to these influences, it identifies the need for guiding principles for integrating religion into therapy, discusses the religious issues that clients bring to therapy, and advocates for major changes in clinical practice, with emphasis on integrity and competence. Building on a large volume of research and using evidence-based conclusions, it clarifies how these two major features of contemporary life can be integrated with integrity and competence. The author maintains that religion should be a feature of the practice of counseling and therapy, so long as it addresses the clinically relevant needs of clients. However, it also explores how the religion of counselors and therapists often expresses the needs of counselors and therapists, instead of addressing the needs of their clients.

In the context of these questions and discussion of contentious challenges, this book provides guidelines for relating religion with clinical practice and recommends needed actions by clinical preparation programs, professional associations, individual therapists, state legislatures, licensing boards, social service agencies, and corporations. All of this stands on the conspicuous need for professional accountability in the delivery of mental health care.

Francis A. Martin is an Adjunct Instructor at Lipscomb University, USA, and Executive Director with The Center for Clinical Training.

Advances in Mental Health Research series

Books in this series:

Schizotypy
New Dimensions
Edited by Oliver Mason and Gordon Claridge

Supervision and Treatment Experiences of Probationers with Mental Illness
Analyses of Contemporary Issues in Community Corrections
Babatunde Oluwaseun Adekson

Mental Wellbeing and Psychology
The Role of Art and History in Self Discovery and Creation
Sue Barker with Louise Jensen and Hamed Al Battashi

Neurolinguistic Programming in Clinical Settings
Theory and Evidence-Based Practice
Edited by Lisa de Rijk, Richard Gray, and Frank Bourke

A Study into Infant Mental Health
Drawing Together Perspectives of International Research, Theory, and Practical Intervention
Hazel G. Whitters

Film/Video-Based Therapy and Trauma
Research and Practice
Joshua L. Cohen

In-Patient Mental Health Care from the Asylum System to the Present Day
A Lived Experience of Policy and Practice
Andrew Colley

The Challenges of Integrating Religion and Spirituality into Psychotherapy

Integrity, Competence, and Cultural Pluralism in Clinical Practice

Francis A. Martin

Routledge
Taylor & Francis Group
NEW YORK AND LONDON

First published 2024
by Routledge
605 Third Avenue, New York, NY 10158

and by Routledge
4 Park Square, Milton Park, Abingdon, Oxon, OX14 4RN

Routledge is an imprint of the Taylor & Francis Group, an informa business

ISBN: 978-1-032-71457-8 (hbk)
ISBN: 978-1-032-75117-7 (pbk)
ISBN: 978-1-003-47246-9 (ebk)

DOI: 10.4324/9781003472469

Typeset in Galliard
by MPS Limited, Dehradun

The recognition of being permanently human and,
therefore, indefinitely unfinished,
sometimes challenges our most basic sensitivities and
beckons us to mask or divert the vulnerability
that comes with this recognition.
But also there are those among us who engage
with their humanity with integrity, courage, and
devotion to the truth of being genuinely human,
while also skillfully inviting others to do this, too.
My friend, Harvey, is one of them.

Therefore, with unspeakable gratitude,
this book is dedicated to
Harvey A. Hester, PhD

Contents

Introduction

Despite efforts to maintain maximal openness to alternate points of view, no one composes a document of this kind in an entirely neutral manner. After all, each one of us is a creature of our culture, including our respective individual family culture. Nevertheless, this book is an effort to share ideas that are open, honest, judicious, welcoming, and helpful. These features of the book are firmly supported by numerous resources. In composing the book, I sought to avoid assumptions and conclusions about the place of religion in the practice of counseling and therapy, while recognizing the importance of searching for ways to understand the issue and demonstrating a readiness to express my points of view. Still, instead of offering only points of view, including mine or others, I have sought to offer ways to think about this issue, based on a considerable body of evidence.

The evidence must be taken seriously. No doubt, the evidence that I have gathered, and the evidence from many others that is cited in this book, may be discomfiting. Probably, when readers see the numerous specifically religious approaches to counseling and therapy throughout this book, they may justifiably wonder how their profession could have reached such a disturbing situation and what, if anything, they may do to improve their profession. And if they count the number of these approaches, they will discover more than 1,000 of them in this book and rightly conclude that there are many, many more than 1,000 specifically religious approaches to counseling and therapy. Then, when they include the multiple, readily available fake academic degrees and licenses that numerous counselors and therapists acquire, they may feel rising cynicism about their profession. Worse, these things and many others may prompt the thought that the book is a product of cynicism about our profession. In truth, the book is just the opposite of cynicism. Instead of cynicism, I aspire to endorse our profession as a significant source of good, healing, optimism, and social change. Having many years of experience in our profession, I am aware of many of my peers who demonstrate their clinical prowess, strength of character, and important personal values that increase the likelihood that

DOI: 10.4324/9781003472469-1

they have delivered and will continue to deliver excellent professional services for their clients.

For example, my professional peer who attends to the intense and prolonged anguish of a suicidal client requires courage from my peer and admiration from me. Similarly, another professional peer who endures insults from an angry and recalcitrant adolescent whose emotional injuries necessitate years of clinical competence and human compassion, likewise, requires my peer's solid grounding in personal mental health and admiration from me. Another professional peer who suffered personal anguish from multiple tragedies that have befallen his family and who believed strongly enough in our profession to utilize it as a guide for his recovery requires faith in his honest and professional understanding of our profession also demands admiration from me. So, instead of thoughts from cynicism that energized the work on this book, thoughts from inspiration, assurance, hopefulness, confidence, and optimism have energized my work. Moreover, these are the thoughts that have led to the necessity of this book.

Aiming to leave no unnecessary ambiguity about my personal views and as readers will repeatedly discover, I have concluded two things that relate to almost everything in this book. One, religion has a place in counseling and therapy. Two, most of the expressions of religion in counseling and therapy should be eliminated because they obviously compromise, if not harm, the profession of counseling and therapy and clients who need professional services from counselors and therapists.

Probably, at this time, the question of the place of religion in the practice of counseling and therapy is more important than the answer. The matter needs widespread discussion and commitments to action, with many of these actions proposed in this book. While each of us has answers, the evidence makes clear that none of our answers is widely accepted. To be sure, the question needs an answer(s). The necessity of answering the question of the place of religion in the practice of counseling and therapy comes from many sources but receives confirmation in this book. Among other consequences of not having generally agreed-upon answers, the basic character of counseling and therapy cannot be known, understood, practiced, and confidently shared, without them. Such consequences necessitate the emphasis on integrity, competence, and pluralism in the clinical practice of counseling and therapy. The much too conspicuous lack of integrity, competence, and ethically solid pluralism in clinical practice places counseling and therapy in peril.

For now, a brief discussion of some relevant numbers may be useful. My research has so far identified more than 5,000 titles of specifically religious approaches to counseling and therapy. Many are identified in this book. Quite apart from every other consideration, the fact of more than 5,000 advertised, specifically religious approaches begs for understanding of how religion may or may not have a place in clinical practice. My hope is that this book may help to create such understanding, recognizing that we must collectively seek it. Without understanding the place of religion in the practice of counseling and therapy, the clinical community will maintain its slide toward irrelevancy, due to its copious avoidance of attempts to define what counseling and therapy are and, therefore, to determine what is or is not an appropriate approach to counseling and therapy, whether the approach is religious or another kind of ideology.

What Is Religion?

Many scholars address the evolving nature of the place of religion in counseling and therapy. While a brief characterization of the evolution may be too simple, it may be briefly characterized, nevertheless. It began with *suspicion* about almost all expressions of religion. After all, for example, Sigmund Freud endured the somewhat painful and prolonged anti-Semitism that understandably skewed his view of religion. Thus, due to Freud's and others' influence, religion was frequently viewed as pathological. From suspicion, the mental health movement evolved into a period when, mainly due to the pastoral psychology and therapy advocated by orthodox Christians, *tension and argument* characterized the relationship between counseling and therapy, on the one side, and religion, on the other side, with proponents of integration being caught uncomfortably in the middle. Then, this morphed into *questions and doubt* about how religion could possibly be a positive feature of treatment. Currently, instead of questioning and doubting whether religion has a place in counseling and therapy, the prevailing view is that it has a place, but that the place is not entirely clear. Thus, the current phase of evolving places an emphasis on *how religion may be clinically and ethically understood* in the conduct of counseling and therapy. Thus, research and opinions about the ethics of the place of religion in counseling and therapy are common.

Because religion is the major focus of this book, particularly in the context of counseling and therapy, a necessary question is "What is religion?" In short, religion among counselors and therapists or in the larger world is whatever an individual or group of individuals says that it is. This answer may be as sufficient as it is disappointing. Surely, a more precise definition of religion could be offered here. However, as this book clearly demonstrates, religion or religion-related ideologies can be almost anything that an individual or group of individuals wants it to be. Sun worship may not be widely practiced, but this could be an expression of religion. Or, Heaven's Gate likely died when its adherents killed themselves, but it was an expression of religion. Much more conventionally than sun worship or Heaven's Gate adherents, "Christian" can mean almost anything. Indeed, as this book confirms, thousands of presumed approaches to counseling and therapy are "Christian."

To mitigate against the appearance of conveniently escaping from answering the question about what religion is, some of the commonly recognized qualities of religion presumably inhere in the numerous expressions of religion that are identified in this book. Among those who are religious, veneration of a person or object, such as Jesus Christ, is common. A set of values, such as holding marriage as a sacred bond, is similarly common. Along with veneration and values, specific beliefs, such as believing that God is good or that the Bible is the Word of God, are common representatives of religion. Also, typically, religion gathers and expresses a wide array of social and cultural norms such as altruistic ministry or sexual purity. For many of those who are religious, their religion gives them positive meaning, enabling them to conclude that life makes sense or that their respective personal lives have important positive meaning. No doubt, religion is more complex than these qualities indicate.

For clarity, this book is not about any particular religious orientation such as a Christian orientation. Whether a Christian approach to therapy or any other religious or clinical approach is preferred by a therapist, the overwhelming presence of Christian-related therapies in the Western World must be considered. As noted elsewhere in the book, I located 278 Buddhist models/approaches to therapy and 3,908 Christian models/approaches. To frame the matter differently, the book is not about whether counseling and therapy are Christian or should be about being Christian. The more fundamental matter is whether therapy can be both clinical and religious. And, if it can be both, what is the place of religion in therapy?

An operative assumption here is that the religious experience of clients may be and often is a feature of helping them. Insofar as clients' religious experience is clinically relevant, it should be a component of treatment. Several of the religion-related issues that clients bring to therapy are addressed in this book. Mostly, though, the focus here is the religious experience and views of counselors and therapists, as Chapters 1–6 indicate. With this in mind, the compelling question here is "If the religious experience and views of counselors and therapists may be applied to their professional work, how and in what ways should this be understood?" Does this understanding strengthen the integrity of counseling and therapy and elevate competence or not? To answer the question, several guidelines are offered in Chapter 6.

To emphasize the significance of religion-related concerns, Chapter 7 gives attention to "Clients' Religion in Therapy." Along with the rest of the book, this chapter is intended to be a strong and clear affirmation of counseling and therapy, on therapists' side of the clinical relationship, and the religion-related concerns of clients, on the client's side. Indeed, while the book describes several important concerns, its unambiguous aim is to affirm clinical work and the clients who are served by it. Therefore, the book includes a chapter on the religion-related issues that clients present. It places a priority on the necessary well-being of clients.

Much of the method of presentation in this book is a descriptive analysis of the current place of religion in the practice of counseling and therapy. However, this analysis receives considerable support from the research of others. As such, instead of standing alone, it joins a large and longstanding conversation. A couple of the voices in this conversation may suffice, for now, as illustrations. Religion is both an accelerant of personal problems and a source of hope and healing. McGraw, Skidmore, Lefevor, Docherty, and Mahone (2023, p. 303) conclude that religion is a contributor to personal problems. In contrast, Jerome, Heath, Williams, Winters, and Cutrer-Pårraga (2023, p. 186) conclude that religion is a contributor to successful coping with trauma.

The primary aim of the book, though, significantly extends beyond analysis and gathering of research. It is to contribute quite specific ways of understanding and practicing integrity and competence in the delivery of professional services and of recommending several specific ways to improve integrity and competence in clinical practice. These ways become manifestly visible in Chapters 6–9. A brief guide to the chapters looks like this.

Chapter 1, Religious Opportunism in Counseling and Therapy, provides details and analysis of the impact of the proliferation of religion-oriented approaches to counseling and therapy. It concludes that this proliferation arises from opportunism, more than anything else.

Chapter 2, Excessive Individualism as Therapy, briefly explains the current proliferation of religion-oriented approaches to counseling and therapy as an expression of exaggerated individualism among counselors and therapists. As such, this chapter partially accounts for the proliferation of religion-related approaches to counseling and therapy.

Chapter 3, Mercenary Organizations, describes in detail the multiple ways that religion-associated organizations have co-opted counseling and therapy. While they have no professional standing, they sell licenses, promote approaches to therapy that have no clinical bases, and allow or endorse treatments that their so-called "licensees" are not qualified to provide.

Chapter 4, Equivocating Allies, presents individuals and institutions that conspicuously presume to deliver counseling and therapy, mostly through their close-mindedness and largely non-clinical approach to counseling and therapy.

Chapter 5, Career Counseling for Therapy, offers conclusions about the current crisis-laden condition of counseling and therapy, with emphasis on the multiple compromises of their integrity and, very likely, their competence. It describes of the current vulnerabilities and compromises in the clinical work of practicing counselors and therapists.

Chapter 6, How To Relate Religion with Therapy: Guiding Principles, initiates ten principles that are intended to facilitate the integration of religion into therapy.

Chapter 7, Clients' Religion in Therapy, includes a discussion of several recent research initiatives about religion in therapy, reports about several useful orientations to understanding religion in therapy, and describes many of the specifically religious issues that clients bring to therapy.

Chapter 8, How To Improve Graduate Preparation for Clinical Practice, aims to analyze specific problems and recommend several actions that should be taken by preparation programs. It includes a detailed discussion of specialized accreditation, with emphasis on several weaknesses in it and ways to improve it. The chapter both affirms the significance of religion-related preparation in preparation programs and emphasizes the need to ensure its professionalization.

Chapter 9, Advocacy among Therapists and Their Constituencies, aims to recommend needed actions by individual counselors and therapists, professional associations, licensing boards and state legislatures, and businesses and corporations. The need for major changes in counseling and therapy receives specific recommendations for actions by these major constituencies.

Chapter 10, Integrity: Aspirations and Encouragement, offers an endorsement of counseling and therapy, with a clear and positive view of therapists and their future.

Integrity, Competence, Cultural Pluralism, and Integration

This book contains a significant volume of evidence. Some of the evidence is truly discomfiting. Nevertheless, the evidence points to the need to argue for integrity, competence, and cultural pluralism in counseling and therapy. This need likely creates a surge of urgency, when the evidence that calls for addressing it is taken into account. The need, though, is no mere discussion that a book like this contains. It is a need that is seen in the faces of tormented individuals who seek help from mental health care providers and, sometimes tragically, receive services that exacerbate their torment. It is a need that begs the question, "Knowing what I know about mental health care—particularly from those whose priority appears to be one of expressing their religious zealotry—would I recommend that my spouse or child seek help, even when both of us recognize the need for help?"

Integrity mandates that counselors and therapists are in reality who they say they are. This is to say that, as the profession evolves based on the best information and evidence available, counselors and therapists persist in their growth toward increasing effectiveness within the demonstrable boundaries of their individual competencies.

As a minimal standard, the necessity of clinically relevant competence is that counselors and therapists are demonstrably capable of engaging their clients in clinically relevant change. Objectively and consistently, they can provide documentation of their ability to achieve desirable and clinically relevant goals with their clients.

Foremost, cultural pluralism acknowledges that each of us is surrounded by others who are different from us. The list of differences is too long to list. Still, whatever differences each of us may see on any given day, they are

The young woman who despises her physique because she was born with *spina bifida* and lacks ability to walk independently.
The stock broker who earns more than she could have imagined when she began her career.
The gathered family who attends a middle school graduation.
The elite athletes who feel confusion from the fans of those who support opposing elite athletes and yell obscenities.
The city councilman who feels and sometimes enjoys the tension of wanting to satisfy all of his constituents.
The elderly man at the fruit counter in the supermarket selecting oranges to take home.
The polite and optimistic wives who nurture their dying husbands, knowing that they have faithfully loved each other until "death do us part."
The icing-smeared one-year-old whose birthday cake is more an adornment than a delicious dessert.
The nine year-old boy who is helping his mother to change a ceiling light bulb.
The expectant, soon-to-be father who cannot stop pacing, as his wife gives birth.
The newly married couple who find fulfillment in their shared joy.
The lineman who installs wires to bring electrical power to a new neighborhood.
The grandmother who silently reads her daily paper and contemplates whom she will vote for in the upcoming election.
The middle-aged jogger whose lungs are burning, causing her to wonder whether she can meet her jogging goals today.
The crowd sitting pensively in the waiting room at a medical clinic.
Mom and dad who vigorously wave at their daughter as she drives away to a distant college.
The weary employee who frequently and eagerly anticipates the nearest possible date for retirement.

The young child who excitedly races into the donut shop ahead of his grandfather.
The bankruptcy judge who continues to wonder how and why so many individuals get themselves in financial trouble.

None of us can be all of these individuals, but we can recognize ourselves in them. We are they! Each one shares our humanity. We are pluralism. Altogether, we are pluralism. While each of us should and will seek to meet our individual needs, pluralism compels us to act toward others as we want them to act toward us. This is pluralism that is well-informed, adaptive, and liberating.

Somewhat naturally, cultural pluralism requires that those who live in it also must make sense of it. Probably, the worst sense that may be made of pluralism is that those who are different from "me" should not have as much as I want or have and that "they" are to be feared, vigorously opposed, and suppressed. The best sense that may be made of pluralism is seen in therapists who do well what competent therapists do. They engage their clients in change. They seek to lower the level of unnecessary conflict or eliminate it. They actively seek to assist their clients with reframing their thoughts and behaviors in relation to clinically relevant problems. Allowing for this, the fact is that some differences can be scary. And, to be sure, some individuals are scary—and dangerous. Most others though are neither scary nor dangerous. Reframing teaches us this. As presented above as individuals, others are pretty much like the rest of us. They get hungry and they eat. They feel lonely and join family or friends. They have aspirations toward achievements and seek to fulfill them. They laugh at jokes. They lose loved ones to death and grieve. Mostly, they seek to live with love and peace, secure in believing that today is okay and that tomorrow may be better. And, they want love and peace with others. This is the heart of pluralism.

In mental health care, the language may not be "love and peace." To get there, though, as outcomes of therapy, therapists exhibit demonstrable commitments to integrity, competence, and cultural pluralism. In the process of fulfilling such commitments, therapists remember and gladly affirm their humanity—all humanity—just as they seek to affirm themselves as individuals. Thus, in the context of discussions about pluralism in mental health care, welcoming of differences is a necessity. In the absence of welcoming differences among therapists, what takes its place? Intolerance? Ideological purity? Clinical incompetence? Alienation? What else? In welcoming differences, clients who are severely depressed are welcome. Chronic substance abusers are welcome. Overanxious students are welcome. Terminally ill clients are welcome. Embezzlers are welcome. Divorcees are welcome. Fragmented, hostile families are welcome. Tightly wound perfectionists are welcome. And so on. Therapists welcome differences. By definition, competent therapists are cultural pluralists.

What could a viable, intellectually honest, and clinically appropriate integration of religion and therapy be? Obviously, given the profession's commitment to pluralism, integration has been and will take more than one form. This ambiguity should not dissuade counselors and therapists from seeking the integration of religion and therapy that responds to the clinically relevant needs of their clients. Toward this, they may adopt the principles of Integrative Therapy. As simple as this may appear, Integrative Therapy has been more than a singular concept, as Hoffart and Hoffart (2014) succinctly report. Drawing from Norcross, they indicate that

> In *theoretical integration*, two or more theories are synthesized. In *technical eclecticism*, techniques are drawn from different and sometimes divergent theories in the approach to a particular case. *Assimilative integration* involves grounding oneself in one single theory of psychotherapy but with a view to incorporating or assimilating practices and views from other systems. Finally, common *factors integration* seeks to determine the core ingredients that different therapies have in common. (p. 263) (Italicized words appear in the original.)

Also, Integrative Therapy has been an evolving and major orientation among counselors and therapists. Norcross, Rocha, and Chrysler (2023, p. 5) report that psychologists who indicate a preference for integrative approaches to therapy rose from 30% in 1981 to 86% in 2022. The several types of Integrative Therapy and its ongoing evolution should not obscure its underlying principles. The principles can serve as a general orientation for integrating religion and therapy. On the one side, Integrative Therapy aims to release counselors and therapists from the constraints of a particular set of methods or self-contained, limiting theoretical orientations. On the other side, it aims to provide treatments that have been confirmed by broadly agreed-upon research about effective treatments. Thus, the significance of integration in the practice of therapy is that it holds these two principles in tension. The anticipated outcomes of maintaining this tension are (1) demonstrable improvement in the efficacy and efficiency of treatment and (2) clinically relevant adaptation to the specific needs of clients. A substantial interpretation of these dynamics appears in Castonguay, Eubanks, Goldfried, Muran, and Lutz (2015), "Research on psychotherapy integration: building on the past, looking to the future."

Just as a medical provider treats specific needs (e.g., broken ankle, diabetes, or sleep apnea), Integrative Therapy clearly embodies the expectation that its treatment is individualized. Based on this orientation, Integrative Therapy almost inexorably also becomes flexible and holistic. As such, it neither excludes religion from clinical practice nor advocates for its inclusion. However, when religion is included, the treatment that includes it should be open to the scrutiny of the professional community in which the therapist is a member, so long as the community advocates for professional accountability, including evidence-based and empirically affirmed treatments.

Guidelines

So far, no one has been able to issue guidelines for relating religion to counseling and therapy with which almost everyone else would agree. The guidelines here very likely maintain this inability. Nevertheless, as an individual who has major interests in both of these major features of being a contemporary therapist, I hope to offer some useful ideas. The guidelines emerge from a professional context that must be described. This description takes much of the book to present, analogous to a detailed case conceptualization.

The guidelines for how to relate religion and the practice of counseling and therapy are relevant and significant for the future of counseling and therapy. However, the future of counseling and therapy likely does not depend on the integration of these guidelines into clinical practice, although they would very likely make a positive difference if they were widely implemented. Instead, if nothing else, this book makes clear the need for integrity and competence in the practice of counseling and therapy, with or without specific reference to the guidelines that this book proposes. The need is immense, pressing, and determinative. Without attention to it, counseling and therapy will exist—or fail to exist—in a perilous future.

Clearly, many individuals have given serious attention to various topics related to the place of religion in the practice of counseling and therapy. For example, both secular and religious counselors and therapists have addressed the psychology of religion. Their contributions are presumed to be relevant to the discussion here, although this discussion is not about the psychology of religion. By analogy, a study of the psychology of parenting is relevant to a discussion of how to view family life, but it is not necessarily useful in the context of conducting therapy.

Much closer to the discussion here is the question of how counselors and therapists may be trained to maintain their clinical effectiveness while also utilizing or not their individual understanding of their religion. Many have given attention to this issue, too. For example, Rupert, Moon, and Sandage (2019) have developed clinical training groups for spirituality and religion in therapy. They have developed "SERT groups" for mental health care providers. They explain the acronym SERT in the following terms. An explanation of their model requires more than this brief mention of it covers. Suffice it to report that the "S" stands for spirituality; the "E" stands for existential; the "R" stands for religion; and the "T" stands for theology and other traditions or systems of thought and meaning-making (Rupert et al, pp. 164–166).

This serious, thoughtful, and practical effort to answer important questions about the place of religion in the practice of counseling and therapy deserves attention and support. Another kind of effort toward understanding the place of religion in the practice of counseling and therapy has been attempts to clarify professional, ethical responsibilities for mental health care providers. One of many valuable resources is the contribution of Barnett and Johnson (2011). While their answers cannot be complete to the degree that they cover all clinical and personal contingencies, they offer a valuable decision-making model. In the end, Barnett and Johnson (pp. 161–162) conclude, "The practice of psychotherapy with religious and spiritual clients can be highly effective and rewarding." However, they continue, "Yet … it can present psychotherapists with a number of challenges and dilemmas that can make ethical and clinically effective treatment difficult to accomplish. These challenging situations often present psychotherapists with a range of options without a clear best course of action. The use of the proposed ethical decision-making process model should be of value to psychotherapists facing these situations." Their decision-making model contributes specific ways to increase ethical propriety with regard to several important features therapists attempt to integrate religion and therapy.

This book adds to the urgency for re-examining ways to integrate religion and therapy, by observing that current clinical practice is characterized by a massive proliferation of specifically religious approaches to counseling and therapy, with surges in numbers that outpace the rapid rise in the number of counselors and therapists. It provides needed details about this proliferation, along with the evidence that clearly shows how this proliferation seriously compromises the integrity and competence of counseling and therapy and likely suppresses cultural pluralism in clinical services.

About the Big List

During the last seven or eight decades, the tension between clinical humanism and religious orthodoxy has been stalemated, from my view. Focusing narrowly on this tension has often precluded awareness of other important social changes during these decades that influence views of the relation between religion and therapy. Some of the other major social changes include widespread economic freedom, rapid redefinitions of sex roles, surges of interest in civil rights, the rise of technology, ongoing revisions in kinds of work and employment, and many others. Surely, turmoil and major advances characterize these decades. Also, note should be made of the fact that mental health care has been another constantly expanding movement during the last seven decades.

Within the mental health movement during the past several decades, the social dynamics referred to above have influenced how counseling and therapy are conducted. Back then, psychoanalysis dominated the practice of psychotherapy. Back then, alternates to heterosexuality were regarded as abnormal. Also, back then, religion lived mostly on the fringes of the practice of therapy. Along with other reports, my research (Martin, 2020) has confirmed the rapid rise in visibility of specifically religious practices in the delivery of counseling and psychotherapy. In this book, the information indicates that there are more than 5,000 titles of specifically religious approaches to counseling and therapy, along with another 10,000 or so that are religion-related. More than 1,100 of these approaches are included in this book.

The religious and religion-related approaches were not located solely for the purpose of including them in this book. Instead, over a period of years, I have compiled a list of approaches to counseling and therapy. Due to its size, I have come to refer to the list as "the Big List." The Big List of treatment orientations is truly big! So far, the number of treatment orientations that have been gathered from the advertising by practicing counselors and therapists is 38,373. This is a staggering number. Fifteen years ago, I could never have imagined that anyone could locate as many as I have found so far. To be sure, it is a staggering number. While the number may be a little less staggering, when specific caveats are added to it, it will likely remain a knee-buckling number. Given its potential significance, a compelling question about the Big List is "How was the information gathered?" Another question is "What, if anything, apart from this book, has been done with the Big List?"

Interest in the research that led to the Big List was ignited by experience with my peers. In short, approximately 14 years ago, following invitations to view their websites, I visited several of them. One of my professional peers had a website that I visited. The information on his website was shocking because it indicated that as a new licensee he advertised his expertise in an unusually large number—38—of treatment models, including models in which he probably lacked expertise. For example, he listed psychoanalysis as one of his models of therapy. He had no expertise in psychoanalysis. Another peer listed Christian Counseling as one of her specializations, although she had no training or other experience that would qualify her as a Christian counselor. A third peer identified eating disorders as one of his specialties, although he had no experience with eating disorders, except for passing glances at them during graduate classes. While these incongruities continue to confound me, they were more confounding back then than they are now.

These experiences prompted me to visit the websites of other peers. With no defined expectations, I easily located other strange features of what counselors and therapists said that they were doing. Believing that my findings needed to be shared with my colleagues, I prepared papers and shared them. I delivered professional presentations about my findings. I prepared two books that reflected some of my findings. With Janet Turner, one was *Clinical Supervision in the Real World* (2020). Much more directly related to aberrant approaches to therapy, the other book was *Therapy Thieves: How To Save Mental Health Care from Its Providers* (2020). Among other things, *Therapy Thieves* provides profiles of therapists' representation of their professional services in analyses of urban v. rural therapists, comparative reports about several major cities, graduates of accredited v. unaccredited preparation programs, gender differences, types of institutions where licensees completed their training, and data about "appropriate" and "inappropriate" approaches to counseling and therapy, among other things. Recently, along with Janet Turner and Jennifer Fugate (Martin, Turner & Fugate, 2023), I prepared a research article, Post-Degree Clinical Supervision in Tennessee: A Report about the Advertising by Supervision Dyads, that is scheduled for publication.

The published analyses of various iterations of the Big List constitute a useful record. However, in this discussion, I should assist readers with their need—insofar as there is a need—to understand the number, 38,373. Some observations about it may be helpful. Each observation stems not only from an interest in candor about the condition of counseling and therapy but also from an interest in judicious openness to the discretion and aspirations of those who advertise their approaches.

First, the number, 38,373 could be and, no doubt, will be larger. It is the number that was reached when the constraints of time indicated that counting approaches to counseling and therapy should stop so that analyzing the gathered evidence could be completed. Without stopping and engaging in analysis, the Big List would be little more than merely counting.

Second, throughout the Big List, some treatment approaches overlap with approaches that are very similar. For example, both Christian Creation Therapy and the Christian Creationist Approach are included. Are they the same thing? Given reasonable doubt about whether they are the same thing, both are included in the Big List. Similarly, are Rogerian Therapy and Person-centered Therapy the same thing? The manner of the presentations of these approaches suggests that they may or may not be the same thing. To extend and further clarify the challenge of what to include on the Big List, are Classical Psychoanalysis and Psychoanalysis the same thing? Recognizing that these two approaches obviously overlap with regard to their probable, similar meanings, both are included on the Big List. In most cases, allowing for inevitable overlapping among approaches to counseling and therapy, both or more are included.

Exaggeration of the number of approaches must be avoided. Therefore, recognizing that many approaches to counseling and therapy that are included on the Big List are closely similar to others that are listed separately, a very liberal estimate of these approaches is approximately 10% or approximately 4,000. Toward attempting to maintain the avoidance of any suggestion that the number of treatment approaches identified by practicing counselors and therapists may be inflated and to ensure that the estimate of overlapping approaches cannot be an issue of concern, the estimate of overlapping approaches is arbitrarily raised to 20% or approximately 8,000. This reduces the total to a number around 30,000 approaches.

Third, many counselors and therapists identify a specific clientele whose mental health needs they seek to meet and refer to the clientele as a treatment orientation. Some examples may help to make this clear. Apparently, "Women's Therapy" is understood to be both a designation of a specific clientele and an approach to therapy. Similarly, another commonly identified treatment orientation is "Christian Counseling." Is this counseling for those who are Christian or a treatment approach that somehow may be "Christian" or both? Some counselors and therapists make clear that it is a service that is intended for Christians, while others advertise it as a clinical orientation. When counselors and therapists say that an approach is clinical, it is included, regardless of my view of it. For example, is Goat Therapy or Chicken Therapy a real thing? For the purpose of accurate representation of what therapists say that they offer, it is included on the Big List.

Fourth, acronyms present a dilemma, because their meaning sometimes cannot be readily determined, although at a glance, their meaning is often taken for granted. However, due to uncertainty about their meaning, they are included. Among numerous others, common and sometimes unidentifiable acronyms are EFT, ACT, and CBT. What are they? Or, are they what most counselors and therapists believe they are? At least, they should not be presumed to refer to Emotion Focused Therapy, Acceptance and Commitment Therapy, and Cognitive Behavior Therapy. Such a presumption may be a mistake—an understandable or even predictable mistake.

What is the meaning of "EFT?" Is it "Emotion Focused Therapy?" Or, is it "Emotional Freedom Techniques?" Or, is it "Energy Field Therapy?" Or, is it "Emotional Freedom Tapping?" Or, is it "Energy Freedom Therapy?" It may be any of these or something else. Similarly, what is "ACT?" As an acronym, ACT is included in the Big List. Probably, ACT is generally understood to be Acceptance and Commitment Therapy, but it may refer to several different approaches. For example, it may refer to Advanced Christian Therapy, Advanced Callahan Techniques, Acceptance and Compassion Therapy, Adolescent Creative Therapy, Action and Commitment Therapy, Advanced Counseling Therapies, Accelerated Compassionate Therapy, and Assertive Community Treatment.

Fifth, no doubt, numerous approaches advertised by counselors and therapists make little clinical sense. These approaches may be reasonably determined to be inappropriate or unethical. Regardless of the conclusion about any one of them, the fact is that they are numerous. Readers will likely have many quizzical, head-scratching moments if they could peruse the Big List. For now, suffice it to report that, taken together, counselors and therapists identify a zoo-like menagerie in their advertising, including

Chicken Therapy	Fishing Therapy	Fly-fishing Therapy
Dolphin-assisted Therapy	Mini-mule Therapy	Llama Therapy
Goat Yoga	Bunny Therapy	Therapy Pigs
Duck Therapy	Goat Therapy	Therapy Lamb
Turtle/Tortoise Therapy	Pigmy Goat Therapy	Geese Therapy
Mini Pig Therapy	Canine Therapy	Equine Therapy

along many with others. What else could compare with such a menagerie? Well, name almost any activity that occupies time and gives enjoyment to human beings. A counselor or therapist somewhere has likely made it into a therapy. For example,

Piano Therapy	Rock Climbing Therapy	Guitar Therapy
Running Therapy	Harp Therapy	Hiking Therapy
Cinema Therapy	Farming Therapy	Culinary Arts Therapy
Sailing Therapy	Painting Therapy	Gardening Therapy
Wire-sculpting Therapy	Punching-bag Therapy	Hockey Therapy
Pet Massage Therapy	Golf Therapy	Ballet Therapy

and hundreds—yes, hundreds—of others. For now, these so-called "therapies" raise questions. Do they demonstrate good clinical judgment? How many therapists utilize these approaches? No doubt, cumulatively, the number runs into many thousands. Do these approaches suggest that there is no way to filter approaches into clinical practice and no way to filter them out of clinical practice? Do these approaches express the individual interests of therapists, not clinical interests? Do these approaches impair, if not harm, the potential of therapy? Insofar as these approaches may be collectively widespread, what definition do they give to the practice of counseling and therapy? All of them are included on the Big List.

Allowing for the fact that the Big List forms the basis for much of the discussion in this book, the larger discussion gives substantial, detailed, and comprehensive evidence that indicates the extraordinary jeopardy with which counseling and therapy live at the present time and into the foreseeable future. The case for this jeopardy is made throughout this book. This view stands with many others who share it. As one of many examples, Nuttgens (2023, p. 29), says, "The proliferation of therapeutic models, with their untold numbers of purportedly unique interventions, serves as a source of division, confusion, and retrogression for the field of psychotherapy." For now, much, if not most, of the jeopardy is likely an expression of exaggerated individualism that manifests itself in tens of thousands of practicing counselors and therapists who make up stuff that they call "therapy."

This book provides details that confirm that those who make up stuff and those who blend therapy with approaches that are inherently hostile to counseling and therapy are grossly blunting, if not bludgeoning, the profession of which they are members. Although religion-like approaches are numerous, most of the non-clinical and likely unethical approaches are not specifically religious, such as those listed, above, including Geese Therapy and Hockey Therapy.

Readers are invited to consider basic and pressing questions that almost inevitably arise from the information in this book. Among these questions, the following ones are offered as encouragements for consideration and discussion.

- If I am an active member of a health care profession in which I cannot recognize thousands of the treatments and treatment approaches that my peers advertise, am I really a member of the profession?
- If I confidently conclude that a very large number of these treatments are unethical, should I be member of the profession?
- Is my profession really a profession?
- If, for good professional reasons, I reject virtually countless approaches to counseling and therapy, what can I do to protect myself and my profession?

These are truly formidable questions. And, no doubt, they arise from studying the place of religion in the practice of counseling and therapy. Regardless of the angst that these questions may evoke, they acknowledge serious concerns about the welfare of the profession and the clients who are served by it. Also, in meaningful, personal ways, I am very affirming of religion, including my own. And, quite apart from the serious abuses of religion that this book describes, I am transparently supportive of others' religion, too.

No one has a "final analysis" of the place of religion in the practice of counseling and therapy, mainly, because they are an ongoing profession that has not yet terminated. However, as a characterization of vast numbers of therapists and their aberrant approaches to their clinical practices, the following, albeit somewhat cryptic, generalization may be apt:

> Anyone can do it! It's merely therapy. And, when I do it, I can do just anything that comes to mind—just whatever I want to do. I want to do what I want to do and, because I want to do it, I am right to do it because I want to do it.

Or, as the lyric from *One Tin Soldier* says, "Do it in the name of heaven, you can justify it in the end" (One Tin Soldier lyrics, 1969).

Mental health care holds the unspeakably large potential for healing and hope. This book is an attempt to advance the cause of this potential. To achieve the immense potential of mental health care, counselors and therapists must energetically address the problems that currently beset it.

References

Barnett, J. E., & Johnson, W. B. (2011, March). Integrating spirituality and religion into psychotherapy: persistent dilemmas, ethical Issues, and a proposed decision-making process. *Ethics and Behavior*, *21*(2), 147–164. 10.1080/10508422.2011.551471

Castonguay, L. G., Eubanks, C. F., Goldfried, M. R., Muran, J. C., & Lutz, W. (2015). Research on psychotherapy integration: Building on the past, looking to the future. *Psychotherapy Research*, *25*(3), 365–382. doi:10.1080/10503307.2015.1014010

Hoffart, A. & Hoffart, A. E. (2014). Psychotherapy integration through general therapy change principles: Missing the core of psychotherapy? *Journal of Psychotherapy Integration*, *24*(4), 263–274. 10.1037/a0038135

Jerome, A., Heath, M. A., Williams, M. Winters, R., & Cutrer-Pårraga (2023). Traversing trauma: Resilient women's religious and spiritual stories of hope and strength. *Professional Psychology: Research and Practice*, *54*(2), 177–187. 10.1037/pro0000491

Martin, F. A. (2020). *Therapy thieves: How to save mental health care from its providers.* New York: Oxford University Press.

Martin, F. A., & Turner, J. P. (2020). *Clinical supervision in the real world: A practical guide to ethics, legal issues, and personal development.* New York: Routledge.

Martin, F. A., Turner, J. P., & Fugate, J. (2023). Post-degree clinical supervision in Tennessee: A report about the advertising by supervision dyads. *Tennessee Counseling Association Journal* (in process).

McGraw, J. S., Skidmore, S. J., Lefevor, G. T., Docherty, M. & Mahone, A. (2023). Affirming and nonaffirming religious beliefs predicting depression and suicide risk among Latter-Day Saint sexual minorities. *Journal of Counseling Psychology, 70*(3),293–306. 10.1037/cou0000659

Norcross, J. C., Rocha, M. N., & Chrysler, A. A. (2023, May 18). Psychologists conducting psychotherapy in 2022: Contemporary practices and historical patterns of the society for the advancement of psychotherapy. *Psychotherapy* Advance online publication. 10.1037/pst0000493

Nuttgens, S. (2023). Of interventive doppelgangers and other barriers to evidence-based practice in psychotherapy. *Journal of Psychotherapy Integration, 33*(1), 20–33. 10.1037/int0000279

Rupert, D., Moon, S. H., & Sandage, S. J. (2019). Clinical training groups for spirituality and religion in psychotherapy. *Journal of Spirituality in Mental Health, 21*(3), 163–177. 10.1080/19349637.2018.1465879

1 Religious Opportunism in Counseling and Psychotherapy

This discussion is not an assessment of religion. It is a discussion of the exploitation of religion and persons of faith. In contrast with what this discussion says about those who exploit religion through their ostensible provision of counseling and therapy, I regard religion as mostly a good thing. I believe that a virtually countless number of individuals find positive meaning in their religion and make positive contributions to their families and communities because of their religion.

This chapter addresses the crisis-laden condition of counseling and psychotherapy that stems from specifically religious issues related to mental health care. Later, looking beyond this chapter, other threats to professionally accountable counselors and therapists will be discussed. For now, merely to give samples of some of the challenges that are relevant to the matter of religion in the practice of counseling and therapy, illustrations may be a good place to begin. On a website, a licensed therapist says, "Contact me today to begin your journey to achieve nirvana" (Licensed Clinical Social Worker, 2021). Nirvana? Really? Similarly, another state-licensed individual (Licensed Clinical Social Worker—Two, 2021) who completed her graduate preparation in a university that is not religious in its philosophy includes the following statements in her description of her professional practice.

> I am a bible believing Christian .... Every counselor, or coach has an ideology, philosophy, point of reference they use when speaking into your life. I choose to be upfront and tell you what mine is. Whatever problem you are experiencing the core of the solution is found in Christ. In all our ways acknowledge Him. Proverbs 3:6.
>
> Prayer is a vibrant part of our therapy session whether audibly heard or silently engaged.

Also, on her website, this social worker offers group sessions for $30.00 for each session.

DOI: 10.4324/9781003472469-2

> Worship Therapy in the Word: For those who find themselves, stressed, anxious, depressed in these COVID times. Centering our own strength on the only one who gives strength is the way out of the feelings of turmoil experienced. The groups are limited to min 3 and max 9 participants per 75 min sessions. Praise, Prayer, Proverbs & Psalms.

Like "volunteer child labor" or "low cost sexual intimacy," the marketing of "worship" likely jolts the senses of many therapists. Also, it provokes questions such as these. Is worship a clinical activity or a clinically relevant activity? Who decides what worship is and how it relates to counseling and therapy? What or who should be worshipped? If worship is appropriately integrated into clinical practice, what are the implications of this for those who do not worship, whether they are the ones who provide professional services or the ones who receive professional services? In what ways does including worship in counseling and therapy influence or redefine professional services? What is the intended or unintended message from this therapist to other therapists?

Marketing worship or many other specifically religious matters may jolt the senses, but it also arouses a critically important issue: If religion, along with the multiple ways of representing God, God-consciousness, and spirituality, can be virtually anything that an individual's interests wish religion and therapy to be, do religion and therapy really matter? Or, more specifically, if God, as an all-encompassing term, can be paired with almost all known forms of counseling and therapy, do either God or therapy mean much of anything of significance? The answers to these questions may not be final and definitive, but they are clear and disturbing. They are explored in this discussion.

The Bragging Buddha

So far, the Big List of titles for approaches to counseling and therapy contains 278 items that contain "Buddhism" or "Buddhist." Many individuals who identify with Buddhism or who study Buddhism may be surprised not only by this number but also by the extraordinary variety of pairings of Buddhism with multiple approaches to counseling and therapy. When they see some of the pairings, they may justifiably ask, "Why is Buddhism paired with this particular approach?" For example, why is Buddhism paired with Aikido-Buddhist Mindfulness Meditation. Or, should Attachment Theory and Buddhism be paired? Or, how about Ayurvedic-Buddhist Therapy? Or, how about Buddha-Christ Healing? Adding to these four Buddhist-related approaches to counseling and psychotherapy, Chart 1.1 draws from the long list of other pairings. The items in Chart 1.1 are copied from the websites of practicing counselors and therapists. Only 40 of the 278 Buddhist-related therapies have been selected for inclusion in the chart.

Chart 1.1 Buddhist Pairings with Clinical Approaches

Asana Buddhist Principles
Buddhism and Christian Spirituality
Buddhism and Diamond Heart
Buddhism and Indigenous Art Therapy
Buddhism-Cognitive Behavioral Therapy
Buddhism-Hinduism
Buddhism/Feminism/and Jungian Philosophy
Buddhism/Hinduism/A Course in Miracles
Buddhism/The Chakra System/The Christ Path
Buddhist and Daoist (Taoist) Philosophies
Buddhist and Earth-Based Beliefs
Buddhist and Existentially Informed Therapies
Buddhist and First Nation Traditions
Buddhist and Law of Attraction Teachings
Buddhist and Shamanic Practices
Buddhist and Sufi Integrated
Buddhist Energy Psychologies
Buddhist Meditation/Soto Zen Tradition
Buddhist Psychology/Hakomi Method
Buddhist Theravada and Vajrayana Traditions
Buddhist Transpersonal & Positive Psychology
Christianity, Islam, Buddhism, Nature-based, Mysticism, Gnosticism, etc.
Dharmacharya—Buddhist
Family Systems Theory-Buddhist Thought
Herbalism/Wilderness Adventures/Buddhist
Indian Buddhist Tantra
Indo-Tibetan Buddhism
Integration of Secular Buddhist Psychology
Japanese Soto Zen Buddhism Style
Jung and Mahayana Buddhism
Kabbalistic and Buddhist Psychology
Nature-based Buddhist-Agnostic
Neurobiology/Neuroscience/Buddhist Practices
Samatha Samadhi (Buddhism)
Shambhala and Tibetan Vajrayana Buddhist Traditions
Tibetan Buddhist Chod Ritual
Tibetan Mongolian Buddhist
Transpersonal-Hypnosis-Body-Centered Psychotherapy-NLP-Trauma-informed
Buddhist and Yogic Philosophy
Zen Buddhist Interpersonal Psychodynamic Psychotherapy

This is a study of counseling and therapy, not a study of Buddhism. Nevertheless, in the context of studying counseling and therapy and their relation to Buddhism, a simple question is raised. What is Buddhism? The question is particularly important in a discussion of the place of religion in counseling and therapy. According to The Buddhist Center (2021, online), "Buddhism is a path of practice and spiritual development leading to

Insight into the true nature of reality. Buddhist practices like meditation are means of changing yourself in order to develop the qualities of awareness, kindness, and wisdom." The frequently expressed outcome of practicing Buddhism is "enlightenment." Thus, The Buddhist Center adds, "An enlightened being sees the nature of reality absolutely clearly, just as it is, and lives fully and naturally in accordance with that vision. This is the goal of the Buddhist spiritual life, representing the end of suffering for anyone who attains it."

Explaining some of the implications of Buddhism, The Buddhist Center adds,

> Because Buddhism does not include the idea of worshipping a creator god, some people do not see it as a religion in the normal, Western sense. The basic tenets of Buddhist teaching are straightforward and practical: nothing is fixed or permanent; actions have consequences; change is possible. So Buddhism addresses itself to all people irrespective of race, nationality, caste, sexuality, or gender. It teaches practical methods which enable people to realize and use its teachings in order to transform their experience, to be fully responsible for their lives.

Practicing Buddhists may wish to modify the view of The Buddhist Center to accommodate their own. However, if the view of The Buddhist Center may be taken as a reliable and useful definition of Buddhism, how may practicing counselors and therapists modify it to accommodate their clinical orientations? Without wrecking the integrity of Buddhism, can counselors and therapists deliver therapy that encompasses the multiple different orientations to counseling and therapy listed above? The appearance is that, taken as a body of approaches that include Buddhism, many of these approaches are wildly incompatible with Buddhism. However, whether they are compatible or not, many of the paired approaches are incompatible with one another. Based on the list above, the treatment approaches with which Buddhism is paired include the ones in Chart 1.2.

Is Buddhism compatible with these approaches? With which ones is Buddhism compatible or incompatible? Are some of the approaches that are paired with Buddhism incompatible with one another? For example, what level of compatibility is there among The Christ Path, Hinduism, Agnosticism, Gnosticism, Feminism, Secularism, Mysticism, and other religious or quasi-religious orientations? Then, when Cognitive Behavior Therapy, Psychodynamic Therapy, Past Life Regression, Transpersonal Therapy, and Neurobiology/Neuroscience are added to the mix, what level of compatibility is there? With an apparent and high level of incompatibility among the ways that Buddhism has been modified by counselors and therapists, the answer to the question of what Buddhism is

Chart 1.2 Buddhism-Associated Therapies

Asana Yoga	Daoist (Taoist) Philosophies
Diamond Heart Approach	Indigenous Art Therapy
Cognitive Behavioral Therapy	The Chakra System
The Christ Path	Hinduism
A Course in Miracles	Christian Spirituality
Earth-Based Beliefs	Existentially Informed Psychotherapies
First Nation Traditions	Law of Attraction Teachings
Shamanic Practices	Integrated Sufism
Soto Zen Tradition	Hakomi Method
Recovery Models	Theravada and Vajrayana Traditions
Energy Psychologies	Transpersonal & Positive Psychology
Jung and Mahayana Buddhism	Dharmacharya
Family Systems Theory	Herbalism
Wilderness Adventures	Shamanism
Past Life Regression	Indian Buddhist Tantra
Indo-Tibetan Buddhism	Christianity
Islam	Mysticism
Nature-based	Gnosticism
Secular Buddhist Psychology	Japanese Soto Zen Buddhism Style
Kabbalistic* Ideology	Mindfulness
Contemplative Psychology	Feminism
Jungian Philosophy	Agnosticism
Neurobiology/Neuroscience	Samatha Samadhi Practices
Tibetan Buddhist Chod Ritual	Tibetan Mongolian Buddhism
Transpersonal Therapy	Hypnosis
Body-Centered Psychotherapy	NLP**
Trauma-Informed Buddhism	Yogic Philosophy
Zen	Interpersonal Psychodynamic Therapy
Shambhala and Tibetan Vajrayana Buddhist Traditions	

Notes

* Kabbalistic (Dictionary.com, 2021) is an esoteric theology and theurgy that involves mystical experiences and insights that come to individuals who are immersed in a mystical method of interpreting Scriptures.

** NLP is likely Neurolinguistic Programming. However, acronyms often mask the item to which the user refers. NLP may refer to Neurolinguistic Programming, New Life Psychotherapy, Native Language Psychotherapy, or others.

may be unanswerable. Buddhism can be anything that an individual wishes it to be. If Buddhism is anything that an individual wishes it to be, is it any longer Buddhism? And, if Buddhism can be paired with multiple variations of clinical orientations that an individual merely prefers, are they any longer counseling and therapy?

More fundamentally, should Buddhism be integrated into counseling and therapy at all? If it may be integrated into counseling and therapy, with what rationale is it included? Who should decide whether Buddhism is integrated into counseling and therapy? And, if Buddhism is a feature of a clinician's approach to counseling and therapy, what are the implications of the clinician's selection of Buddhism, particularly when it is paired with approaches that are incompatible with Buddhism? What are the ethical implications of practicing Buddhism as a stand-alone clinical orientation? If Buddhism as a philosophy or as a religion may be integrated into counseling and therapy, any and all other philosophies and religions may be integrated into counseling and therapy, too. After all, if one religion or quasi-religion is acceptable as an orientation to counseling and therapy, almost all other religions or quasi-religions are acceptable too, transforming therapy into a profession without a minimally reasonable basis for its existence, based only on individual proclivities.

Siddhartha Gautama—or Buddha—lived approximately 2,600 years ago. Buddha is a title, not a name. The title identifies the person as "the one who is awake" (Buddha, 2021). The teachings of the Buddha called for individuals to relinquish personal impurities, such as greed, hate, and other forms of avariciousness, and to seek personal integrity, emotional attunement, peace of mind, and humility—to use contemporary, American terms—but also "nirvana." Nirvana was/is a transformed existence, encompassing a thorough and intense perception of reality, the most basic blending of nature with human consciousness (Buddha, 2021). The significance of this overly brief, but relevant, description of the Buddha and Buddhist teachings is to ask, "If this is Buddhism, why are so many counselors and therapists making many things of it that it clearly is not?" Compromising both mental health care and Buddhism, at least, they have transformed the Buddha into an unnatural, nicely managed braggart—the Bragging Buddha.

Jesus Barely Survives

In the Prologue to his book, *Christ in Crisis: Why We Need to Reclaim Jesus,* Jim Wallis wrote, "It's always amazing to me how Jesus has apparently survived all of us Christians" (2019, p. 2). Near the end of his book, Wallis adds, "It is time to be followers of Jesus before anything else—nationality, political party, race, ethnicity, gender, geography—our identity in Christ precedes every other identity" (p. 283). In this discussion, as valuable as Wallis' comments may independently be, they should be modified, with apology, of course. If the first comment were slightly adapted so that it comfortably fits in this discussion, Wallis' comment would say, "Jesus has apparently survived all of us who are Christian counselors and therapists." If his second comment were similarly adapted, it would read, "It is time to be followers of Jesus before anything else, including nationality, political party, race, ethnicity, gender, geography and/or counseling and therapy."

To be clear about this discussion, it is not about theology or genuinely held religious beliefs or broadly accepted practices of personal faith or any particular religious point of view. It is a discussion about counseling and therapy. As such, it acknowledges that countless individuals experience their life of faith as meaningful, positive, and relevant to many aspects of the way they live, including the socially contributing values that they seek to express through their faith.

No doubt, while some Christian or other religion-oriented counselors and therapists pose threats, if not harm, to counseling and therapy, they alone cannot cause the demise of counseling and therapy, let alone kill them. To effectuate such consequences, those who advance harmful religious approaches as therapeutic need help from others. And, they get it. Confirmed by many other researchers and writers, this book shows that numerous individuals and groups have harmed and will likely continue to harm counseling and therapy, largely because of their poor professional judgments including leaders of major professional associations and preparation program faculty and leaders. For now, the evidence clearly indicates that religion-oriented therapists, along with both overt and tacit support from many others, threaten the potential of counseling and therapy. Self-identified Christian therapists may be the largest group of mental health care providers, but many others advertise specifically religious approaches to their therapy that represent a religion other than Christianity. Many of these other approaches appear to be demonstrably inappropriate. As partial confirmation of this, some of these approaches appear in Chart 1.3.

To refer to these approaches as ones that compromise the integrity of counseling and therapy or that cause harm needs elaboration. In the first place, the compromise of integrity and potential harm should be separated

Chart 1.3 Thirty Questionable Approaches to Counseling and Psychotherapy

African Epistemology	Alchemical Hypnotherapy Approaches
Alien Abduction Therapy	Ancestral Regression Therapy
Ancient Shamanic Drum Journeys	Angelic Massage
Animal Spirits Guidance	Archangel Life Coaching
Ceremonial Magic	Christa Energy Attunement
Clearing Past Life Relationship	Color Silk Therapy
Divine Channeling	Foot Reflexology
Geode Therapy	Herd Meditation
Luminous Life Maps	Mary Queen of Angels Cards Readings
Mesa-Building	Missionary Worldview
Mystery School Teachings	Quantum Angel Healing
Radiant Moon Reiki	Shamanic Drumming Circle
South American Toltec Shamanic Traditions	Spiritual Stargates
Spiritual Mentoring (Order of Melchizedek)	Tarot and Mediumship Readings
Therapeutic Chickens	Throne Room Therapy

from the intentions of those who practice these approaches. Among those who seek to help others, good will almost always motivates them to express their care for others. Their good intentions need to be supported, not suppressed. In the second place, while compromise or potential harm may appear to be unduly pejorative, it says at least that those who practice these approaches fail to understand that they represent far more than their individual preferences. They represent every other member of the professional community that delivers counseling and therapy. Thus, they should ask and answer a few simple questions.

How may I select the best approaches to counseling and psychotherapy?
What questions or objections could be raised about my selected approach?
What relevant training and experience do I bring to my practice of this approach?
What broadly recognized and approved criteria do I use when I select an approach to counseling and therapy?
Should I gain professional endorsement of approaches that are not generally recognized and approved, maybe, by consulting with recognized leaders and colleagues who are capable of helping me?
How do I best represent the professional community of which I am a member?

In the third place, those who reject the 30 approaches to therapy in Chart 1.3 must bear the accountability to which they wish to hold others. Whether they reject these approaches or hold relevant and seriously doubt about their appropriateness, they should also carefully scrutinize their own decision-making when it comes to selecting approaches to therapy. This is particularly critical when they are selecting well-known and commonly accepted approaches to therapy. After all, while Cognitive Behavioral Therapy, Acceptance and Commitment Therapy, or Applied Behavior Analysis may have research-based support, they should be utilized in counseling and therapy because they meet the needs of clients, not because of the interests or preferences of the provider alone. Further, while they may be research-based, counselors and therapists who practice them must also scrutinize their clinical abilities to practice them.

The assertion that many therapists may be providing specifically religious approaches to therapy that are demonstrably inappropriate may appear to be an audacious one. However, in the context of this report about the multiple ways religious views have penetrated every aspect of mental health care, the assertion may be hardly noticeable. As Chart 1.3 indicates, numerous non-religious and inappropriate approaches to therapy are practiced, too. Thus, the assertion about many specifically religious approaches to therapy as

Chart 1.4 Unusual Approaches to Therapy

Alchemy	Aqua massage
Arbinger Facilitation	Aroma Freedom Technique
Aromatouch (massage)	Astrology
Bach flower therapy	BSFF—be set free fast
Chakra Balancing	Circus Arts Therapy
Clairvoyance	Comedy Therapy
Diamond Approach	Emotional Freedom Technique
Essential Oils	Fairy Tale Model
Feline-Assisted Therapy	Heathen Therapy
Hermetic Philosophy	Hormone and Amino Acid Therapy
Kalish Practice	Law of Attraction
Light Touch Therapies	Mud Therapy
Past Life Regression Therapy	Power Animal Retrieval
Radix Neo-Reichian Approach	Time Travel
Vibrator Therapy	Wicca

inappropriate may be lost in the larger fog of non-religious inappropriate approaches. The unusual and non-religious approaches to therapy are much too numerous to include here, but a small list of 30 of such approaches represents them, as identified in Chart 1.4.

There are numerous ways that the advertised approaches of counselors and therapists have sliced therapy into very small pieces, according to only therapists' individual preferences, with little apparent positive regard for the welfare of their clients or the profession in which they are members. Further, these approaches establish a picture of the extraordinary randomness and carelessness of many mental health care providers. As such, religious in character or not, many thousands of preferred approaches to therapy are more like the imaginary and "real" identities of many three-year-old children who believe that they are princesses or transformers than serious and adult contributors to providing mental health care. They are more ideological than clinical. They are more individual expressions by presumptive clinicians than professional accountability. They are more commercial than authentically religious, spiritual, and clinically relevant. And, paradoxically, they opportunistically exploit the almost universal and longstanding support of pluralism and diversity.

From the approaches to counseling and therapy on the Big List that have so far been gathered, many of the words and the number of each one are identified in Chart 1.5. Conceivably, many approaches on the Big List could be included here as Christian-related approaches, with further investigation. These would include approaches such as Divine Essence of God, Embrace God's Perspective, Empowerment and Application of God's Word, Focus on God, GNA-God Named Authenticity, God Loves You!,

Chart 1.5 Christian-Related Words in Treatment Orientations

Percent Christian-Related Word	*Total*	*Specifically Christian*	*Adjusted Total*
Apostolic	3	100%	3
Archangel/archangelic	2	100%	2
Baptist	1	100%	1
Bible-related	466	100%	466
Bibliotherapy	21	26%	6
Catholic	33	100%	22
Celebrate Recovery	3	100%	3
Christ/Christian	1,246	100%	1,246
Church	12	100%	12
Discipleship	12	100%	12
Divine	76	32%	24
Evangelical	6	100%	6
Faith	350	98%	343
God	118	86%	96
Gospel	12	100%	12
Grace	34	53%	18
Heaven	7	100%	7
Holy Spirit	47	100%	47
Immanuel	5	100%	5
Inspired/Inspiration/Inspire	59	17%	10
Jesus	19	100%	19
LDS (14)/Mormon(9)	23	100%	23
Light	118	18%	21
Lord	10	100%	10
Love	137	20%	31
Loving	25	20%	5
Ministry	31	100%	31
Mission/Missional	20	100%	2
Nouthetic (7) Nauthetic (2)	9	100%	9
Pastoral	79	74%	58
Prayer	136	100%	136
Redemption	4	100%	4
Religion/Religious	79	17%	20
Sacred	79	58%	46
Salvation’	4	100%	4
Scriptural	50	100%	50
Shepherd/shepherding	2	100%	2
Soul	429	28%	120
Spirit-related	1,842	47%	866
Splankna	49	100%	49
Word of God	37	100%	37
Worship	6	100%	6
		TOTAL	3,908

God Wonderful Counseling, God-Person Bonding Counseling, or God's Life Design. No doubt, the number of Christian approaches to therapy exceeds the number above.

To reiterate, these words appear in the titles of treatment orientations that licensed mental health professionals advertise on their websites and that they identify as "Christian." Some of the words, such as "Bible-related" (i.e., Bible, Biblical, Biblically), "Christian," and "Spirit-related" (i.e., spirit, spiritual, spiritually, spirituality), are quite common. The number of Christian-related titles likely comes as a surprise to most practicing mental health care professionals. The surprise emanates from the fact that they have seen none of the titles of therapies that include these words, but also that their history has told them that the total number of clinical orientations likely includes far fewer than the number of Christian approaches. Both published and conversational comments suggest that there may be 400 or 500 approaches to counseling and psychotherapy and that most of them lack evidentiary support and clinical efficacy (e.g., Bradley Erford, former President of the American Counseling Association, cited by Shallcross, 2012). However, the number of 3,908 for Christian-related approaches alone is just the tip of the proverbial iceberg. The total number of so-called "therapies" is larger than the 38,373 that have been located, so far.

Also, significantly, Christian-related titles of specifically religious approaches to counseling and therapy may surprise, if not shock, those who have not contemplated the potential variety of Christian-related titles. After all, 3,908 is a very large number. However, the number of specifically religious titles of approaches to counseling and therapy far exceeds 3,908. So far, the number of collected titles of titles for specifically religious approaches to counseling and psychotherapy that are not Christian-related exceeds 1,600. Combined, the specifically religious titles for counseling and therapy reach far more than 5,000. The number of providers who offer these titles is much larger than this.

So far, more than 5,000 titles of some form of specifically religious counseling and psychotherapy have been located, although it should be noted that there are, no doubt, many more that have not yet been located. These are titles, not the number of therapists. Because an unknown, large number of therapists usually advertise a particular religious approach, the number of therapists who allege to practice it is many multiples of 5,000. The overwhelming majority of those who advertise their specifically religious approach to counseling and therapy have almost nothing to support their offerings. Most of those who advertise a specifically religious approach to their clinical work have no theological training, having completed their training in public universities, for-profit universities, or private secular universities. Analysis of information gathered for the Big List indicates that most of them—87%—do not indicate in their advertising that they have relevant training or certifications or associated memberships that would support their presumed offering.

A theme of this presentation is that personal and sometimes group ideologies have overcome and frequently redirected clinical practice from professional accountability. The ideologies that have overcome professional accountability often take the form of religious ideologies. Chapter 2 addresses the diminution of professional accountability and the simultaneous ascendancy of religious ideologies as expressions of exaggerated individualism. As such, it holds a mirror to the face of counseling and therapy, much more than judging the adequacy of inadequacy of the ideologies that appear in this chapter, although the inadequacy of some of the ideologies is necessarily implied. More broadly than religious ideologies, all approaches to counseling and therapy should be evaluated. Outside the scope of such evaluations, the adequacy of the religious beliefs that may be held by counselors and therapists should almost always be accepted. They should be free to claim a religious and/or spiritual orientation, along with preferred attending beliefs, that they wish to have. Neither their beliefs nor freedom to hold such beliefs is in question here.

As noted earlier in this discussion, the need to report the information in this chapter should be clear. It is not a refutation of religion or religious beliefs or personal faith. I have a well-documented personal history of involvement with my faith and religion. As noted in the References, I have expressed my personal faith in several books, among other ways. Just as I reject anyone's attempt to deny my prerogative to believe what I believe—with regard to religion—I also reject anyone's attempt to deny the religious commitments of others.

However, to support the right of each of us to hold religious beliefs is not an endorsement of an individual's prerogative to equate their religious beliefs with clinical, professional accountability. These things are fundamentally different. To illustrate this, a counselor or therapist is free to hold strong beliefs in the sanctity of marriage. However, a belief in the sanctity of marriage should not give the counselor or therapist the prerogative to expect clients to see marriage as a sign of their mental health, their lack of marriage as a sign of their mental illness, a divorcee as deficient because of this status, or a troubled marriage as an expression of hostility toward God. No doubt, many counselors and therapists believe in the sanctity of marriage. However, based on a strong belief in the sanctity of marriage and the belief that adults should commit only to church-sanctioned heterosexual partnering, holding clients to this standard should be rejected by practicing counselors and therapists. Similarly, a deeply and sincerely held devotion to a religion is not a qualifier for integrating it into counseling and therapy. Alone, personal religious faith is not a qualifier for conducting counseling and therapy. This discussion emphasizes the necessity of a sustained, inclusive, and serious exploration of the integration of religion and spirituality into the practice of therapy, with competence, integrity, and healthy pluralism.

References

Buddha (2021). *Who was the Buddha?* https://www.lionsroar.com/who-was-the-buddha/

Buddhist Center (2021). *What is Buddhism?* https://thebuddhistcentre.com/buddhism

Dictionary.com (2021). *Kabbalah.* https://www.dictionary.com/browse/kabbalah

Licensed Clinical Social Worker. (2021). *Achieving Nirvana, LLC.* https://www.psychologytoday.com/us/therapists/achieving-nirvana-llc-pennsauken-nj/778632

Licensed Clinical Social Worker—Two. (2021). No title. https://www.psychologytoday.com/us/therapists/i-regina-gourdine-saint-louis-mo/327277

Shallcross, L. (Compiler) (2012, March). What the future holds for the counseling profession. *Counseling Today.* https://ct.counseling.org/2012/03/what-the-future-holds-for-the-counseling-profession/

Wallis, J. (2019). *Christ in crisis: Why we need to reclaim Jesus.* New York: Harper Collins.

2 Individualism as Therapy

In whatever way it may be conceived, the entry of religion and spirituality into health care is not news. In various forms and accompanied by numerous beliefs, religion and spirituality have presumably been involved in health care, very likely from the beginning of health care, although such an assertion confronts the fact that neither the beginning of health care nor religion's relation to such a beginning is known. Certainly, recent decades have included the needed, visible, and widespread inclusion of specifically religion-trained professionals in the delivery of health care. For example, many hospitals have chapels and chaplains. More than merely a local phenomenon, though, this is a longstanding, formal, and institutionalized feature of hospital life. One of the exemplars of this phenomenon is the Healthcare Chaplains Ministry Association. On its website it states, "God's heart in Healthcare since 1939" (Healthcare Chaplains Ministry Association, 2022). Another example of the presence of specifically religion-trained professionals in health care is seen in hospice care. As Davis (1988, p. 100) notes, when the Medicare Hospice Benefit became a funded service in 1982, it specified that hospice patients would have access to "a pastoral or other counselor," usually a chaplain.

The concept or belief that religion has a role in health care is almost universally taken for granted. No one argues against having chaplains in health care. They—or similarly trained and titled individuals—work with physicians, nurses, and other health care providers to respond to the identified needs of patients. In many medical facilities, spiritual assessments of patients are routine features of medical care.

In mental health care, the inclusion of religion is different from what is described above. Generally, the difference is that, in mental health care, the inclusion of religion or "God" comes mostly from individuals who are not trained and whose services relate only tangentially, at best, to the needs of clients. As the information in this book confirms, numerous individuals who hold state-issued licenses and advertise their specifically religious services as health care usually have no relevant training and utilize their religion as an instrument of mental health care. This individualism and presumptuous

DOI: 10.4324/9781003472469-3

utilization of specifically religious approaches to counseling and therapy pose threats to clients and to the well-being of counseling and therapy. It is more about advancing a point of view and the interests of counselors and therapists than responding to clients' needs.

Another critical differentiation of therapy is that therapists are accountable for managing transference-related issues in their practice of therapy. This is a longstanding ethical and legal principle. Commonly, this principle has been associated with the sexual victimization of clients by their therapists. Too often, such victimization happens when a therapist fails to appropriately manage transference and countertransference in the therapeutic relationship. Much less attention and research have been given to transference and countertransference in the therapeutic relationship as it relates to religion and spirituality. This is a category of needed research. However, authors who give attention to this issue often provide valuable insights about how transference issues that involve religion may be managed (e.g., Cohen 2019; Kehoe & Gutheil 1993; Malark, 2017; Peteet 2009; White 2023).

This chapter is more an acknowledgment of the proliferation of specifically religious approaches in counseling and therapy than an explanation of it, but includes explanations, nevertheless. Explanations of this phenomenon, though, require more than the aims of this book encompass. Suffice it to say that the massive proliferation of religion-oriented and quasi-religious approaches to counseling and therapy manifests the severely underregulated individualism that has characterized the mental health movement from its beginning. Exaggerated individualism is the door through which religion enters the practice of counseling and therapy.

I Am Unique. Really. I Am. Really.

Numerous titles have been given to others who occupy a special, usually intimate adult relationship with another person. Many of these titles could be listed, somewhat readily, just because they are known. And, although many of them have accrued meaning that gives them a small distinction from the others, almost all of the ones listed in Chart 2.1 are commonly used.

In this list, "soul mate" and "husband" are not necessarily the same person, but could be. Likewise, "girlfriend" and "wife" are not necessarily the same person, but could be. Some, such as "groom" and "bride" are not the same person, will almost never be combined into a reference to one person. And, while couples may have private titles that they assign to one other, all of the 30 titles in the list above are widely, if not universally, recognized and accepted.

However, as a thought experiment, another list that refers to the same kind of relationships that are suggested in the list above could be easily assembled. Each of the titles refers to an individual in an adult, intimate relationship (Chart 2.2). Readers are encouraged to read the column on the left side of the page and then read the column on the right side of the page.

Chart 2.1 Common Titles for Adult Intimate Partners

Better half	Boyfriend	Bride
Bridegroom	Companion	Consort
Domestic partner	Girlfriend	Groom
Helpmate	Helpmeet	Hubby
Husband	Lady	Man
Mate	Missis	Missus
Mister	Old lady	Old man
Old woman	Other half	Partner
Roommate	Significant other	Soul mate
Wife	Wifey	Woman

Chart 2.2 Contrived Labels for Intimate Relationships

Column One	*Column Two*
Allopreen	Divine Allopreen
Boctyl	Godly Boctyl
Coutle	Muslim Coutle
Donitz	Christian Donitz
Elemental Lover	Jesus' Elemental Lover
Attachment Woman	Sacred Attachment Woman
Frixolen	Lordly Frixolen
Fumetind	Faith-Based Fumetind
Grifford	Holiness Oriented Grifford
Hewetted	Biblical Hewetted
Ivoso	Solutional Ivoso
Jemembrate	Catholic Jemembrate
Kandrid	Kandrid Biblical Principals
Lamitol	Lordly Lamitol
Mylone	Spiritual Mylone
Nilicious	Nouthetic Nilicious
Oxlandre	Son of God Oxlandre
Pairprect	Archangel Family Pairprect
Para-Sync	Prayer-Focused Para-Sync
Quandrodle	Quandroldle Christ Oriented
Ruccess	Apostolic Ruccess
Sistinctor	Religious Sistinctor
Sprack	Evangelical Sprack
Telegor	Telegor Discipleship
Utility Man	Gospel Utility Man
Valtue	Valtue Grace Approach
Worthy One	Heavenly Worthy One
Xullyl	Pastoral Xully
Yon-Soul	Ministry of Yon-Soul
Zoweller	Zoweller Holy Spirit

The list in Chart 2.1 contains only 30 labels for intimate partners, while Chart 2.2 contains 30 labels for intimate relationships. Each label refers to an adult, intimate relationship. The obvious difference between Charts 2.1 and 2.2 is that the titles for intimate partners in Chart 2.1 are commonly recognized, while the labels for intimate relationships in Chart 2.2 are contrived and surely almost completely unrecognizable. As a thought experiment, these two charts indicate how easily titles and labels can be invented. Further, Chart 2.2 illustrates how easily religious labels can be applied to virtually anything that comes to mind. At least, an implication of this thought experiment is that religion-related titles of approaches to therapy have been invented on a massive scale, with the preponderant majority of them having no relevant connection to professionally accountable counseling and therapy.

As noted in the Introduction to this book, more than 38,000 titles of approaches to counseling and therapy have been located, so far. They are approaches that are advertised by licensed counselors and therapists. The number indicates that individualism among mental health care professionals has become a primary conceptualization of the profession. Enlarging the view of individualism, the thought experiment invites consideration of the possibility that very large numbers of random and non-clinical, and non-evidentiary approaches are thrown into the professional clinical world. Also, the inclusion of very large numbers of made-up approaches to mental health care irrationally and irresponsibly accommodates exaggerated individualism and accelerates the decline of mental health care.

The caricature of approaches to therapy and religion in Charts 2.1 and 2.2, expresses the current reality of mental health care. In short, any approach to counseling and therapy, including the truly absurd ones, may be adjectivized with any and every term, title, or concept that an individual therapist may wish to add to it. Anything can become "Christian," merely by adding the adjective, "Christian," to it. While incomplete as an explanation of the adjectivizing phenomenon, rampant, widespread, and dangerous individualism among counselors and therapists accounts for almost all of it. The next chapter adds to the discussion of ways through which counseling and therapy have become an adjectivized profession.

Quite apart from the thought experiment above, tens of thousands of titles of counseling and therapy orientations, many of which are identified in this book, do not come into professional practice because of professionalism; they come because of exaggerated individualism. As much as individualism may be an inviting personal ideal, a prerogative and desirable condition for living in a complex and often depersonalizing world, it does not and cannot confirm and sustain professionalism. Through a countless number of irrationally selected and advertised, anti-scientific, anti-intellectual, highly personalized, and merely contrived approaches to therapy, individualism demonstrably threatens the viability of counseling and therapy.

In their ongoing survey of the websites of practicing counselors and therapists, Martin and Turner (2023) have identified thousands of sites in which counselors and therapists promote their uniqueness. The examples appear in such quantities and forms that a simple accounting of them is not possible. Suffice it to say that the explicit reference to being "unique" appears with shocking frequency. The accrued, considerable volume of advertised "uniqueness" prompts the question, "If other health care providers, such as cardiologists, pediatricians, or pharmacists, advertised unique treatments, would they be credible and trustworthy?" Or, as readers review each of the statements below, copied as is, does therapy seem more or less credible and trustworthy? Or, what message(s), if any, does it convey to readers? The small sampling of only 40 selected examples of "unique" represent tens of thousands of very similar statements.

I bring a unique perspective from an Eastern worldview that includes Self Compassion and Neuroscience.

My entire practice is unique from top to bottom. My personality, my training, and my perspective, all the way to the unique approaches I take and the constant innovations I bring.

Solid grounding in Christian theology and doctorate [sic] level training in clinical psychology give me a unique perspective on the human soul and relationships.

My current and ongoing training in play therapy makes me uniquely qualified to help younger children ages 5–11 and adolescents ages 12–18.

I am uniquely qualified to address issues of personal improvement and due to my preceptive skills, patience and compassion for others, my clients feel comfortable and at ease working with me.

My years of experience as a counselor, in the school-based setting, as well as church ministry and community services, provide me with a unique insight for helping people navigate their life journey.

My unique approach integrates psychological, philosophical and spiritual concepts to "custom fit" each client with the most effective treatment.

I provide a unique counseling experience, validating the humanity in each of us.

My unique approach to psychotherapy encourages a balanced integration of the physical, emotional, mental and spiritual aspects of your wellbeing.

Because I have worked in a variety of settings, I am able to bring diverse experience and a unique perspective to every case.

My clinical and educational background make me uniquely qualified to help others to achieve their potential.

My style and experience have given me a unique way of relating to adults, adolescents and their parents that empowers them to make changes that are desired to find happiness and the life they imagined.

I provide an encouraging therapeutic approach where I use a combination of Cognitive Behavior Therapy, Solution-Focused Brief Therapy, Person-Centered Therapy, and Dialectical behavior therapy (DBT), Art Therapy; in which I'm able to offer a unique perspective on life challenges.

I specialize in a unique brand of equine therapy that I have developed through my in-depth studies of the horse-human relationship.

My unique style of working with clients combines all of my expertise in the field of counseling and positive psychology along with deep wisdom and intuitive insight.

I offer unique & dynamic experiences in mindfulness & boundary work. Results can be felt immediately.

I have personal unique insight for those individuals struggling with eating disorders.

My practice is unique because I encourage the use of mindfulness and yoga.

My unique therapeutic approach utilizes the principles of EMDR, yoga, and nervous system regulation with emphasis on the mind-body connection.

My experience in treating hospice patients has given me a unique point of view—life is too short not to enjoy each day with the people you love.

Over the last 13 years, I've worked to help normalize the therapy process with a unique and individual approach.

As a counselor, I am uniquely positioned to be your person, and there needn't be a diagnosable problem.

Those searching for help from any hurt, habit, or hang-up, will find a unique approach utilizing both psychological and biblical perspectives with a Process Based Therapy (PBT).

I embrace a wide-range of Eastern and Western religions/philosophies resulting in a unique depth of perspective, allowing you to openly and freely access your own inner resources and wisdom.

I believe I bring a unique blend of compassion, wisdom, humor and love of storytelling to the psychotherapy experience.

My unique ability to bridge the traditional scientific healing model with alternative methods allows me to synthesize multiple methodologies in my approach for each client.

Unique to my practice is using equine assisted psychotherapy from a Jungian perspective when and as deemed appropriate.

My practice is unique because it takes place outside. I have a unique model and approach that incorporates nature in every step.
I developed a unique integrated treatment model, in which I combine my broad clinical training with ancient healing modalities.
I provide a unique blend of techniques from a variety of the world's wisdom traditions, along with methods from a number healing modalities from contemporary psychology, energy medicine and neuroscience, used with individuals and in group settings.
My approach integrates a unique combination of support practices from my studies in Psychology, Counseling, EBT, CBT, DBT, Ayurveda, Meditation and Yoga Philosophy.
I hold a strong belief in Biblical principles and the power of Christian faith and prayer in an individual's life and incorporate these principles in therapy. Along with deeply caring for my clients, this makes my practice truly unique.
I use a unique blend of awareness and improvisation tools that get you out of your seat, into your body, out of your head, and into a creative flow.
I am unique in the that integrate Christianity into my counseling sessions.
What makes me unique? I feel like I combine caring, knowledge, acceptance and a sense of humor to help people through their most difficult times. Another thing I feel separates me from some therapists is my ability to personalize treatments specific to the person and what they are going through. My ability to apply knowledge to create the perfect treatment plan has helped me to help individuals that other therapists could not.
I am an experiential/Client-Centered/Self Actualization type of therapist, this is unique from other therapists.
Our practice is unique in that we offer massage and aromatherapy as a complementary and alternative approach to comprehensive care!
My practice is unique due to my compassion and warmth. I live with a servant's heart. I love helping clients from all walks of life. I am unique because I provide feel everyone has value.
The most unique thing about me or my practice is that I listen, talk, and consider you as important. A person of value.
Our practice is a unique practice where we care about our clients.

Taken together, these statements appear to be frustrated pleas for recognition and significance. As such, they almost erupt from the websites where they are posted by counselors and therapists. Readers of their websites—presumably, prospective clients—may or may not wonder why counselors and therapists believe that they, each one, are unique. Are they hungry for validation? Do they really believe that their treatment(s) is unique? If they are unique, do they really belong to a profession? Are their claims beyond the range of good sense and reason? How many of them are truly unique? And, if any of them is unique, should they be practicing counseling and therapy at all? After all, if one is or many of them are unique, they are declaring that they practice in ways that no one else practices. If this is correct, maybe, they should not be practicing. Prescribing a blend of lemon gelatin, soy sauce, and chocolate chips for herpes is unique, but it is not likely legal, let alone effective. Are these "unique" counselors and therapists effective?

At least, the profusion of "unique" therapies and therapists refers to excessive individualism. The reality of rampant individualism in counseling and therapy cannot be and should not be disregarded. Currently, it commonly characterizes clinical practice, as this book makes clear. However, this book is not the beginning of the discussion of individualism in counseling and therapy, nor will it be the end. Martin (2020) gives a detailed account of the long conversation about critical issues, including individualism, in therapy. More recently, others such as Constantino et al. (2023) have addressed this matter, too. They discuss the persistent overestimation of clinical effectiveness and explain it mostly in terms of the overconfidence bias, the belief that therapists are much more effective than the outcomes of their therapy indicate. Nuttgens (2023) describes contemporary psychotherapy as characterized by a massive proliferation of therapeutic models. Nuttgens (2023) describes contemporary psychotherapy as characterized by a massive proliferation of therapeutic models and as regressing into ineffectiveness.

No doubt many practicing therapists wish for a profession that exhibits coherence, research support, and nearly universal procedures among its members, among other broadly agreed upon features of their profession. And, likely with chagrin, they recognize that there is no minimal coherence, research support, or universal procedures among its members. Instead of minimal coherence among counselors and therapists, individuals practice what they wish to practice, without regard for the larger profession of which they are members. They express their individualism, as if to say, "I believe what I believe and because I believe what I believe, I am right to believe what I believe and, therefore, I can do what I want to do when I practice counseling and therapy." This leaves counseling and therapy as a profession without standards and, consequently, in danger.

As already indicated, the discussion of counseling and therapy as expressions of individualism has been a long one. The scope of its length lies beyond what needs to be covered here. No doubt, exaggerated individualism obviates judicious clinical decision-making and minimally competent clinical actions of counselors and therapists, inherently rejecting appropriate respect for clients' needs, autonomy, and individualism.

As a partial context for discussing the exaggerated individualism among counselors and therapists, brief attention should be given to clients' autonomy and preferences. On the side of generally showing deference to client's autonomy and preferences, Swift, Callahan, Cooper, and Parkin (2018), provide a comprehensive review of relevant research and conclude, "Based on the meta-analytic results, we conclude that accommodating client preferences exerts a positive influence on therapy dropout and treatment outcomes" (p. 1935). Extending this conclusion, they offer several specific clinical recommendations, including this one: "Seek to accommodate client preferences in psychotherapy—especially when strong preferences are held. Preference accommodation should be the default choice, at least initially, unless there are clinical or legal reasons not to" (p. 1935). While nothing in their analysis abrogates appropriate clinical attention to systems of which clients may be members, their recommendations demonstrate not only the importance of respecting clients' autonomy but also the importance of research as a source for understanding clinical decision-making. A significant implication of this meta-analysis is that therapists' preferences, with specific reference to religious preferences, may impair the possibility of positive treatment outcomes.

The clinical and presumed belief in client autonomy and preferences appears to be an almost universal one. Among others, Anderson (2020) attests to the importance of client autonomy in the context of family therapy. However, client preferences and autonomy should not be taken to mean that counselors and therapists should sanction unqualified self-interest—either their clients' or their own. The cautions around this are clear. For example, Tredinnick and Fowers (1999) discuss individualism and psychotherapy and conclude, "From this perspective, relationships are based not so much on loyalties, duties, and obligations, but on an instrumental understanding of what will maximize one's self-interest" (pp. 310–311). They emphasize the high potential for unhealthy, even selfish, approaches to therapy. With this emphasis, they conclude, "Unfortunately, if we as psychologists [and other counselors and therapists] promote the utilitarian perspective we may unwittingly exacerbate the endemic isolation, alienation, anxiety, and depression in the United States" (p. 311).

Expressed Individualism

This book includes an appendix in which 400 religion-oriented approaches are listed. As large as the list is, it is a small, partial list of such approaches. Altogether, they represent a number of religious approaches to counseling and therapy that likely surprise, if not shock, most readers. Read carefully and taken seriously, the list of titles for some sort of religion-oriented therapy may be understandably mind-numbing. The list includes only 400 items. While the number and variety of approaches may be shocking, it comes from the larger endeavor of collecting information from the websites of practicing licensed counselors and therapists. As large as it is, it is a small sampling of religious approaches to therapy, taken from the Big List. So far, research has located more than ten times the number of religious therapies (e.g., Islamic Integrated Psychotherapy, Recovery of Soul-Mind Fragmentation (RSF) Therapy, Soul Biofield Tuning, Mary Queen of Angels Cards Readings, and RoHun Soul Alignment) that appear in this book. Further, in addition to the number of specifically religious approaches, another much larger number of religion-related approaches (e.g., Archangel Life Coaching, Divine Channeling, Nature-based Mysticism, or Throne Room Therapy) exceeds 10,000. A careful reading of the Appendix may be mind-numbing, but those who read it should consider whether the practice of these therapies may be profession-numbing, too. As asked several times in this book, "Can you be a member of a health care profession, when you cannot recognize most of the treatments that your peers advertise?"

If counseling and therapy can be all of the approaches that appear in this book—even if these were the complete list—can counseling and therapy sustain viability? Framed differently to inquire about religion-specific approaches, when "Christian" is used by licensed counselors and therapists as an adjective for almost every conceivable approach to counseling and therapy, what does "Christian" mean? When it becomes an adjective attached to Gestalt, EMDR, Natal Charts, Narrative Therapy, Eclecticism, Feminist Therapy, Cognitive Behavior Therapy, Mysticism, LDS Therapy, Psychoanalysis, Buddhism, Yoga, Dream Interpretation, and almost 4,000 other approaches, what does "Christian" mean? These questions are not simply about what Christianity is? Each individual who wishes to identify as Christian may define it simply according to personal preference. With regard to religion in general or Christianity in particular, individual personal preferences express religious freedom. This is the way it should be. In this discussion, however, the more fundamental question is "What are is counseling and therapy?" Can counseling and therapy truly be all of these things? Can counseling and therapy be all of the 38,373 approaches to counseling and therapy that we have so far located on the websites of practicing counselors and therapists? If therapy can be all of these things, an understanding and effective practice of it may be impossible.

Can counseling and therapy be all of the 400 approaches listed in the Appendix. For now, as a partial context for understanding the approaches in the Appendix, Chart 2.3 indicates the number of approaches that include some form of the selected words. The chart includes two numbers for each word(s) that is used in a title for an approach to counseling and therapy.

Chart 2.3 Number of Six Selected Approaches in the Appendix and Big List

Selected Word	*Number in Appendix A*	*Total Number Collected*[*]
Shaman/Shamanic	17	112
Bible/Biblical[*]	25	466
Spirit/Spiritual/Spiritually	31	1,842
Buddhism/Buddhist[*]	43	278
Christ/Christian[*]	113	1,246
Soul	114	429

Note
[*] This refers to the number of times that these terms appear on The Big List.

The first number comes from the list in Appendix A. The second number comes from the Big List—the one with 38,373 titles of therapies in it—that has so far been gathered.

The selected words in the chart do not encompass all of the words that may be associated with them. Each of them closely relates to other words that are reported as treatment orientations. "Biblical" closely relates to Word of God. "Buddhist" closely relates to Contemplative Therapy. And, "Christian" closely relates to numerous approaches to counseling and therapy, including Apostolic Counseling, Catholic Counseling, Ministry, Gospel, Holy Spirit, Church, and Prayer. All of these words appear on the Big List, but none of these related words are accounted for in Chart 2.3. Many of the Christian-related words appear in Chart 1.5.

The number of religion-oriented approaches to counseling and therapy may be compared with the number of approaches that are not religion-oriented. Such a comparison avoids the easy temptation to think incorrectly about how skewed counseling and therapy have become because of religious interests alone. Similar to the extraordinarily large number of specifically religious approaches to therapy, numerous others that are not religious also evoke skepticism about therapy. Therefore, just as six religion-oriented approaches are listed in Chart 2.3, Chart 2.4 contains another six

Chart 2.4 Frequently Use Words in Advertised Treatment Orientations

Word	*Number of Appearances on the Big List*
Body-Related	1,168
CBT (479)/Cognitive Behavioral Therapy (1,012)	1,491
Coaching	1,119
Integrative/Integrated	1,608
Mindful	1,134
Trauma	1,205

words that are commonly advertised approaches to counseling and therapy. They are not religion-oriented. Also, they are a mere sampling of a much larger list and much larger numbers. Taken together, these two short lists of only 12 treatment approaches refer to an astonishing number: 12,098 treatment approaches. One of the non-religious words is "coaching." A large list of coaching-related, advertised approaches to counseling and therapy appears later in this chapter. Charts 2.3 and 2.4, along with Chart 2.5, later in this chapter, compel concern about the status of counseling and therapy, while the emphasis on exaggerated individualism out of which these advertised approaches have been invented is the energizing factor from which these numbers come.

These numbers give the appearance of many approaches to counseling and therapy as being normal. The appearance may be misleading. The Big List includes numerous approaches that professionally accountable counselors and therapists would deem to be abnormal and possibly harmful. Among the numerous approaches that have been gathered and appear in The Big List, 34 contain the word, "Alchemy." Another 103 contain the words "Past Life," (e.g., Advanced Past Life Memory Access Therapy, Age/Past Life Regression Therapy, Ancestral Past Life Healing, Bio-genic Past Life Regression Therapy, Clearing Past Life Relationships, Past-Life Regression Meditation, Past Life Partner Regressions, and Past Life Soul Retrieval). Taken together, the list of past life-associated approaches to therapy may be as alarming as they are entertaining, allowing for the observation that they are almost entirely non-clinical and non-relevant but also potentially harmful to clients. The Big List also includes numerous quasi-religious approaches to counseling and therapy, including Divine Destiny Therapy and Divine Metaphysics.

This book gives attention to religion and related matters in the practice of counseling and therapy. As a necessary aside, some of the absurdity that characterizes specifically religious approaches to therapy may be easily seen in a large number of other approaches. This may be illustrated if coaching-related approaches are taken from the Big List. As noted in the chart above, "Coaching" appears more than 1,100 times in the Big List. Usually, the presence of "coaching" in counseling and therapy is presumed to be common and acceptable—as something normal. The number and variety of coaching-related approaches are not normal, though. As an analog to the profligate, specifically religious approaches to therapy, the presentation of a sampling of coaching-related approaches helps to establish a view of counseling and therapy as activities that are, at least, out of appropriate control, due largely to exaggerated individualism. While all of the terms in Charts 2.3 and 2.4 suggest that virtually limitless ways of thinking about counseling and therapy have been selected and/or invented, the list of coaching-related approaches in Chart 2.5 further confirms how very out of

Chart 2.5 Coaching-Related Approaches to Counseling and Therapy

24/7 Laser Confidence Coaching
Alternative Spirituality Coaching & Counseling
American Natural Wellness Coaching
Angelic Life Purpose Coaching
Anodyne Coaching
Archangel Life Coaching
Authentic Happiness Coaching
Avis-R Skill Coaching Protocol
Bible Life Coaching
Bible Studies Coaching
Biblical Marriage Coaching
Body-Centered Transformational Coaching
Boundaries in Dating/Coaching
Brain-Informed Empathic Coaching & Training
Buddhist Coaching
Business Strategies and Life Coaching
Catholic Coaching
Ceremonial Practices Coaching
Character Champions Self-Leadership Coaching
Christ-Centered Coaching
Christian Biblical Coaching
Christian Conflict and Relationship Coaching
Christian Soul Coaching
Christian-God Focused Coaching
Co-Active Coaching Gestalt
CoacHer
Coaching and Hypnotherapy
Coaching and Inspirational Services
Coaching for Trauma
Coaching in The Law of Attraction
Coaching Kiva
Coaching Wisdom
CoachVille Life Coaching
Collaborative Journey Coaching
Collaborative Law Divorce Coaching
Complicated Pain Recovery Coaching
Comprehensive Spiritual and Life Coaching
Complicated Pain Recovery Coaching
Comprehensive Spiritual and Life Coaching
Confidence Life Coaching
Conscious Uncoupling Coaching
Contemplative Coaching
Core Energy Coaching
Couples Principals [sic] Coaching
CRAFT/Parent Coaching
Creative Prescriptions Coaching
Creativity & Imagery Coaching/Movement
Culinary Health Coaching
Cultural Competency Coaching
Cutting Edge Laser Coaching

control counseling and therapy are. From a total of 1,119 on The Big List, the Chart includes only 50 approaches.

Obviously, allowing for several exceptions, most of the Coaching approaches in Chart 2.5 are not related to religion. Including the ones that are related to religion, though, the list, at least, makes the point that numerous counselors and therapists invent approaches that have little or no basis in clinical reality. Also, the list reinforces the fact that, like religious approaches to counseling and therapy, coaching can be anything that an individual wants it to be. If coaching can be anything that an individual or subset of individuals say that it is, is it anything of relevance that can be defined and utilized with minimal understanding, appropriateness, and effectiveness? Thus, whether the topic is coaching or religion, those who observe the vast array of advertised approaches to them must wonder whether either of them can endure with minimal credibility.

Readers who may want to take time to reflect on the list of advertised approaches in Chart 2.5 consider the following questions.

How many of them do you recognize as treatment approaches?
How many of them would you want to adopt as treatment approaches?
How many counselors and therapists who advertise and practice some of these approaches do you know?
If you recognize only a few of them or, maybe, none of them, what do you conclude about our profession?
If you recognize few, if any of them, are you really a member of the profession in which these treatments are advertised by your presumed peers?
Or, possibly, more consequentially, if individuals or subsets of individual can invent so very many coaching-related approaches to counseling and therapy, do counseling and therapy really exist?

As this book develops, several observations will be added to those already made. For now and in anticipation of presentations of information and analyses throughout this book, only four observations will be made here. They are intended to be invitations to consideration of and dialogue about significant challenges for counselors and therapists.

One, the profession of counseling and therapy is massively under-regulated. As evidence is further presented in this book, this observation will be confirmed. For now, suffice it to report that we have so far located more than 5,000 specifically religious approaches to counseling and therapy.

Two, the proliferation of specifically religious ideologies, along with other ideologies, is transforming counseling and therapy into religious or quasi-religious activities. As such, rising numbers of those who provide mental health care do not struggle with ways to include agreed-upon, research-validated evidence into their clinical work; they oppose it.

Three, on a nearly incomprehensible scale, individuals who have been trained in conventional and universally accepted preparation programs "just make up stuff" and call it "therapy." Such "made up stuff" needs no basis in anything appropriately related to counseling and psychotherapy (e.g., Holy Spirit-Guided Psychotherapy or Laying-on-of-hands Healing). Possibly, the most important implication of this is that preparation programs for licensing and practice appear to contribute little toward the professional and effective practice of counseling and therapy, as the evidence in Chapter 8 shows. Instead, they appear to manifest the exaggerated individualism that was discussed earlier.

Four, counseling and psychotherapy are not healthy. Insofar as this observation describes the current condition of counseling and therapy, questions arise: What, if anything, is being done about this? What should be done about this? Why would major professional associations not seek to protect clients from the onslaught of treatments that are likely ineffective and easily conceivably harmful—to clients and to the profession? Chapters 6–9 recommend urgently needed actions by preparation programs, individual therapists, professional associations, state legislatures, licensing boards, businesses and corporations, and social service agencies.

The self-serving, magical thinking that facilitates conspicuous and exaggerated individualism into counseling and therapy betrays clinical judgment and subordinates professional accountability to individuals and practices that deny the immense, positive potential of counseling and therapy. Such thinking seems to follow a child-like trajectory: "I believe what I believe and because I believe it, I am right. And, because I am right—and righteous—I can integrate my beliefs into my practice of therapy."

Rampant individualism has shaped client care, almost from the beginning of the mental health movement. Discussions of individualism refer to it as an impairment in the way therapy is conducted, accentuating clinical distortions of individuals. This is to say that individual clients are often treated as if they are not members of families or larger systems. For example, Vermes (2017) posits that individualism and individual therapy models have seriously and unnecessarily limited the potential of psychotherapy. Along with Vermes, others have reported similar conclusions (e.g., Fowers, Tredinnick, & Applegate, 1997; Richardson & Zeddies, 2001; Walfish, McAllister, O'Donnell, & Lambert 2012). Instead of an emphasis on individualizing treatment, but not in opposition to it, the view here is that individualism has saturated the decision-making of counselors and therapists and that this saturation has come to be expressed in a virtually countless number of approaches to counseling and therapy. Translated into a common idea, the ubiquitous meaning is that numerous counselors and therapists have concluded, "It's about me!" And, their "me-ism" appears as tens of thousands of specifically religion or quasi-religious approaches to therapy.

Significantly, the view here is that whatever personal beliefs an individual may wish to claim, they are likely to be entirely respectable beliefs. May an individual wish to claim Native American spirituality? Well, of course. May an individual wish to claim Christian fundamentalism or liberalism? Again, of course. May an individual wish to claim Sufi mysticism? Again, of course. Any or all of these beliefs may not appeal to many others, but an individual may find appropriate meaning in them. These beliefs should not be targets for denial or elimination. Each of us is entitled to pursue and hold beliefs that give us meaning, a social place, useful values, and other life-affirming assets. However, when these personal beliefs, along with many of the ones identified in this book, become the reason and cause for conducting counseling and therapy, they have breached a boundary. A strongly and sincerely held personal belief is not in itself a sufficient basis for integrating it into the practice of counseling and psychotherapy, any more than a sincerely held personal belief in one's own approach to parenting is a sufficient basis for integrating it into counseling and therapy.

Among those who identify as Christian, who is right, when one of them who is a therapist holds an opposing view that is held by another Christian therapist? Who is right, if the question relates to racial animus or racial justice? Who is right, when the questions relate to sexual orientation? If one Christian argues for abortion and another Christian argues against it, who is right? Can both of these individuals be therapists? To what extent should either of them have the prerogative to advance their point of view as therapeutic? More fundamentally, do their respective views have relevance to the practice of counseling and therapy? If they have a view, such as the rightness or wrongness of abortion, by what credible and professional rationale may they conclude that they can pursue an approach to therapy that confirms their rightness? And, as therapists, if they need to be right about such issues, to what extent have they abandoned clinical judgment? Generally, a therapist's role does not require the vindication of rightness; it requires clinical effectiveness. To choose rightness instead of effectiveness leads to ineffectiveness and, worse, potential harm.

The current suffusion of religion into counseling and therapy may be justifiably characterized as a war against counseling and therapy. As war, it is not an aggressive, bloody, militant, angry, explosive war. Instead, it is a clean, gentle, or even empathic, ideological, fragmented, extremely variegated, sometimes self-righteous and self-serving war. It is waged largely through the means of a borrowed identity, an affiliation with health care that betrays the rigor, evidence, clinical neutrality, and openness of nearly all, if not all, other kinds of health care. This war is sustained by huge numbers of "clinical troops" who pose as counselors and therapists.

Confident in their ideological causes, they wage war, to be sure. Their warfare, though, perpetuates the irrational and harmful commitment to pre-scientific, anti-intellectual, and highly individualized "therapies." Their therapies have become "weapons," implemented as numerous forms of assault on counseling and therapy. As wagers war, their commitment is this: "If I believe it, it's true. If I believe it's true, I can use it as therapy. And, if I am doing it as therapy, I am doing something therapeutic." Such a commitment lacks clinically relevant evidence to support it. Worse, it may harm clinical practice and clients who receive it.

More broadly, the massive proliferation of specifically religious approaches to counseling and therapy supports numerous, presumed clinical initiatives that join with at least two other supports for these initiatives. If the first one emphasizes exaggerated individualism, the other is the conspicuous fragmentation among counselors and therapists, depriving the profession of desperately needed coherence and credibility. These three symptoms of the critical, tenuous condition of counseling and therapy appear as themes or subthemes throughout this book.

However, the present discussion accounts for rampant individualism as only one major, deleterious influence on counseling and therapy. Individualism alone cannot explain everything that may characterize the ongoing decline of mental health care. The other influences—explored later in this book—should not be ignored. For example, several theological schools prepare prospective licensees within programs that are heavily ideological and oppressive, grossly out of sync with normative academic standards and standards of professional mental health care. Similarly, another source of serious harm to counseling and therapy are organizations that issue non-state licenses to clearly unqualified individuals who presume to practice counseling and therapy. And, as noted later, professional associations, credentialing organizations, and other influences likely contribute to the seriously compromised condition of counseling and therapy. Individualism, then, is clearly a problem, but it does not stand alone in its ongoing, expanding, and deleterious impact on counseling and therapy.

References

Anderson, J. R. (2020). Inviting autonomy back to the table: The importance of autonomy for healthy relationship functioning. *Journal of Marital & Family Therapy*, *46*(1), 3–14.

Cohen, M. (2019). Working with religion: Often neglected aspects of transference and countertransference. *The American Journal of Psychoanalysis*, *79*(1), 103–113.

Constantino, M. J., Boswell, J. F., Coyne, A. E., Muir, H. H., Gaines, A. N., & Kraus, D. R. (2023). Therapist perceptions of their own measurement-based, problem-specific effectiveness. *Journal of Consulting and Clinical Psychology*, *91*(8), 474–484. 10.1037/ccp0000813

Davis, F. A. (1988). Medicare hospice benefit: Early program experiences. *Health Care Financing Review*, *9*(4), 99–111.
Fowers, B. J., Tredinnick, M., & Applegate, B. (1997). Individualism and counseling: An empirical examination of the prevalence of individualistic values in psychologists' responses to case vignettes. *Counseling and Values*, *41*(3), 204–217.
Healthcare Chaplains Ministry Association. (2022). Healthcare Chaplains Ministry Association. https://www.hcmachaplains.com
Kehoe, N. C., & Gutheil, T. G. (1993). Ministry or therapy: The role of transference and countertransference in a religious therapist. In M. L. Randour (Ed.), *Exploring sacred landscapes: religious and spiritual experiences in psychotherapy* (pp. 55–80). New York: Columbia University Press.
Malark, A. (2017). Sexuality, religion, and atheism in psychodynamic treatment. *Psychology of Sexual Orientation and Gender Diversity*, *4*(4), 412–421.
Martin, F. A. (2020). *Therapy thieves: How to save mental health care from its providers.* New York: Oxford University Press.
Martin, F. A., & Turner, J. P. (2023). Healthy helping: Confronting impairments and creating a new vision for counseling and psychotherapy (Unpublished manuscript)
Nuttgens, S. (2023). Of interventive doppelgangers and other barriers to evidence-based practice in psychotherapy. *Journal of Psychotherapy Integration*, *33*(1), 20–33. 10.1037/int0000279
Peteet, J. R. (2009). Struggles with god: transference and religious countertransference in the treatment of a trauma survivor. *The Journal of the American Academy of Psychoanalysis and Dynamic Psychiatry*, *37*(1), 165–174.
Richardson, F. C., Zeddies, T. J. (2001). Individualism and modern psychotherapy. In B. D. Slife, R. N. Williams, & S. H. Barlow (Eds.), *Critical issues in psychotherapy: Translating new ideas into practice* (pp. 147–164). Thousand Oaks, CA: Sage.
Swift, J. K., Callahan, J. L., Cooper, M., & Parkin, S. R. (2018). The impact of accommodating client preference in psychotherapy: A meta-analysis. *Journal of Clinical Psychology*, *74*, 1924–1937.
Tredinnick, M., & Fowers, B. J. (1999). Individualism and psychotherapy: Are psychologists leading or following individualistic trends. *Counselling Psychology Quarterly*, *12*, 303–313. doi: 10.1080/09515079908254100
Vermes, C. (2017). The individualism impasse in counselling psychology. *Counselling Psychology Review*, *32*(1), 44–53.
Walfish, S., McAllister, B., O'Donnell, P. & Lambert, M. J. (2012). An investigation of self-assessment bias in mental health providers. *Psychological Reports*, *110*(2), 639–644.
White, R. S. (2023). An antisemitic transference and countertransference. *International Journal of Applied Psychoanalytic Studies*, *20*(1), 55–69.

3 Mercenary Organizations

Almost nine of ten of those who advertise some form of "Christian Counseling" do not give any indication of preparation for providing Christian Counseling where they advertise their services, according to the survey of tens of thousands of websites. They completed their clinical preparation programs in institutions that are not "Christian," including state-sponsored, for-profit, or non-religious private institutions. Also, most of those who offer some form of "Christian Counseling" do not indicate that they have any relevant training such as a professional and broadly recognized certification. However, the apparent failure of self-identified Christian counselors to complete professional preparation for the services that they advertise is not exceptional, with regard to incomplete or no such preparation. Similar to this failure, those who advertise sex therapy, Eye Movement Desensitization and Reprogramming (EMDR), or play therapy exhibit less preparation and fewer indicators of their professional competency to deliver it than those who advertise some form of Christian Counseling.

Expressions of or Exploitations of Faith?

Although they may be appropriately trained and licensed, individual counselors and psychotherapists who advertise services for which they appear to be unqualified to provide do not stand alone. For one thing, they are accompanied by an unknown but large number of individuals who have little or no training and, obviously, no license, but who claim to deliver the therapies that appropriately trained and credentialed individuals also deliver. In addition, they are augmented by institutions and organizations that undermine professional accountability and integrity in counseling and therapy. The number and size of these institutions and organizations are not clearly known. However, there are many of them that advertise their various certifications, licenses, degrees, and other offerings. A brief discussion of some of these organizations surely includes the five of them that are included below. They are

DOI: 10.4324/9781003472469-4

National Association of Christian Counselors (NACC)
Association of Certified Biblical Counselors (ACBC)
Pastoral Medical Association (PMA)
Ministry International Institute (MII)
National Christian Counselors Association (NCCA)

National Association of Christian Counselors

The National Association of Christian Counselors (NACC) offers certifications and licenses. The NACC provides licenses to individuals whose training is, at best, minimal. Although the NACC says that its licenses are "applicable to Counseling and Therapy performed under the covering of a church, ministry, or other religious non-profit corporation" (National Association of Christian Counselors, 2021), some of their licensees utilize their licenses as if they are state-issued licenses and some of the titles of their licenses are identical to state-issued licenses. Wisely, it advises its licensees, "The NACC does not compete with state licensing. We do however offer an alternative for those 'Pastors' and other Ministers who choose to make counseling their 'ministry' and cannot for some reason pursue state licensing" (NACC, 2021). Does NACC's "alternative" to state licenses indicate that those who hold its alternative license are somehow equal to or approximately the same as state-issued licenses? Apparently, the implication is that NACC promotes its licenses as having the same—or maybe superior—status as state-issued licenses. It adds, "Please check with your state to determine the use of the words 'Clinical,' 'Therapist,' and the term 'Licensed.' If your state does not allow you to use these terms you need to know this information." The NACC defines its role as a "ministry." One can only imagine the volcanic fury that would erupt among professional associations and state legislatures, if, say, the National Association of Christian Cardiologists (NACC), a fictional organization, advertised that it issued licenses to those who for some reason cannot pursue state licensing, but who, despite this serious limitation, practice Christian cardiology. The NACC explains,

> The National Association of Christian Counselors is a Christian ministry established in 2008 to train Biblical counselors and teachers to assist local churches and to help meet related needs. Our purpose is to bridge the gap between faith and life so that as the individual's relationship with God grows, they begin to live for God's glory. As change takes place, they experience His peace and joy. The main purpose of NACC is to provide adequate training for local Pastors and Christians who feel the call of God to counsel. Once trained, counselors are provided with

> credentials through the National Association of Christian Counselors. (National Association of Christian Counselors, 2021)

A response to the NACC's issuance of certifications and licenses should include questions such as these. If the services that individuals are encouraged to deliver are intended "to assist local churches," why is a license necessary? Why is a license issued that involves so very little training and no clinical supervision? If the license has minimal merit and/or integrity, why are some licenses not revoked, based on the fact that license holders engage in practices for which they are conspicuously unqualified? The advertising of the licenses at the NACC website strongly suggests that little more than a fee of $450.00 is required. Apparently, no clinical supervision is required. Apparently, no specific clinical coursework or continuing education is required.

Despite the obvious and serious limitations of those who are credentialed by the NACC, the organization promises to provide services that appear to be very similar to the services offered by those who are professionally trained, holders of credible state-issued licenses, and subject to professional ethical standards. The NACC says,

> NACC provides counseling for men, women, adolescents, and children. We also provide individual, family/group, and marriage counseling. All of our counselors are equipped to deal with abuse issues, depression, addictions, anxiety, and the many complex counseling needs of individuals and couples living in today's society.
>
> NACC provides Christ centered, biblically based professional counseling to individuals and families in a way that brings encouragement, understanding and healing. (National Association of Christian Counselors, 2022)

If NACC licenses are presumed to qualify their holders to provide counseling and therapy, as they apparently presume is the case, why is this not misleading and fraudulent? Apparently, the NACC and similar organizations are protected from prosecution for practicing a major health care service (i.e., counseling and therapy) without proper training or licensing because it is a "Christian" organization. Analogously, the possibility that an organization such as the NACC could issue licenses that presumably authorizes and qualifies individuals to practice dentistry or neurosurgery would inevitably and justly receive immediate condemnation and prohibition.

Association of Certified Biblical Counselors

Began in 1976, the Association of Certified Biblical Counselors (ACBC) says that its members (i.e., certified individuals) have risen to many thousands. The ACBC defines its role and mission, stating, "We seek to strengthen the Church to speak the truth in love by providing a quality training and certification process, a global network of like-minded individuals and institutions, and a source of practical and biblical resources for the Church" (Association of Certified Biblical Counselors, 2021). To extend and clarify this, it also says, "In short, we seek to bring biblical solutions for the problems people face, upholding that the method God has given to do this is truth in love." Naturally, this assertion opens the question about whether God has given ACBC certificate holders the counseling and therapy methods that are needed for effective counseling and therapy.

ACBC's expressed determination to bring biblical solutions to problems through "the method God has given to do this is truth in love." To "speak the truth in love" in love rests on a massively self-indulgent assumption. Namely, that those who are certified by the ACBC know "the truth." They may not be as loving or consistent as the idea of being loving may imply. When it speaks about those who are not "like-minded," it says,

> As state governments continue to encroach upon the religious liberties of individuals and groups, ACBC recognizes that this is particularly noticeable within the discipline and practice of counseling. As Christians, we affirm that it is inconsistent to withhold biblical morality and mandates in counseling and soul care, in deference to state statues and codes of ethics which regulate Christian principles and truths. With these concerns in mind, ACBC welcomes those currently holding state licensure for professional counseling to engage in our Phase One training, to further discern the philosophical and theological underpinnings that distinguish biblical counseling from other approaches.
>
> Since counseling is fundamentally theological in nature, ACBC reserves the right not to approve current Licensed Professional Counselors, Licensed Mental Health Counselors, or those holding equitable licenses for counseling services, from continuing the certification process due to the growing ethical and moral restrictions placed upon state licensed practitioners. However, those who have completed Phase One and wish to continue in progression with ACBC certification may make an appeal for consideration with the ACBC Membership Services department. (Association of Certified Biblical Counselors, 2021a)

ACBC imposes a critically important restriction on those who are licensed by state governments. It holds that "state governments continue to encroach on religious liberties," but offers no explanation of this, let alone evidence for it. Also, with the apparent intention of constraining state-issued licensees who are Christian, but who disagree with the ACBC, the ACBC affirms "that it is inconsistent to withhold biblical morality and mandates in counseling and soul care, in deference to state statues and codes of ethics which regulate Christian principles and truths." The conclusion that those who hold state-issued licenses "withhold biblical morality and mandates in counseling and soul care" appears to express grandiosity and a judgmental view, as if its ideas about biblical morality and mandates hold more significance than all others.

The ACBC makes a "Commitment to Purity" (Association of Certified Biblical Counselors, 2021b). It defines "purity" in the following manner "God created sex to be enjoyed in the context of the marriage relationship between one man and one woman." Based on this commitment, the rest of ACBC's commitment to purity is somewhat predictable. It says, "All other sexual expressions constitute sexual immorality and are heinous sins, bringing pain into the lives of all who are engaged in them. Counselors have a biblical responsibility to foster sexual purity in their attitudes, actions, and speech." If this standard of purity demands the approach that it clearly demands, every child around the age of, say, 14 is led to conclude that her or his heightened and sometimes extraordinarily compelling interest in sex expressed through masturbation has committed a "heinous sin." Do ACBCers hold equal concern about overeating, excessive alcohol consumption, or other indicators of human fallibility and vulnerability? If not, does this suggest that they are excessively preoccupied with sex and sexual activities, along with a denial of their humanity?

If "Counselors have a biblical responsibility to foster sexual purity in their attitudes, actions, and speech," what are the real-life implications of this, particularly in the lives of those who are targets of such a standard, including counselors who intend to deliver professional services to their clients? What is "sexual purity?" What is the meaning of "foster sexual purity?" What should counselors do to foster sexual purity in their clients' "attitudes, actions and speech?" What should counselors do when they are confronted with clients whose lives have been destroyed by the promotion of sexual purity? [Refer to Chapter 9 for examples of the possible destructive consequences of promoting sexual purity.] And, what should counselors do for clients whose attitudes, actions, and speech contradict the views of such counselors? The view here is that professionally accountable counselors and therapists more likely than not create an unfriendly, cynical, non-clinical, and judgmental clinical relationship with clients when they promote their preferred ideology, regardless of the specific needs and values of their clients. Is this what the ACBC does?

Apparently, ACBC's beliefs about purity come entirely from the views of men about women. Again, somewhat predictably, its views about women are clear and rigid. Under the heading, "Female Pastors," the question,

"Can I become certified if my church has a female pastor?" is raised and answered on its website, ACBC says,

> The local church is indispensable in the ministry of counseling. We believe our counselors must pursue the closest possible connection to their church for accountability and ecclesiastical authority. In light of the importance of ecclesiastical oversight, we require our counselors to serve under biblically qualified leadership in their church. At ACBC, we hold a complementarian view, recognizing that while women may serve the church in a myriad of ways, the Bible requires that an elder/pastor be a man meeting specific qualifications (1 Timothy 2:11–15; 1 Corinthians 11:1–3; 1 Timothy 3:2–7; Titus 1:5–9; 1 Peter 5:1–3). Because of these beliefs, both of which are reflected in our guiding documents, we cannot certify an individual who has joined fellowship with a church that has a female given the role or title of elder/pastor, regardless of their oversight responsibilities. (Association of Certified Biblical Counselors, 2021c)

The ACBC appears to advocate for a non-human understanding of being human, presuming such understanding to be divine. Including its apparently closed-minded and cynical, if not hostile, view of those who prepared for and received a license from a state, the ACBC advances a view of counseling that defies a minimally reasonable view of human beings. It seems to want the human experience to regress into a primitive style of life that ACBC-related devotees are unlikely to accept. What is ACBC's "biblical solution" to the challenge of climate change, with specific reference to how its adherents allegiance to "the truth" heat their homes? Have ACBC certificants opted to live in homes without electricity? How many of them are divorced? Can a divorced man be certified through ACBC? How many of them have masturbated? How precisely does ACBC monitor sexual purity? Does "biblical solution" involve pediatric dentists, when maybe the dentist is not Christian, let alone certified by ACBC? Do "biblical solutions" include avoidance of buying products that were produced in various oppressive, tyrannical countries? More generally, where does "the truth" begin and end, in the lives of those who are certified through ACBC? Are Biblical morality and its mandates limited mostly to sex-related aspects of being human?

Additional questions inevitably arise, with regard to ACBC's specific biblical instructions for treating sickness. Are ACBC certificants truly "biblical," "Christ-centered," "gospel-centered," or other specifically religious ways of framing their alleged clinical approach? In James 5:15 ESV, The Bible says, "And the prayer of faith will save the one who is sick ..." Or, more narrowly, with regard to trauma and distress, The Bible says, "Give strong drink to the one who is perishing, and wine to those in bitter distress" (Proverbs 31:6 ESV). As Biblical mandates, adherents of ACBC's approach to life would necessarily not seek medical care and, when distressed, drink wine. This is "good news" for everyone who lives with compulsions to medicate their distress with alcohol. And, wryly construed, if taken seriously, those who practice counseling and therapy or almost any other form of health care should know that they should encourage others to take "strong drink" and "wine" as their medicine. These actions are, after all, Biblical mandates.

Apparently, the ACBC believes that training in counseling and therapy, particularly when it leads to a state-issued license, is not only necessary but also an act of disobedience to God. After all, as another reminder for those whose "biblical" views guide their healing-related behaviors, "Is anyone among you sick? Let him call for the elders of the church, and let them pray over him, anointing him with oil in the name of the Lord" (James 5:14 ESV). Examined carefully, this statement may refer only to boys and men, not to women and girls, as in "let him call for the elders." Again, taking their views seriously—maybe, more seriously than ACBCers do, training as a counselor/therapist is not necessary and may be a betrayal of clearly stated biblical teachings. Indeed, instead of training to be counselors, everyone who shares in their like-mindedness should go to church leaders and pray for healing and, then, of course, have plenty of oil on hand. Apparently, the ACBC intends to co-opt a professional service for its ill-equipped and rigidly ideological predation toward and acquisition of counseling and therapy. As such, observers of the ACBE must wonder whether it harms counseling and therapy and those who need services from professional counselors and therapists.

Pastoral Medical Association

The Pastoral Medical Association (PMA) has issued licenses and degrees for at least 25 years, although the exact beginning of the PMA could not be easily located. While the beginning of the PMA may not be clearly known, its truly unusual work has not eluded notice. In 2016, NPR—National Public Radio—provided an analysis of PMA's work. It reported,

> You've probably heard of the credentials M.D. and R.N., and maybe N.P. The people using those letters are doctors, registered nurses and nurse practitioners. But what about PSC.D or D.PSc? Those letters refer to someone who practices pastoral medicine—or "Bible-based" health care.
>
> It's a relatively new title being used by some alternative health practitioners. The Texas-based Pastoral Medical Association gives out "pastoral provider licenses" in all 50 states and 30 countries. Some providers call themselves doctors of pastoral medicine. But these licenses

> are not medical degrees. That has watchdog organizations concerned that some patients may not understand what this certification really means. (NPR, 2021)

Steven Barrett (2018) wrote a detailed and compelling analysis of the Pastoral Medical Association, "Some Notes on the Pastoral Medical Association and other 'Private Membership Associations.'" Writing from the view of a physician, Barrett closes his article with a list of "My Concerns." Introducing his list of concerns with the statement, "The 'PSc.D.' credential and the claims made for private membership associations have considerable potential for harm," he continued with his list of concerns. He wrote,

> Consumers may mistakenly conclude that the PSc.D. credential signifies doctoral-level training.
>
> Consumers may mistakenly conclude that PMA's "license" reflects competence and government approval.
>
> Licensed practitioners may be encouraged to expand their scope into areas beyond their competence.
>
> Unlicensed practitioners, including some who have had their real state license(s) revoked, may think that the PMA's offerings will exempt them from government regulation.
>
> Marketers of supplements and bogus devices may think they can get away with making bolder claims for their products.
>
> Dealing with PMA's credentials may be burdensome to regulators and the courts. (Barrett, 2018)

Barrett's judgments may be regarded with suspicion, because he writes from the view of a physician who, just because he opposes the activities of the PMA, feels compelled to judge the PMA negatively. However, insofar as Barrett judges the PMA negatively, the PMA itself provides clear bases for doing so. For example, one of the PMA's allied associations says,

> Not long ago Colorado became the 17th state to provide legal recognition for naturopathic doctors; however, the law recognizes them only if they have completed a 4-year post-graduate program at an accredited naturopathic medical school and have passed a national science and clinical board exam. If this law were to pass in Oklahoma the non-licensed naturopathic doctors would not be recognized.
>
> Although Dr. Menzel is a Board Certified Naturopathic Doctor, she is not a licensed medical doctor, so the PMA allows her to share freely her suggestions under an ecclesiastical membership association. This also gives you the assurance you are getting a qualified naturopathic doctor.

> To receive her license she went through an extensive background check along with written and oral interviews. (Energetic Wellness, 2023)

The view of Energetic Wellness and the Pastoral Medical Association is that, if regulatory laws were passed, "the non-licensed naturopathic doctors would not be recognized." They add that "she is not a licensed medical doctor," but that she may "share freely her suggestions under an ecclesiastical membership association." Converted into its licensing for mental health care providers, the idea is that they may practice "under an ecclesiastical membership association." The PMA is clear about this. It defines itself, stating, "The Pastoral Medical Association (PMA) is an established ecclesiastical association developed over a decade and a half ago to restore bible based wellness and counseling services, to provide a constitutionally sound path for licensing of spiritually oriented practitioners that desire to offer those services, and to connect the millions seeking such services with our licensed providers" (Pastoral Medical Association, 2021). With narrowed specificity, it adds, "First and foremost, PMA practitioners have taken a vow to uphold scriptural principles when interacting with clients and providing services" (Pastoral Medical Association, 2021).

In its description of the services that its licensees provide, the PMA uses several, somewhat synonymous phrases, including "scriptural principles" and "biblically-sound natural processes," to establish its ideological foundation. In addition, decrying its opposition to conventional medicine, it claims that its providers can effectively treat a large number of physical and mental-emotional problems. Its list of problems (Pastoral Medical Association, 2021) includes

Abnormal bumps	Aggression	Binge eating
Blurred vision	Bone fracture	Brain fog
Chest tightness	Changes in appetite	Chronic cough
Congestion	Constipation	Difficulty communicating
Digestive distress	Dizziness	Excessive thirst
Excessive urination	Fainting	Fatigue
Fever	Food allergies	Forgetfulness
Heartburn	Headaches	Inability to concentrate
Inability to exercise	Inability to lose weight	Incoherent speech
Indigestion	Insomnia	Irritability
Irritable bowel	Jaundice	Lightheadedness
Limited social skill	Loss of height	Malaise
Memory loss	Nausea	Night sweats
Obsessive interests	Pain	Pot belly
Rapid heartbeat	Reduced range of motion	Repetitive behaviors
Recurrent infections	Shortness of breath	Skin rash

Snoring	Social isolation	Stiffness
Swelling	Thoughts of suicide	Unexplained fever
Unexpected weight gain	Unintentional weight loss	Wheezing

The list of problems that PMA's licensees presumably and effectively treat evokes questions. Do PMA's licensees need training to treat "thoughts of suicide," "aggression," "limited social skill," "obsessive interests," or "shortness of breath?" Is the commitment to vaguely defined biblical principles sufficient for treating these important personal problems? What exactly do PMA licensees do to treat these problems? No doubt, other questions could be raised. And, no doubt, minimally well-trained counselors and therapists recognize that 'PMA's commitment "to restore bible based wellness and counseling services" lacks a credible basis upon which to deliver professionally accountable, effective clinical services to the patients and clients whom they allege to serve.

Ministry International Institute

Ministry International Institute (MII) reports that it "offers fully accredited courses where students can earn an Associate through Doctorate in Ministry. We offer in class and online courses." MII adds, "Qualified individuals can open a satellite campus in their church or facility. Ministry International Institute (MII) has a vision of training and empowering ministers with proven Bible courses that are accredited with the prestigious Accrediting Commission International (ACI)" (Ministry International Institute, 2021).

Unusual among degree-granting institutions that prepare individuals for licensing, MII requires regular, ongoing payment. It says, "Licensed ministers are required to Partner with MII for a minimum of $25.00 per month ($35.00 if seeking married couple credentials) or you may choose to tithe (10% of your income) monthly to MII" (Ministry International Institute, 2021) However, among institutions of this kind, regular payment, well beyond the time of receiving a degree or a license, as a way of doing business, is common.

As a significant feature of this discussion, MII states that it is an "accredited" institution. Along with many other "like-minded" organizations, MII is accredited by the Accrediting Commission International. Although the number of unaccredited or "fake" licensing agencies is unknown, most of them refer to the Accrediting Commission International as the agency that accredits them. Sadly, the Accrediting Commission International is well known as a sham organization. [Refer to the note in Chapter 8.]

Referring to a long list of accrediting agencies that includes the Accrediting Commission International, Barrett says, "In addition to nonaccredited schools, there are also nonrecognized agencies. The following entities are not approved by the U.S. Department of Education. Therefore any so-called 'accreditation' by these entities should be considered meaningless" (Barrett, 2016). Barrett's conclusion received reinforcement from others, including GetEducated.com. Providing a very long list of "fake colleges," GetEducated.com, issued the following warning:

> Consumers Beware: NONE of these accrediting agencies are recognized as college accreditors in the U.S. by the Council on Higher Education Accreditation or the U.S. Department of Education. As such, colleges claiming "accreditation" by these agencies are not accepted as valid providers of online degrees and should be approached with great caution if college credibility is important to you. (GetEducated.com, 2021, *List of Accreditation Agencies Used By Fake Colleges*)

Fake colleges that issue meaningless degrees are easily located and appear in large numbers. Likewise, fake accrediting agencies appear in large numbers and are easily located. Almost without exception, these fake entities are emphatically and specifically religious. Often, in the context of their "like-minded" universe, they express a large consensus around their belief that state-issued licenses and those who hold them have been grossly compromised by their lack of commitment to the like-mindedness that holds their fake world together. Under the heading, "MII Beliefs," its first ten asserted beliefs are these:

> The Bible is the inspired and only infallible and authoritative written Word of God.
>
> There is one God, eternally existent in three Persons: God the Father, God the Son, and God the Holy Spirit.
>
> We believe in the Deity of our Lord Jesus Christ, His sinless life, His miracles, His shed Blood, His atoning death for us on the cross, so that we might be saved and forgiven of all sin, and His resurrection from the dead.
>
> We believe in salvation by grace through faith in our Lord Jesus Christ.
>
> We believe in the ministry of the Holy Spirit in people today, including the conviction of sin, revealing Christ and showing things to come.
>
> We believe in the Baptism of the Holy Spirit and the God-given ability to speak in spiritual languages.
>
> We believe in the nine gifts of the Holy Spirit operating in the Body of Christ today.

> We believe in the Biblical practices of baptism in water, the Lord's Supper, foot washing, laying on of hands, and anointing with oil.
>
> We believe that there is one Church of our Lord Jesus Christ. We believe in fellowship among all true believers and Church bodies.
>
> We believe in the second coming of our Lord Jesus Christ. (Ministry International Institute, 2021a)

These beliefs may be sincerely and strongly held by those who choose to believe them. This is not a problem. Nor should they be challenged as sincerely held beliefs. However, when these beliefs are presumed to be the necessary and sufficient beliefs that direct the activities of counselors and therapists or pretend to be medical providers, they are truly inappropriate. At least, they presume to require providers and clients to succumb to close-mindedness and massive shaming. For example, if these beliefs are enacted by providers, the providers would apparently be expected "to speak spiritual languages" and to practice "baptism in water, foot washing, laying on of hands and anointing with oil." This is not health care of any kind, including mental health care. These presumptions qualify the MII as promoting disingenuous and harmful approaches to counseling and therapy.

National Christian Counselors Association

The National Christian Counselors Association (NCCA) advertises, "Looking to advance your education with a degree in Christian Counseling? View our comprehensive licensing and degree programs today!" (National Christian Counselors Association, 2022). Emphasizing its orientation to training and its approach to counseling, the NCCA also says, "The staff of the Association has committed themselves to the Lord Jesus Christ and believes that counseling is in vain, unless it is founded upon, and directed by, the Word of God" (National Christian Counselors Association, 2021a).

The NCCA issues certifications and licenses. As confirmed later in this chapter, aggregated data from 30 NCCA-related individuals indicate that a significant proportion of those who receive certifications and/or licenses to practice counseling and who advertise on internet platforms shared with those who have state-issued licenses to practice need a bachelor's degree or less for certification. Further, they pose as counselors and therapists who provide services for which they are conspicuously unqualified to provide.

NCCA raises and answers the question, "Can I be licensed as a Christian (Faith-based) counselor without having a B.A. degree?" Its answer is "No, you can only be certified. However, we can help you qualify for your B.A., M.A. and/or your Ph.D. through one of the several colleges that have partnered with the N.C.C.A." (National Christian Counselors Association,

2021b). Those who hold NCCA certificates often represent themselves as trained therapists, based on locating them at their *Psychology Today* websites. Strangely, as a "licensing and degree granting" association, the NCCA disavows its licensees and degree holders. The NCCA emphasizes that it does not endorse "any individual, company, program, or organization referenced" and denies "the accuracy, completeness, adequacy or currency of the Content" on its website (National Christian Counselors Association, 2023). Thus, on the one side, the NCCA can offer high assurance that it equips and affiliates with others whose training and counseling are solidly based on the Word of God, apparently endorsed by the Lord Jesus Christ, while, on the other side, it cannot endorse their work.

The NCCA is careful to distinguish its licensing from state licensing. However, based on reviewing numerous websites where its licensees advertise their services, they usually do not clearly indicate the source of their license nor the low standards for receiving their license. Instead, sometimes, they report that they are licensed, leaving an unsuspecting public to believe that they hold a state-issued licenses. Compared with the licensing requirements for state-issued licenses, the licensing requirements through the NCCA are extremely low, falling critically below minimal professional standards. Nevertheless, they often provide services as if they are well-trained, including approaches to therapy that require considerable training such as Acceptance and Commitment Therapy, Cognitive Behavioral Therapy, Career Counseling, Sex Therapy, Person-Centered Therapy, Trauma-focused Therapy, and EMDR. Also, they advertise treatment specializations that they lack qualifications to treat, including most of the personality disorders, depression and other mood disorders, video game addiction, anxiety, substance abuse, and many others.

The NCCA expresses its view of state-issued licensing, in a self-validating manner that excoriates state licensees for their lack of fidelity to NCCA's beliefs.

> The major difference between state-licensed professional counselors and Pastoral or Christian counselors, who are licensed by the N.C.C.A. and under the authority of the Church (Body of Christ), is clear and well-defined. Counselors who have been licensed by the state are held to strict ethical standards which mandate an individual's right to be free from religious influence. The state licensed professional counselor in certain states is forbidden to pray, read or refer to the Holy Scriptures, counsel against things such as homosexuality, abortion, etc. Initiating such counsel could be considered unethical by the state. In most states in the U.S., state licensed counselors "must not promote their personal religious beliefs" according to the code of ethics in each respective state.

> The only time a state licensed counselor can involve religious (Christian) principles, morals, activities, instruction, etc., is if the counselee initiates or requests counsel in this area. The state-licensed counselor may not have the education, experience and knowledge of Scripture that the N.C.C.A. counselor provides. (National Christian Counselors Association, 2021a)

From the NCCA, the messaging to culturally conservative individuals is that "the state will deny your beliefs and your opportunity to express them as you wish." This appears to be fear inducing, at least. It is also misleading. Underlying the NCCA's attempts to mislead others is the tragic misunderstanding of the necessity of training and careful, scrutinizing oversight for those who aspire to deliver counseling and therapy. Instead of recognizing the obligation to train for a professional role, the NCCA apparently encourages its licensees and unaccredited degree holders to provide professional services that they are unqualified to provide. As noted elsewhere, no other kind of health care provider (e.g., pediatrician, pharmacist, or physical therapist), legislators or others would allow such dubious approaches to health care to exist. To make this clear, no accountable adult would allow an inexperienced, untrained—albeit faith-based or faith-oriented—to advertise and deliver any other form of health care and to openly claim that it is really health care. For example, the individual who holds no degrees of any kind and reports no relevant training, but who advertises that she provides breast augmentation surgery based on her faith orientation alone would likely face necessary, immediate, and adverse consequences from criminal prosecutors.

A Sharper Picture

A discussion of these five organizations that issue licenses should be extended to include details about what their licensees and affiliates report that they advertise. The following details come from a sampling of licensees and affiliates associated with the NCCA.

A profile of 30 randomly located individuals who identify as credentialed by the NCCA indicated that only one of them held a degree from an accredited academic institution. Thirteen of them did not report on their *Psychology Today* website that they held a degree of any kind. Lacking training of any professional consequence or standing, many of these 30 individuals advertise treatment approaches that well-trained counselors and therapists advertise with a total of 131. The following 40 approaches (Chart 3.1) appear in their advertising. Naturally, the necessary question is whether untrained individuals should be attempting to provide any or all of these therapies.

Chart 3.1 Treatment Approaches Advertised by NCCA Affiliates

Acceptance and Commitment (ACT)	Adlerian Therapy
Art Therapy	Biofeedback
Career Counseling	Child and Adolescent Therapy
Clinical Supervision and Licensed Supervisors	Cognitive Behavioral (CBT)
Coherence Therapy	College & Career Counseling
Compassion Focused	Crisis and Abuse Therapy
Dialectical (DBT)	EMDR
Emotionally Focused	Forensic Psychology
Gestalt Therapy	Gottman Method
Humanistic Therapy	Mindfulness-Based (MBCT)
Motivational Interviewing	Music Therapy (Guitar)
Music Therapy (Playing Bass)	Narrative Therapy
Neuro-Linguistic Therapy	Neurofeedback
Parent-Child Interaction (PCIT)	Play Therapy
Psychoanalytic	Psychodynamic Therapy
Psychobiological Approach Couple Therapy	Reality Therapy
Psychological Testing and Evaluation	Sex Addiction Treatment
Rational Emotive Behavior (REBT)	Sex Therapy
Solution Focused Brief (SFBT)	Somatic Therapy
Structural Family Therapy	TREM, MTREM, MRT

The lack of relevant credentials also refers to the total lack of a state-issued license. In addition, only one of the 30 individuals held a professional certification of any kind such as a certification in EMDR, play therapy, or sex therapy.

The list of approaches to therapy above likely astonishes well-trained and appropriately credentialed individuals who have sought to achieve clinical effectiveness in their professional services. Then, when these 30 NCCA-affiliated individuals identify the problems—127 in total—in which they presume to have expertise, the level of astonishment likely rises significantly. Their treatment specializations include the following ones (Chart 3.2). From the list of 127 problems that 30 NCCA-affiliated individuals presume to treat, only 40 are listed here.

The identified concerns about NCCA-affiliated individuals could easily be expanded to include other issues. For example, three of the 30 individuals reported that they earned the degree, Ph.D. The three institutions that they named do not offer Ph.D. programs. However, quite apart from numbers and lists that may help to establish a profile of NCCA-affiliated individuals, their narratives about their services may be more revealing. As representatives of a larger body of narratives, the selected comments from the advertising of NCCA-related counselors and psychotherapists are intended only to communicate the sentiments of those who posted them in their advertising. The selected comments appear in no particular order.

Chart 3.2 Treatment Specialization among NCCA Affiliates

ADHD	Alzheimer's
Antisocial Personality	Anxiety
Asperger's Syndrome	Bipolar Disorder
Borderline Personality	Chronic Pain
COVID-19	Depression
Developmental Disorders	Dissociative Disorders
Eating Disorders	Elderly Persons Disorders
Hoarding	Impulse Control Disorders
Infertility	Internet Addiction
Medication Management	Mood Disorders
Narcissistic Personality	Obesity/Weight Loss
Obsessive-Compulsive (OCD)	Oppositional Defiance
Personality Disorders	Porn Addiction
Psychosis	PTSD
Self-Harming	Sex Therapy
Sexual Abuse	Sexual Addiction
Substance Use	Suicidal Ideation
Thinking Disorders	Transgender
Traumatic Brain Injury	Video Game Addiction
Wives	Women's Issues

I help individuals from a Christ Centered Therapy Model, addressing the body, soul, and spiritual factors from the science of psychology integrated with theology to treat chronic disorders, marriage problems, premarital initiatives, human development, gender dysphoria, sexual addiction, alcohol addiction, drug addiction, sexual abuse, conflict factors. My style of practice is Christ Centered, Jesus is the chief counselor, meaning that we will use the word of God and the APS Temperament Analysis as our treatment tools to identify internal problems and deep-seated blocks, circumventing the surface, or mask (personality).

https://www.psychologytoday.com/us/therapists/philemon-ministry-of-counseling-academy-jacksonville-fl/838750

Growing up broken I never thought God would use me to help bring restoration to others. After years of healing and also seeing so many injustices in the world God spoke to me about the brake (sic) down of families. Family can bring much joy but also pain, such as divorce, abuse, neglect, entanglement and more. Gods (sic) hope is to restore the Christian home. Often, we want a redo with where we came from but God wants to start the process of healing with you in order to not continue the generational sin, and pain.

https://www.psychologytoday.com/us/therapists/ciara-mcdowell-moorestown-nj/353800

I rely on the Holy Spirit to help my clients find forgiveness for the past, strength and comfort for the present, and hope for the future by trusting the Lord to meet needs and heal emotional wounds. By using an integrated approach to counseling that combines temperament theory, scientific knowledge, and Biblical truth, I create a non-judgmental and safe place for families, couples, and individuals to share their issues and fears with the goal of attaining healing and hope.

https://www.psychologytoday.com/us/therapists/margie-negri-christian-family-counseling-clinton-nj/276428

[Name of therapist] works with people who have been deeply wounded on emotional, spiritual and physical levels. His capacity for empathy, extensive clinical pastoral training, and his relationship skills serve as an excellent tool in God's hands.

https://www.psychologytoday.com/us/therapists/higher-appeal-counseling-coaching-milwaukee-wi/346631

I use a non-secular model called Temperament Therapy, which allows you to better understand your uniqueness. You will receive an expert clinical scientifically based temperament assessment, using the Arno Profile system to help direct Spirit led Biblical guidance.

https://www.psychologytoday.com/us/therapists/debra-picarello-strawberry-plains-tn/774026

Observations about the Websites of NCCA-Related Counselors and Therapists

The observations below emerge from a heightened ambivalence about the information that NCCA-related individuals posted on their websites. On one side, their apparent sincere interest in helping others stands as a clear and important indicator of their intentions. On the other side, their lack of clinical sophistication evokes worry about their clients, along with serious concern about the implications of the potentially deleterious impact on the future of professionally accountable mental health care. Acknowledging this ambivalence, observations about the information they share should be offered.

The NCCA-related counselors and psychotherapists appear to have a genuine interest in the well-being of their clients.

Instead of contributing to professional competence, cultural pluralism, and professional integrity, NCCA-affiliated individuals appear to have retreated into an ideological enclave where their rigidly held religious interests are not likely to be challenged.

NCCA-affiliated individuals seem not to understand the clinical world in which they seek to participate. Without apparent relevant training, they advertise many treatment issues for which their training has not prepared them.

Some of their identified treatment issues evoke confusion about their understanding of mental health care. Without professional training and appropriate credentialing, should NCCA affiliates be treating any of these problems: Alzheimer's, Asperger's Syndrome, Developmental Disorders, Medication Management, Porn Addiction, PTSD, Alzheimer's, Traumatic Brain Injury, Psychosis, Antisocial Personality, Dissociative Disorders, Personality Disorders, Eating Disorders, or Sexual Addiction, along with almost all of the others on the longer list above?

They advertise treatment orientations that belie their individual and collective inadequacies. While this may appear to be overstated, these NCCA-related counselors and psychotherapists advertise several approaches to their work for which professional certifications are well-known, commonly pursued, and markers of expertise for those who have these certifications. Of all the certifications that are available—for such treatment approaches as Art Therapy, Biofeedback, Music Therapy, SYMBIS, Sex Therapy, EMDR, Play Therapy, and Career Counseling—only one certification appeared in the advertising of these 30 individuals. It was a certification for EMDR.

NCCA provides another indicator of the severe lack of regulations of mental health care and its extreme vulnerability from the lack of regulations. The practice of a phlebotomist, pharmacist, psychiatrist, pulmonologist, or pediatrician, who meets no minimal professional standards for professional practice defies imagination and, surely, meets immediate and effective interventions that would prevent them from practicing. Such reasonableness simply does not exist within the large body of mental health care providers.

Finally, along with other similar organizations, the NCCA itself should be scrutinized by professional associations and legislative bodies. The primary question, but surely not the only one, is whether the NCCA promotes and institutionalizes poor "professional" mental health care, possibly perpetrating harm on clients who receive their services.

Consequences of Deception

No doubt, collectively, the licenses and certifications issued by the organizations briefly described above, along with their numerous followers, represent a large and apparently rapidly growing interest in riding the wave of expressed needs for mental health care. Unfortunately, despite their rising influence and increasing size, they pose serious challenges to the viable future of mental health care. They promote ideologies much more than professional health care. They present mental health care as a religious activity, not a professional clinical service. Preferring to operate within the boundaries of tightly constructed ideologies, they appear to oppose mental health, including their misogyny and homophobia. They appear to offer solutions to mental health care needs that are not solutions, but more likely are instruments through which they feed and sustain the problems that they seek to solve, insofar as their absolutist views implemented as therapy appear to be perfectionistic and shaming. Their rigidly held beliefs, as if they know with certainty what God thinks, strongly imply that those who disagree with them also disagree with God. They betray the best of what is known about how counseling and therapy are understood and conducted and how religion is often experienced. Opportunistically, they take advantage of individuals who believe that their personal religion qualifies them to provide counseling and therapy.

In short, these organizations undermine the care that serious, responsible, professional, duly supervised, and well-trained individuals seek to provide. Collectively, these organizations promote ancient and contemporary biases and bigotry. In varying degrees, they are anti-scientific, anti-intellectual, homophobic, misogynist, and close-mindedly ideological. In addition to their various misrepresentations, this alone makes them more of a menace than a ministry. Further, they falsely claim that their understanding of a major and desperately needed health care service (i.e., counseling, therapy, and/or mental health care) is a faithful adaptation of 2,000-year-old social habits and beliefs. In any form of health care, including dentistry, pediatrics, massage therapy, and pharmacy, this kind of adaptation is and should be unacceptable. Likewise, their commitment to deliver services that are based on ancient social mores and beliefs, such as holding that women are inferior to men, also misrepresents scientific, reliable, and evolving understandings and treatments of numerous deeply personal problems. They fail to see or want to see that clinical depression is not a sign of separation from God or of sinfulness, any more than ordinary eye strain is a sign of an individual's failure to "see God." Instead, with clear and high levels of absurdity, they wish to see that prayer alone effectively treats almost anything or that faith in God can cure almost any mental disorder such as ADHD, OCD, or personality disorders. Their presence in mental health care should disturb and alarm professionally accountable counselors and therapists. Also, probably, their presence in mental health care reveals their personal, but sternly and rigidly suppressed, unresolved fears and anxieties. Insofar as this may be correct, they need treatment—mental health care.

An examination of these groups, along with other similar groups, leads to seeing their commitment to homophobic, misogynist, and mostly anti-clinical points of view. Still, in addition to their potentially harmful approaches to counseling and therapy, untold and very large numbers of appropriately trained and licensed counselors and therapists advertise their services with very similar language. They, too, advertise counseling and psychotherapy based on "Biblical Principles" or "Basic Christian Values," or many other similar labels. At least, they concoct a dangerous mixture of personal sincerity with presumed professional accountability.

The organizations briefly profiled here demonstrate that they commit to provide much more than they deliver. They espouse values that they obviously refuse to live by. They avow their ownership of truth that they fail to grasp. They deceive those from whom they collect money and to whom they make promises. They assault the health care community, as if their unhuman, rigidly held, largely commercial, self-indulgent righteousness gives them superior capabilities in health care. As they perpetrate their close-minded ideology on others, they deny their own humanity and the humanity of those whom they allege to serve. And, through their carefully pruned beliefs and stealthy manipulations of others' beliefs, appear to have sought to create God in their nicely groomed image.

What is the difference between the MII that partners with those whom it licenses "for a minimum of $25.00 per month ($35.00 if seeking married couple credentials) or you may choose to tithe (10% of your income)" in perpetuity and state-licensed individuals who are untrained to provide their services based on Biblical Principles or Christ-Centered Therapy? Probably, very little. Both are charlatans. Unfortunately, the likelihood is that, by manipulating the beliefs of others, they are also securely positioned to maintain substantial incomes. However, MII is one of many similar businesses.

References

Association of Certified Biblical Counselors. (2021). *Speaking the truth in love.* https://biblicalcounseling.com/about/beliefs/statements-from-the-board/licensure/

Association of Certified Biblical Counselors. (2021a). *Licensure.* https://biblicalcounseling.com/about/beliefs/statements-from-the-board/licensure/

Association of Certified Biblical Counselors. (2021b). *Our beliefs.* https://biblicalcounseling.com/about/beliefs/statements-from-the-board/licensure/

Association of Certified Biblical Counselors. (2021c). *Female pastors.* https://biblicalcounseling.com/about/beliefs/statements-from-the-board/licensure/

Barrett, S. (2018, May 4). *Some notes on the Pastoral Medical Association and other "Private Membership Associations."* Credential Watch: Your Guide to Health-Related Education and Training. https://quackwatch.org/credential/reports/pma/

Barrett, S. (2016, November 25). *Be wary of nonrecognized accreditation agencies.* Credential Watch: Your Guide to Health-Related Education and Training. https://quackwatch.org/credential/non/agencies/

Energetic Wellness. (2023). *Pastoral Medical Association.* https://energeticwellnessok.com/naturopathic-appointments/about-dr-menzel/pastoral-medical-association/

GetEducated.com. (2021) *List of accreditation agencies used by fake colleges.* https://www.geteducated.com/college-degree-mills/204-fake-agencies-for-college-accreditation/

Ministry International Institute. (2021). *Ministry certification/credentialing.* Retrieved from https://ministryinternational.tv/ministry-info/ministry-certification/

Ministry International Institute. (2021a). *MII Beliefs.* Retrieved from https://ministryinternational.tv/contactu/

National Association of Christian Counselors (NACC). (2021). *About: Who we are.* Retrieved from https://nacconline.org

National Association of Christian Counselors. (2022). *Counseling.* Retrieved from https://nacconline.org/counseling/

National Christian Counselors Association. (2021). *Code of ethical standards.* Retrieved from https://docs.google.com/document/d/1OZuiUJftOr592arU8GRieUMoUXuzeWJke5VDYz1i4Os/preview

National Christian Counselors Association. (2021). *We train, certify and license Christian counselors.* Retrieved from https://www.ncca.org

National Christian Counselors Association. (2021a). *Licensing program for Christian counselors.* https://nccachristiancounseling.com/pdfs/NCCA_Catalog_07012014.pdf

National Christian Counselors Association. (2021b). *Frequently asked questions.* Retrieved from https://www.ncca.org/faq

National Christian Counselors Association (2023). *Disclaimer and Terms of Use of NCCA Directory.* Retrieved from https://auth.ncca.org/NCCA/Members/Directory/Terms.aspx?database=2&edit=

NPR. (2021). *Pastoral medicine credentials raise questions in Texas.* https://www.npr.org/sections/health-shots/2016/04/25/475165193/pastoral-medicine-credentials-raise-questions-in-texas)

Pastoral Medical Association. (2021). *Working for providers and the public.* https://www.quantumhealing.club/18989-2/#0

4 Equivocating Allies

Religious life around the world has been beset with conflict. Among Americans, the conflict falls short of warfare. Instead, it has been characterized by incessant, ubiquitous, and sometimes intense controversies around ideas, with each proponent or group of proponents of an idea confidently concluding that their understanding of God and Truth is correct and that, of course, all others are incorrect. Along with incessant controversies, divisions and fragmentations have also occurred. A similar characterization also describes the world of counseling and therapy in general, but also with regard to the place of religion in this world, more narrowly.

Religious Zeal Wins

Professionally accountable counselors and therapists should feel disturbed and alarmed by the threats posed by poorly trained and ineffective "peers" who practice within the terrible limitations of their rigidly held religious beliefs and under the authority of organizations that have no appropriate standing in the mental health care community. The sources of disturbance and alarm should be carefully scrutinized and neutralized, if not eliminated, if possible. They should also be scrutinized, affirmed, and encouraged, when this is appropriate. The lack of scrutiny appears to be what they readily and copiously desire. The organizations discussed in the previous chapter illustrate the lack of openness to evidence and scrutiny and avoidance of accountability all too well.

When organizations such as the National Association of Christian Counselors, Association of Certified Biblical Counselors, Pastoral Medical Association, Ministry International Institute, National Christian Counselors Association, or other similar organizations come to the awareness of those who seek to be as professionally accountable as possible, the observers may feel smug or even sneer at the ignorance and close-mindedness that they see. Along with other such responses, the respondents may also conclude that their superior training and strongly felt good will elevate their clinical

DOI: 10.4324/9781003472469-5

effectiveness well beyond those whose training emerged from rigid religious environments. Such responses may be misguided.

Their misguided responses to those who advertise their services—validated by their rigid, religious training and licensing—may not recognize that, quite apart from these kinds of providers of mental health care services, there are many others that require similar analyses and responses. For example, the Professional Wellness Alliance offers its "PWA License Program," inviting others to "learn more about the benefits of becoming a licensed provider and protecting your alternative services and clients" (Professional Wellness Alliance, 2021b). Promoting its license, the PWA adds, "The reality is that if you don't have a defendable legal basis for your holistic services, then you run a high risk of legal troubles. This is true whether you recommend supplements for nutritional health, practice crystal healing, reiki, or provide any other sort of holistic services." And, then, PMA makes an astonishing claim. "Legal Protection: Your holistic services will have the best defense possible from state regulatory board concerns—no matter which state you're from, or which areas you specialize" (Professional Wellness Alliance, 2021a). The idea that a purchased license gives the holder and his "clients" legal protection is an alarming one. These so-called "licensees" cannot protect their clients' confidential information. Because their clients have no legal privilege that associates with such licensees, they have no more protection than "clients" who may speak with a barber, bartender, ski instructor, basketball coach, plumber, or landscaper about their personal problems. The important difference between these so-called "licensees" and, say, a plumber is that the plumber is not likely to advertise and attempt to deliver mental health care.

The significance of the several organizations that have so far been briefly presented is that they are there. Because they are there, they seriously compromise and threaten professionally accountable counselors and therapists and the clients whom they serve. However, professionally accountable counselors and therapists may want to look around their professional environment and ask what licensees are doing with their respective licenses. For example, as noted earlier, an individual who holds the same license that I hold advertises that she practices witchcraft. Another practices ceremonial magic. Another practices astrology. And so on. While they hold the same license that I hold, I conclude that their advertised services are inappropriate and that they violate state regulations and professional ethics. Despite this, they are there, doing things that are associated with the licenses that many of us hold. Clearly, those who practice witchcraft, ceremonial magic, astrology, or numerous other approaches must be neutralized, if not eliminated from practicing such so-called "therapies."

As many appropriately trained and licensed counselors and therapists choose to depart from their training as a foundation for their respective practices, practicing outside the scope of practice that their licenses authorize, and commit to practice in unethical ways, they should receive much more than the disappointment of their peers as a response. When they promote their services and practice their respective, so-called "therapies," they corrode professional accountability and credibility of those who are professionally accountable and generally diminish the image and influence of counseling and therapy. They may well be weighting the imbalance of the future of counseling and therapy toward extinction.

Questionable Allies

Graduates of non-religious universities and licensed by the states in which they practice, counselors and therapists describe their practices in ways that are often transparently and unambiguously religious. Apparently, similar to the organizations described above, they conclude that their religious beliefs qualify them to provide mental health care that they appear to be unqualified to provide. Here are some examples, from the virtually countless number available.

> As a believer in the Lord Jesus Christ, I consider it an honor to help you navigate the storms of life with an approach that builds confidence, trust and hope using time-proven techniques. My counsel is based on the combination of both my Christian faith and my psychodynamic understanding of how people heal and mature. My goal is to build with you a trustworthy, empathetic and clarifying relationship, and to rejoice with you in the healing process. With God's good help, for over 30 years, I have walked alongside individuals, couples, and families, seeking resolution to a wide range of life challenges and psychological issues. As a Christ-Centered clinician, I combine sensitivity and compassion with insight and feedback to aid my clients in reaching their goals. I rely on my faith in the Risen Savior, who desires freedom for His people, to inform our time together in session, as we walk through the myriad of life-transforming stressors that have contributed to your seeking help.
>
> https://www.psychologytoday.com/us/therapists/joy-gayle-pasadena-tx/751089
>
> Graduate of the University of Houston and licensed as a clinical social worker.

> As a therapist, I focus on client-needs from both a Christian and evidence-based perspective.
>
> https://www.psychologytoday.com/us/therapists/chantele-mercier-ferguson-lees-summit-mo/3651
>
> A pre-licensed psychologist who practices under the supervision of another psychologist and who is a graduate of the University of Missouri-Kansas City

As an Orthodox Christian Psychologist, Dr. Xenia is deeply committed to a therapeutic practice that flows out of her Orthodox Christian faith and abides in the teachings of the Holy Fathers. She received her Ph.D. from Colorado State University.

https://patristicnectar.org/dr_xenia_serena_enke

As a Christian counselor, I help those that are hurting, pointing them to the cross of Jesus Christ by offering spiritual direction and formational prayer. Spiritual direction is helping people discern the presence and leading of God in their lives, while formational prayer is inviting the healing presence of Jesus Christ into places of pain and brokenness within a wounded person.

https://www.psychologytoday.com/us/therapists/lydia-johnson-milwaukee-wi/258770

Graduate of Drexel University. Licensed Professional Counselor

My personal and professional experience combined with the most empowering element—faith in the positive energy of our universe comes from a loving Heavenly Father and His Son, Jesus Christ and continues to lead me and others to find that peace we are all look for. I want to share it freely with those who are curious and open to expanding their knowledge.

https://www.psychologytoday.com/us/therapists/kirstine-keel-draper-ut/875341

Graduate of Argosy University, a for-profit university, and a Licensed Mental Health Counselor

I combine sound biblical principles with proven, professional counseling practices to help you discover the hope, healing and growth that's possible through Jesus Christ. I earned my B.A. in Psychology from the University of Missouri and Master's in Counseling from the University of Colorado.

https://www.psychologytoday.com/us/therapists/triumph-christian-counseling-columbia-mo/257037

A licensed professional counselor.

Linda deals with family issues, parenting concerns and child development. She works with divorce recovery and grief. Solution-focused, brief therapy allows Linda to see many hurting families and individuals over short periods of time with successful results. Her specific focus is Christian counseling believing the need for every one of God's children to have a personal relationship with Jesus Christ. Linda has been a licensed therapist since 1983. Her training is in Psychology, Social Work, receiving a BA in both at Western Connecticut State University. She earned her MA in counseling at the University of West Florida, Pensacola.

https://www.psychologytoday.com/us/therapists/linda-s-reynolds-fort-myers-fl/37574

I am a Licensed Professional Counselor and Christian Counselor who enjoys working with preteens/teens, adults and couples in office and online .... Christian counseling sessions are a Biblical perspective focused on renewing the mind to the truth of God's character, your identity in Christ and discovering how to walk in the Spirit to find peace.

https://www.psychologytoday.com/us/therapists/lauren-duren-valdosta-ga/330871

Graduate of Valdosta State University

Ladies, God's desire is for you to thrive in every area of your life, in spirit, soul and body .... I provide a God-centered total health approach to healing that nurtures the spirit, soul and body. Using Biblical truths, clinical skills and the science of proven protocols, we will work together to create an individualized wellness plan to meet your mental and physical health needs. During our time together, I may recommend prayer, meditation, nutritional therapies, herbal medicine, detoxification, talk and coaching, and specific exercises.

https://www.psychologytoday.com/us/therapists/minister-rekishia-mcmillian-christian-health-coach-trenton-nj/315052

A licensed clinical social worker who is a graduate of Rutgers University

I am a bible believing Christian .... Every counselor, or coach has an ideology, philosophy, point of reference they use when speaking into your life. I choose to be upfront and tell you what mine is. Whatever problem you are experiencing the core of the solution is found in Christ. "In all our ways acknowledge Him".. Proverbs 3:6.

(https://www.psychologytoday.com/us/therapists/i-regina-gourdine-saint-louis-mo/327277)

A graduate of Washington University and licensed as a clinical social worker.

I approach counseling from a Christian perspective. I believe the word of God has many remedies for improved quality of life.

https://www.psychologytoday.com/us/therapists/clear-path-counseling-virginia-beach-va/470477

A licensed clinical social worker and graduate of Norfolk State University

Karen believes the most effective healing occurs when psychological change comes alongside spiritual transformation found through a personal relationship with Jesus Christ.

https://www.babbcenter.org/staff/
A licensed psychologist who graduated from the Illinois School of Professional
Psychology (M.A. and Psy.D.)
https://apps.health.tn.gov/Licensure/Practitioner.aspx

Each of these statements by counselors and therapists who advertise their services online indicates that they bring Christian commitments to their professional work and that, to a visible and large degree, define their professional work in specifically Christian terms. Significantly, also, all of them offer no indicators of their professional training that would qualify them to define their work in this way, let alone to provide professional services based on such a definition. They appear to be saying "I am a Christian. Therefore, I provide Christian treatment." Far fewer individuals would or could, with integrity, say, "I am a man. Therefore, I provide man-specialized treatment."

As noted earlier, almost nine of ten of those who offer some form of Christian Counseling have no training indicated on the websites where they advertise their services. They completed their clinical preparation programs in institutions that are not "Christian." The institutions are state-sponsored, for-profit, or non-religious private. Those who offer some form of "Christian Counseling" do not indicate that they have any relevant training such as a professional and broadly recognized certification. However, the apparent failure of self-identified Christian counselors to complete professional preparation for the services that they advertise is not exceptional, with regard to incomplete or no such preparation. Similar to this failure, those who advertise sex therapy or play therapy exhibit less preparation and fewer indicators of their professional competency to deliver either sex therapy or play therapy than those who advertise some form of Christian counseling.

A ubiquitous habit among counselors and therapists is that they attach their a favored adjective to any approach to therapy to which they wish to attach it. The word, "Christian," along with many closely related terms, has been associated with numerous other approaches to counseling and psychotherapy such as Christian EMDR, Christian Buddhism, Christian Gestalt Therapy, and Christian Cognitive Behavior Therapy, along with thousands of others. Again, this is not and should not be seen as an argument about Christian beliefs. As I have noted elsewhere in this book, I have published books that bespeak my Christian faith. It is an argument, though, that stands on the view that Christian faith is not a clinical orientation to counseling and therapy. Further, while the appearance is that numerous so-called "Christian Counselors" utilize the fact of their religious ideology as a marketing device, they also appear to assume that their individual set of beliefs are likely to be compatible with the religious ideology of their clients. This is likely a false assumption that accompanies weak approaches to counseling and therapy. From their study of Christian therapists and clients, Prout, Kim, Magaldi, and Cha (2021, pp. 8–9) conclude, "… important differences exist between Christian clients and Christian therapists in terms of how they engage in religious practices and experience their faith." Moreover, "These differences, in the internal experience and external practice of faith, exist, despite Christian therapists and their clients rating themselves similarly in terms of their level of overall religiosity and spirituality."

Institutionalizing Equivocating Alliances

An unknown but large number of academic institutions promote ideologies that their administrators, faculty, and graduates offer as clinical orientations, as if their respective ideologies suffice as clinical orientations. This discussion serves to illustrate the presence of some of these academic institutions. It is not a discussion that evaluates the ideologies of these institutions. No matter whether its ideology is, whether it is specifically religious or another ideology, each institution is entitled to hold whatever beliefs it selects. The individuals who affiliate with these institutions may also believe whatever they wish, just as anyone else. Within the obvious boundaries of this discussion, each institution will be briefly represented mostly as it represents itself, recognizing that such a representation is, indeed, brief. Anticipating that additional, similar institutions will be discussed in Chapter 8, the representatives of many such institutions, the ones discussed here include

Missio Seminary (formerly, Biblical Theological Seminary)
Reformed Theological Seminary
Moody Theological Seminary

Missio Seminary (Formerly, Biblical Theological Seminary)

In multiple ways, the Missio Seminary identifies itself as "a missional seminary." Its mission statement defines its general reason for being and emphasizes this commitment.

> Our Mission Statement
> To incarnate and communicate the story of Jesus with …
> Humility and authenticity
> Fidelity to Scripture
> Appreciation of the Christian tradition
> Sensitivity to the needs and aspirations of postmodern culture.
> (Missio Seminary, 2022)

All academic institutions have mission statements. Such statements serve to shape the priorities of institutions and guide many of its programming decisions. This is the way it should be, just as it is for social service agencies, government agencies, businesses, churches, and other institutions. Surely, the decision-makers who composed the mission of Missio Seminary have sought to be clear about why the Seminary exists. Further, the Seminary has carefully composed its Convictions Statement, to give added detail to its reason for being.

> Convictions Statement: Missio Seminary
> Missio Seminary is an evangelical seminary committed to the gospel of Jesus Christ and a generously orthodox Christian faith for the purpose of preparing missional leaders to serve the church. We are intent on maintaining the following convictions in the life and work of our community.
>
> Together they [two individuals who founded the Seminary] represented two passions that would become hallmarks of Biblical Theological Seminary (renamed Missio Seminary in 2018)—a deep desire to search and understand the Scriptures and a keen interest in effectively reaching people with the hope of the gospel. We believe God heard their prayer. We aspire to continue manifesting God's answer to that prayer in our current endeavors, including through the unanimous adoption of this missional convictions statement. (Missio Seminary, 2022a)

For anyone, including counselor and therapists, whose personal history has not brought them into an acquaintance with or understanding of conservative, evangelical Christian institutions, and who reads the mission statement and conviction statement likely wonders about how academic professionals could invent such things. Following such a reading, they will likely wonder with focused intensity, when they read about the Seminary's approach to preparing its students and graduates for state-issued licensing. The Seminary says that its "60-hour Master of Arts in Counseling (MAC) degree is designed for students who wish to pursue licensure in the Commonwealth of PA" (Missio Seminary, 2022b). Following its mission statement, conviction statement, and its provision of an academic program that prepares students and graduates to pursue licensure, the necessary question is "How are these things expressed through the licensure preparation program?" The Seminary offers the following description of its licensure preparation program.

> Our MAC students are those who are drawn to walk alongside hurting people, seeking to be conduits of God's healing to emotional and relational brokenness. Missio prepares them to skillfully apply the grace

and truth of the Gospel first to their lives and then to those of their counselees.

At our Philadelphia campus, MAC students come to class one night a week, one Saturday a month, for three years and learn to engage science and culture from a Christian perspective, with wisdom and discernment. Students are equipped for professional and non-professional counseling contexts, as they learn effective evidence-based counseling skills from faculty who are practicing clinical counselors. The MAC program is tailored to Pennsylvania state licensure requirements.

What Do Our Graduates Do with Their Degree?

The MAC program trains Christians for a broad spectrum of service. Missio's Graduate School of Counseling program meets the needs of students in a variety of career and avocational settings. MAC graduates serve on pastoral teams or in counseling ministries in their local churches, in social service and mental health organizations, in para-church ministries, in specialized counseling services, and more. MAC's curriculum is designed to provide students with the knowledge, skills, and self-awareness needed for effective, Christ-centered counseling. Courses, retreats, and fieldwork experiences address key professional counseling areas of study while maintaining a biblical and ministry focus. [Bolding added] (Missio Seminary, 2022c)

The phrase, "Christ-centered Counseling," is common, among institutions that self-identify in a manner that is similar to Missio's. It is used by widely disparate advertisers. It has no agreed-upon definition. The necessary question from this is "If a Christ-centered life is what you seek and wish to practice as counseling, why is a state-issued license needed?"

Reformed Theological Seminary

With nine campus locations in the United States, the Reformed Theological Seminary introduces its licensure preparation program with these statements:

The CACREP accredited Master of Arts in Counseling program exists to train distinctly Christian and exceptionally competent Professional Counselors. The 78-credit curriculum integrates clinical mental health counseling coursework and clinical experience with a Reformed theological foundation, equipping graduates to counsel both churched and non-churched populations in multicultural and pluralistic societies. (Reformed Theological Seminary, 2022)

Avowing its commitment to the *Westminster Confession of Faith* [refer to discussion, below], the Reformed Theological Seminary holds a compatible mission. "The mission of Reformed Theological Seminary is to serve the Church by preparing its leaders, through a program of graduate theological education, based upon the authority of the inerrant Word of God, and committed to the Reformed Faith" (Reformed Theological Seminary, 2022a). With this mission, does the Seminary also express this view in its curriculum, with particular expression in its licensure preparation program? The Seminary says, "Since the Bible is absolutely and finally authoritative as the inerrant Word of God, it is the basis for the total curriculum" (Reformed Theological Seminary, 2022b). Making this more specific, it also says, "Students are equipped with the necessary skills to understand and teach the Scriptures, developing above all a burning desire to know and do the will of God as revealed in the Old and New Testaments, for the essence of Reformed theology is a willingness constantly to conform all of life to the Word of God. Our primary distinctives are a commitment to historic Reformed theology and the Bible as God's inerrant Word" (Reformed Theological Seminary, 2022b).

If the inerrant Word of God, as the Reformed Theological Seminary sees it, incorporates the *Westminster Confession of Faith* as an absolutist doctrinal attachment to the Word of God, what, if anything, does the *Confession* say about the work of counselors and therapists? Directly, the *Confession* says nothing about the work of counselors and therapists. However, insofar as the *Confession* apparently forms the substance of much of the preparation for counseling, the *Confession* becomes a critically important source of guidance for the Seminary and its intended influence on its future licensees. As a lengthy document, the *Confession* may be construed to have numerous specific ideological influences on the Seminary's future licensees. Also, without much need for construing its meaning, the *Confession* makes some of its guiding messages quite clear. For example, under the heading, Of Marriage and Divorce, the *Confession* says,

> Of Marriage and Divorce
> Marriage is to be between one man and one woman: neither is it lawful for any man to have more than one wife, nor for any woman to have more than one husband at the same time.
>
> Marriage was ordained for the mutual help of husband and wife; for the increase of mankind with a legitimate issue, and of the church with an holy seed; and for preventing of uncleanness.
>
> It is lawful for all sorts of people to marry who are able with judgment to give their consent. Yet it is the duty of Christians to marry only in the Lord. And, therefore, such as profess the true reformed religion should not marry with infidels, papists, or other idolaters: neither should such as

are godly be unequally yoked, by marrying with such as are notoriously wicked in their life, or maintain damnable heresies.

Marriage ought not to be within the degrees of consanguinity or affinity forbidden in the Word; nor can such incestuous marriages ever be made lawful by any law of man, or consent of parties, so as those persons may live together, as man and wife.

Adultery or fornication, committed after a contract, being detected before marriage, giveth just occasion to the innocent party to dissolve that contract. In the case of adultery after marriage, it is lawful for the innocent party to sue out a divorce, and after the divorce to marry another, as if the offending party were dead.

Although the corruption of man be such as is apt to study arguments, unduly to put asunder those whom God hath joined together in marriage; yet nothing but adultery, or such willful desertion as can no way be remedied by the church or civil magistrate, is cause sufficient of dissolving the bond of marriage; wherein a public and orderly course of proceeding is to be observed; and the persons concerned in it, not left to their own wills and discretion in their own case. (*The Westminster Confession of Faith*)

Originating in 1647, *The Westminster Confession of Faith* may hold important meaning for its adherents. As a demonstrably pre-scientific or, maybe, anti-science, somewhat primitive and unsophisticated document that lacks obvious relevance for the practice of counseling and therapy and a minimally relevant understanding of several decades of research about mental-emotional problems, child development, marriage and family issues, and other related topics, an academic institution that shows extraordinary deference to preparing licensees for a major health care service appears to promulgate a grossly inconsistent approach. On one side, it aspires to prepare its students and graduates for service in a major health care service, while, on the other side, aspires to live by beliefs that betray the interests of those to whom mental health care will be provided by confining itself to an ideology that lacks relevant connection to mental health and mental health care as these matters are understood in the twenty-first century.

Moody Theological Seminary

Commonly referred to as "Moody," the Moody Bible Institute was founded by famed evangelist Dwight L. Moody. As the Seminary reports, "Moody is driven by the belief that people committed to living and declaring the Word of God can actually change the world. Since our founding by D. L. Moody in 1886, Moody Bible Institute has been committed to equipping people across the globe, cultures and generations to take the next step toward spiritual maturity" (Moody Theological Seminary, 2022). Somewhat naturally, given its rich and long history, Moody declares its mission in these words: "Moody exists to Proclaim the Gospel, and equip people to be Biblically grounded, practically trained, and to engage the world through Gospel-centered living" (Moody Theological Seminary, 2022a). To emphasize its biblical grounding, Moody specifies beliefs that guide its programs. Among these beliefs, "Everything we do at Moody falls under the authority of the Bible, which declares timeless truth that is relevant today and throughout every generation. We believe that understanding and sharing God's Word is a lifelong journey. And we're committed to providing encouragement for you in your walk with Christ" (Moody Theological Seminary, 2022b). And, as if this declaration may not be as clear as it should be, Moody further declares, "The Bible is without error in all it affirms in the original autographs and is the only authoritative guide for faith and practice and as such must not be supplanted by any other fields of human learning" (Moody Theological Seminary, 2022c).

Moody has taken great care to voice its beliefs and values. These should be respected as beliefs and values. Then, following appropriate respect, a good question is "How are Moody's beliefs and values implemented?" In this discussion, as a partial response to this question, the implementation refers to three items: gender, sexuality, and licensing for mental health care providers. However, preparing its students to address these issues should be understood to stand in the shadow of Moody's commitment to The Bible as inerrant and to its refusal to allow this commitment to be "supplanted by any other fields of learning."

No doubt, a single statement about gender issues hardly says everything that an individual or an institution may believe or practice. Allowing for this, Moody appears to have adopted a view of gender and gender roles that follows biblical injunctions. Notably, Moody states, "Moody distinguishes between ministry function and church office. While upholding the necessity of mutual respect and affirmation as those subject to the Word of God, Moody understands that the biblical office of elder/pastor in the early church was gender specific. Therefore, it maintains that it is consistent with that understanding of Scripture that those church offices should be limited to the male gender" (Moody Theological Seminary, 2022d). However, while some of its views appear to be absolutist, Moody includes women in leadership roles. Specifically, while men fill the majority of faculty positions, women fill approximately 36% of its faculty positions (Moody Theological Seminary, 2022e). Still, allowing for an approach to gender roles that is paradoxically open and closed, Moody seems to avoid numerous biblical injunctions about other lifestyle issues such as those Biblical injunctions that prohibit wearing gold and pearls (1 Timothy 2:9–10 ESV), along with many others. Are Moody's commitments faithful to The Bible or statements of personal or cultural preferences?

Moody promotes heterosexuality as the "Christian" view and approach to human sexuality. As such, alternate sexual orientations are "sinful." Moody's website features an article, "Sexuality and the Gospel: How to share Christ with the gay community." Authored by Christopher Yuan, it concludes, "We must live the gospel before we preach the gospel. I would never have considered the gospel if I had not seen the gospel lived out in my parents' lives first. In fact, I did not stop pursuing same-sex relationships because my parents convinced me such relationships were sinful. I stopped because they showed me something better—and His name is Jesus" (Moody Theological Seminary, 2022f). Implicit in this view is that the Gospel and sexual orientations other than marital heterosexuality are simply incompatible, with the other orientations regarded as sinful.

With all of these views of various aspects of being human, including Moody's view of the Bible, gender roles, human sexuality, and its avowed mission, it also prepares its students and graduates for licensing as professional counselors. Moody says, "The Masters in Clinical Mental Health Counseling program at Moody Bible Institute is designed to meet the licensure standards set by the state of Illinois for a Licensed Professional Counselor" (Moody Theological Seminary, 2022g). As many such programs do, Moody adds caveats, indicating that it cannot ensure that its preparation for licensing meets the requirements of other legal jurisdictions. Allowing for its compliance with "the licensure standards set by the state of Illinois," a critically important question is whether it meets compliance with normative professional standards. In various places on its website, Moody refers to its belief that its students learn "to apply clinical training and biblical insight to the counseling field" (Moody Theological Seminary, 2022h). Are "biblical insights," "biblical principles," and related beliefs compatible with a profession that provides a major health care service? In short, is Moody's apparent absolutist approach to preparing counselors and therapists compatible with a broadly defined research-based profession, but also a profession that is based in cultural pluralism?

This discussion of theological schools includes details about only three of them (i.e., Missio Seminary, Reformed Theological Seminary, and Moody Theological Seminary). These three institutions are representative of a large number of similar institutions. The total number of them is unknown, but it is likely to exceed 150 in America. Just as their number is not precisely known, the impact of their presence in mental health care is also not precisely known. Comments about their potential impact appear below. For now, an important observation is that they are numerous and easily located. For example, in addition to the three that are briefly discussed, others could include the following ones.

Trinity Evangelical Divinity School

TEDS says, "Trinity has been entrusted with the Gospel since 1897, and every day we are called to live with purpose. Our purpose as a divinity school is to know the Gospel, live the Gospel, and make the Gospel known" Trinity Evangelical Divinity School, 2023). As an evangelical divinity school, its belief about its purpose is understandable. However, those who complete its preparation program for becoming state-licensed and practicing mental health care providers may not understand that counseling and therapy are not evangelical activities, let alone specifically fundamentalist, Christian, activities.

Dallas Theological Seminary

Founded in 1924, the Dallas Theological Seminary says, "The mission of Dallas Theological Seminary as a professional, graduate-level school is to glorify God by equipping godly servant-leaders for the proclamation of His Word and the building up of the body of Christ worldwide" (Dallas Theological Seminary, 2022) Further, the Seminary states, "As a faith-based institution, students are required to agree with these seven Christian essentials" (Dallas Theological Seminary, 2022). The seven essentials are not included here. Similar to the other institution profiled here, the Dallas Theological Seminary poses as an academic, intellectual community that begins and ends its academic and intellectual pursuits with its understandings and conclusions firmly set and apparently immutable religious beliefs, beginning in 1924. Again, this institution and any other may believe what they want to believe. Their challenge and dilemma come in the question, "Can it effectively prepare its students and graduates to be minimally competent counselors and therapists who also qualify for state-issued licensing as mental health care professionals?"

Grace College

"We are a Christ-centered community of higher education applying biblical values in strengthening character, sharpening competence, and preparing for service" (Grace College, 2022). Its licensing preparation program is represented as "Scripturally grounded, professionally skilled, interpersonally competent. These are the distinctives of our Clinical Mental Health Counseling program at Grace College" (Grace College, 2022a).

To the six institutions identified in this discussion, many others could be added. Preceding additional observations and conclusions about them, they should be respected as broadly defined faith-based institutions. Unambiguously, the religious beliefs of these institutions described above should not be challenged, even when others may strongly disagree with or reject their faith commitments. With commensurate clarity, those who hold the beliefs that these institutions hold should not be challenged. The right to freedom of religion applies to all individuals and the institutions with which they choose to affiliate. The necessary challenges to these institutions and an unknown but large number of others arise from their audacious and sometimes dangerous preparation of mental health care providers. Almost without exception, they persist in boasting about their preparation of competent counselors and therapists. The evidence for such boasting appears to stand only on the acquiescence of the faculty, students, and graduates to the doctrinal positions of the institutions that prepare them.

Among many observations, the following ones are compelled by the intrusive presumptuousness of these institutions in their preparation of counselors and therapists.

> They advance pre-scientific, anti-intellectual thinking that predates the mental health care movement. They cannot both advance "biblical principles" as mental health care and mislead others with the incompatible view that they support the massive and relevant outcomes from recent decades of research. They cannot cling to rigid beliefs about sex roles, marriage, parenting, and other presumed biblical truth and provide effective mental health care.
>
> They advance their belief in the Bible as "God's inerrant Word," as if they can know absolute inerrancy when they see it. None of us is gifted with such divine intellect or insight. Yes, to be sure, they may accept inerrancy as a matter of faith, but can they do this without their irrational expectation that the rest of the world should accept their view as their own, with particular reference to their simultaneous commitment to be counselors and therapists?
>
> They have no outcome studies that provide clues about the possible effectiveness of what their graduates as mental health care licensees provide. They appear to conclude that they do not need outcome studies to confirm the effectiveness of their professional work because their presumed attachment to their truth immunizes them from having to be effective, from having to assure their clients of effectiveness, and from their non-clinical conflation of faith with clinical effectiveness.
>
> They advocate for first-century sex roles, leadership, sexuality, and many other culturally sensitive issues, failing to adapt their views and practices to a science-based, evidence-based approach to health care in the twenty-first century. Are such views compatible with any other health care profession? Cardiology? Pharmacy? Physical therapy? Obviously, the answer is "No." They may practice their religion in many ways, but not as mental health care, if they are intellectually and ethically honest. Practicing religion is not health care, including mental health care,

although it may be an understandable motivation to provide health care. To practice mental health care as religion means that it is the practice of religion, not mental health care.

While some of their graduates and state-license holders may achieve an appropriate level of professionalism and accountability, the implicit aim of these institutions appears to one of producing intellectual muggles, as if thinking the same thing forever—throughout their respective careers—permits them to pretend to be something that they, by definition, cannot be. They cannot be growing, developing, learning, skill-enhanced, ethical, and truly professional individuals who, above almost everything else in clinical work, place the highest priority on clients' welfare and not their own. After all, from their point of view, they are absolutely "right," because they identify with God's inerrant Word.

Most of these institutions define themselves clearly and consistently as advocates for tightly held and detailed ideologies with which their faculty, staff, and students must agree. This alone is a position that mandates against their potential for having a professional presence in mental health care. They fail to recognize that freedom of religion also means freedom from religion. Professionally accountable mental health care strives to affirm this freedom, knowing that it is neither ideological nor evangelical.

To the extent that their presumed clinical approach is evangelical, it is harmful as an expression of mental health care. These institutions appear to deny the well-documented potential of harming others. Among many examples of this, their belief in so-called "sexual purity" may be admirable while it also evokes shame in others who fail to be sexually pure.

Individually and collectively, these institutions freeze mental health care in a pre-scientific, anti-intellectual era, as defiance of honesty and real intellectual muscularity, with approaches that not only represent the much larger community of counselors and therapists but also pose the likely potential of inflicting significant damage on properly trained and licensed individuals who aspire to achieve professional accountability and clinical effectiveness. As such, they may be one of the largest sources of unethical behavior among mental health care providers.

Alexandrova (2023) argues for "construct pluralism," in her book, *A Philosophy for the Science of Well-being*. In mental health care, construct pluralism is inevitable. After all, almost all counselors and therapists have their own thoughts—or constructs—about what their professional service may involve. However, accommodating Alexandrova's argument, very few counselors and therapists can articulate their science of well-being or other features of their professional service. Further, religionists are less capable than most others, in this regard.

These institutions promote tacit disapproval of virtually all other institutions that prepare mental health care providers, along with regarding those who are not "like-minded" as inferior colleagues. They appear not to recognize that, as institutions that prepare mental health care providers, they represent all other mental health care preparation programs and providers.

The goals and attitudes of these institutions, insofar as institutions may have attitudes, appear to be much like those that are seen in disturbed clients. There is considerable overlap between clients who exhibit intolerance of ambiguity, the desperate need for certainty beyond human capacity, rejection of logical and emotional reasoning, closed and narrow views of normative human experiencing, and fear-suffused thinking, and the therapists who emerge from these institutions. Likewise, there is considerable overlap between these features of disturbed clients whose paradoxical and delusional thinking asserts the thought that they can control their environment because they are sincerely aligned with their absolutely correct understanding of "the situation" and the features of the so-called "therapists" who emerge from these institutions. Are they therapists or frightened individuals parading as therapists?

Christian-Related Clinical Orientations

Based on The Big List that forms the basis for the lists of approaches to therapy in this book and among the treatment orientations that have been gathered so far, the words, "Christ" and "Christian" are used in 1,246 titles—just titles. These titles represent an unknown but obviously very large number of practicing counselors and therapists. The words, "Christ" and "Christian," are also associated with many other treatment orientations. As an adjective, "Christian," precedes numerous other treatment orientations. Chart 4.1 makes this clear. To illustrate the pervasive assignment of the adjective, "Christian," to numerous treatment orientations, only 50 are listed here. They are much more illustrative than complete. The complete list of "Christian" approaches to counseling and therapy would occupy much more space than should be permitted here.

Obviously, the approaches to counseling and therapy listed above are conditioned by the adjective, "Christian." While the list could be much longer, it enables a clear conclusion: almost any conceivable approach to therapy, including ones that may be antithetical to "Christian," may be labelled "Christian." All of the approaches to counseling and therapy listed above begin with the word, "Christian," but numerous others contain the word, "Christian," in their titles, but begin with other words. Many of them appear in this book, but for now, Animal Assisted Christian Counseling, Behavioral Christian Counseling, Brain-Based Christian Counseling, and Whole Christian Life Integration illustrate those that begin with another word.

Chart 4.1 "Christian" Treatment Orientations

Christian Acceptance and Commitment Therapy
Christian Archetypical Psychology
Christian Art Therapy
Christian Auditory Meditation Therapy
Christian-Based Belief Therapy
Christian-Based Existential Therapy
Christian Based Treatment (CBT)
Christian Behavioral Analysis
Christian Bible-based Morality Orientation
Christian Body-Based Modalities
Christian Buddhism
Christian Client-Centered Techniques
Christian Coaching
Christian Cognitive Behavioral Play Therapy
Christian Cognitive Processing Therapy
Christian Control Mastery Therapy
Christian Counseling—Shamanic Processes
Christian Counseling—Holy Spirit Guided
Christian Creationist Approach
Christian Dialectical Behavior Therapy
Christian Diamond Approach
Christian Dream Interpretation
Christian Eclecticism
Christian EMDR
Christian Experiential Therapy
Christian Family Solutions
Christian Feminist Therapy
Christian Gestalt
Christian Gospel-Based Therapy
Christian Healing Process
Christian Hypnotherapy
Christian Identity Therapy
Christian Integrated Approach
Christian Integration with Depth Psychology
Christian Jungian Therapy
Christian Life Coaching
Christian Marriage Sex Therapy
Christian Mysticism
Christian Natal Charts
Christian Person-Centered Therapy
Christian Philosophy
Christian Psychodrama
Christian Recovery Model
Christian Reiki
Christian Romantic Compatibility Counseling
Christian Sex Addiction Therapy
Christian Sex Therapy
Christian Solution Focused
Christian Soul Attachment
Christian Yoga

Further, many of the approaches to counseling and psychotherapy listed above singularly represent hundreds of individuals. Collectively, these approaches represent many thousands of individual counselors and therapists. However, these thousands of individuals are ideologically related to several other approaches to therapy that do not include the word, "Christian," such as Apostolic, Biblical, Catholic, Divine, God, Gospel, Holy Spirit, Prayer, and others. When they are added and reasonable estimations of the number of counselors and therapists who advertise them, the number rises to tens of thousands. Contemplating that the number of "Christian" approaches to counseling and therapy runs into the thousands and that those who advertise these approaches run into tens of thousands likely feels like a much too heavily weighted professional cargo. If not to ease the burden of such cargo, but to confirm the reality, another list is provided here. Chart 4.2. enlarges the list of "Christian" approaches, confirming the massive proliferation of religion-oriented approaches. While it may not be desirable material to contemplate, such contemplation, along with possible actions, is necessary for professionally accountable counselors and therapists.

Chart 4.2 Additional "Christian" Approaches to Counseling and Therapy

Christian God-Focused Counseling
Christian LDS Counseling
Abundant Life Christian Counseling
Actualized Christian Truth
Adlerian Christian Counseling
Adolescent Sex Offender Christian Counseling
After-Life Christian Affirmative
Analytic Christian Spiritual Therapy
Ancient Christian Wisdom
Animal-Assisted Christian Counseling
Applied Christian Theology
Art-Based Christian Counseling
Attachment-Based Christian Counseling
Authentic Christian Compassion (ACC)
Behavioral Christian Counseling
Bible-Based Christian Principles
Biblical Christian Counseling and Prayer
Biblical Christian Sex Therapy
Bibliotherapeutic Christian Counseling
Brain Health Assessments—Christian
Brain-Based Christian Counseling
Buddhist, Christian, Earth-Based, and other Therapies
Buddhist, Christian, Sufi, and the Innerwork of the Diamond Approach
Calvary Care—Christian
Caring Christian Model
Catholic Christian Faith Oriented
Celtic Christian Orientation

(*Continued*)

Chart 4.2 (Continued)

Centering Christian Prayer and Meditation
Charismatic Christian Psychology
Child-Centered Christian Play Therapy
Distinctive Christian Point of View
Nouthetic Counseling
Twelve-Step Christian Approach
Whole Christian Life Integration
Whole Person Christian Approach
Wise Christian Counseling
Women's Christian Therapy
Word of God Christian Counseling
Your Life Christian Counseling
Transformational Christian Therapy

The abbreviated lists of Christian-related approaches to counseling and psychotherapy may, just because there are so many of them, prompt cynicism, helplessness, anger, surprise, or any number of other understandable responses. The abbreviated lists above contain only 90 of the 3,908 Christian-related approaches that have so far been located. Whatever the responses to the lists and the numbers may be, the list and the numbers come from those who advertise them and who completed training in mostly accredited programs and received licenses from their respective states. While these licensees frequently step outside the appropriate professional constraints of state regulations and professional ethics, they are not outliers. They are normative. They are common. They are widely dispersed. And, as discussed later, instead of showing ambivalence toward research, science, and evidence-based approaches to counseling and therapy, they actively oppose the utilization of these important professional assets.

This chapter has presented individuals who advertise specifically Christian approaches to therapy, but who appear to be unqualified to provide such therapy. It presented several representative institutions that promote preparation programs that defy minimally appropriate professional standards of professional mental health care. And, it presented lists of numerous approaches to Christian counseling and therapy that collectively appear to be random and unrelated to professional mental health care. These three presentations constitute a travesty and a serious injury to professionalism.

Whether the enshrined beliefs of the individual, institutions, or numerous specific presumed clinical approaches are those of Dwight L. Moody, the *Westminster Confession of Faith*, *The Baptist Faith and Message*, or thousands of other rigidly constructed orientations to faith, they are masquerading as counseling and therapy. There are more political views than clinical mental health care, more authoritarian than authentically religious, and more fixedly ideological than humanitarian.

Individualism? Does the information in this chapter represent the rampant and exaggerated individualism that impairs the effectiveness of counseling and therapy and casts a pall over their future? In a word, "Yes." The themes in this book include an emphasis on the conformity to rigid and doctrinaire thinking and an equally strong emphasis on the empowerment of prospective licensees or practicing licensees to think and act as if they hold superior personal, powerful, and clinical potency because of their presumed close relationship with God. Individually and collectively, they may have the relationship with God that they claim to have. No one needs to argue with them about this. When they report that this relationship gives them a special kind of therapy or a special kind of effectiveness in their conduct of therapy, they are simply mistaken. Instead of debating whether their understanding and practice of counseling and therapy are correct, professionally accountable mental health care providers should pursue ways to enable them to reform their approach to their profession or eliminate them from clinical work and from representing the larger and complex community of mental health care providers.

The material in this chapter, along with other parts of this book, exposes these individuals, institutions, and approaches to counseling and therapy as holding widespread, powerful, and possibly dangerous ideologies that undermine the considerable potential of counseling and therapy. As stated elsewhere, the conclusion here is that a common view of tens of thousands of practicing counselors and therapists is "I believe what I believe and what I believe is right and because I am right about what I believe, I can practice what I believe and call it 'counseling and therapy.'" Interpreted differently, they seem to be saying, "I can know the Truth and the Truth can set me free, but, instead of knowing freedom of the Truth, I will lock my mind and spirit in an emotional-mental-relational cage in which I will sooner or later become quite comfortable."

References

Alexandrova, A. (2023). *A philosophy for the science of well-being.* New York: Oxford University Press.

Dallas Theological Seminary. (2022). *What we believe.* https://www.dts.edu/about/what-we-believe/

Grace College. (2022). *About.* https://www.grace.edu/about/grace-college/our-mission/

Grace College. (2022a). *Master of clinical mental health counseling.* https://online.grace.edu/programs/master-of-arts-in-clinical-mental-health-counseling/

Missio Seminary. (2022). *Our mission statement.* https://missio.edu/mission-and-vision/

Missio Seminary. (2022a). *Convictions statement: Missio Seminary.* https://missio.edu/convictions-statement/

Missio Seminary. (2022b). *Counseling licensure.* https://missio.edu/counseling-licensure/
Missio Seminary. (2022c). *Master of arts in counseling (MAC).* https://missio.edu/master-of-arts-in-counseling/
Moody Theological Seminary. (2022). *Heritage.* https://www.moodybible.org/about/#values
Moody Theological Seminary. (2022a). *Values.* https://www.moodybible.org/about/#values
Moody Theological Seminary. (2022b). *About.* https://www.moodybible.org/about/
Moody Theological Seminary (2022c). *Beliefs.* https://www.moodybible.org/beliefs/?_ga=2.231465500.202564335.1656616125417978350.1656616125
Moody Theological Seminary. (2022d). *Gender roles in ministry.* https://www.moodybible.org/beliefs/positional-statements/gender-roles/
Moody Theological Seminary. (2022e). *Moody Bible Institute Faculty Female/Male Ratio.* https://www.collegefactual.com/colleges/moody-bible-institute/student-life/diversity/chart-faculty-gender-diversity.html
Moody Theological Seminary. (2022f). *Sexuality and the gospel: How to share Christ with the gay community.* https://www.moody.edu/alumni/connect/news/2020/sexuality-and-gospel/
Moody Theological Seminary. (2022g). *Eligibility for licensure (LPC).* https://www.moody.edu/academics/grad-programs/clinical-mental-health-counseling/
Moody Theological Seminary. (2022h). *MA in clinical mental health counseling.* https://education.moodybible.org/ma-clinical-mental-health-counseling-request-info?utm_campaign=program_ongoing&utm_content=macmhcad1&utm_source=gads&utm_term=edu&utm_medium=pc&gclid=EAIaIQobChMIp9OL2tHY-AIVdRXUAR2Vjg0UEAAYASAAEgIw7vD_BwE
Professional Wellness Alliance. (2021a). *About licensure.* https://www.pwai.us/about-licensure
Professional Wellness Alliance. (2021b). *Let's protect the future of holistic health.* https://www.pwai.us
Prout, T. A., Kim, E. E., Magaldi, D., & Cha, J. (2021). Christian therapists and their clients. *Spirituality in Clinical Practice*, *8*(1), 1–15. 10.1037/scp0000238
Reformed Theological Seminary. (2022). *Master of arts in counseling (MAC).* https://rts.edu/degree/mac/
Reformed Theological Seminary. (2022a). *Mission.* https://rts.edu/about/purpose/
Reformed Theological Seminary. (2022b). *Beliefs.* https://rts.edu/about/beliefs/
The Westminster Confession of Faith. (2021, May 12). https://www.ligonier.org/learn/articles/westminster-confession-faith
Trinity Evangelical Divinity School. (2023). *Mission and values.* https://www.tiu.edu/mission-core-values/

5 Career Counseling for Therapy

Obviously, this discussion gives attention to the urgency of "career counseling" for the profession of counseling and therapy. If counseling and therapy have a viable future, the profession must reckon with its current condition, with particular emphasis on deliberative and definitive ways to settle the matter of the place of religion in the practice of counseling and therapy. In such a reckoning, counselors and therapists must raise and answer basic questions about what their profession is and is not. A feature of this reckoning is that those who promote their individual version of religion in counseling and therapy very likely and urgently need career counseling. Unfortunately, with the abetting support of most of their colleagues, they protect themselves from this need by apparently rationalizing that their work is God's work. In this context, "career counseling" refers to those who misuse their religion and abuse the clinically relevant needs of their clients, but it also refers to all members of the professional mental health care community.

Those who misuse their religion and abuse the clinically relevant needs of clients should pursue major adjustments in their practice of counseling and therapy—mainly, toward integrity, competence, and pluralism. And, with regard to those who immerse in approaches to therapy that deny integrity, competence, and pluralism, they should be actively pursued by everyone who is a member of the professional mental health care community and held to account. They should be accountable to the profession in which they are members and to the clients whom they serve, regardless of particular professional positions held, type of licensee held, years of experience completed, income level, or other markers of association with the profession. The need is simple: Without such a reckoning, the potential of a viable future of counseling and therapy is in serious doubt.

Such a reckoning should include the idea that religion—broadly defined—has a place in mental health care. The place, though, should stand among other important views of life and therapy as a viable alternate, not as the only outlook or point of view. At least, a serious and urgently

DOI: 10.4324/9781003472469-6

needed reckoning will likely eventuate in ways to include clinically relevant responses to the religion-related needs of clients, but will also conclude that untrained, bigoted, ill-informed, rigidly held dogmas, and other deleterious features of religion must be excluded from the practice of counseling and therapy. Without such an exclusion, counseling and therapy will continue to feel its pending closure through Salvation Divine Therapy, Charismatic Christian Psychology, Gospel-Centered Therapy, and many similar approaches. Along with numerous other approaches, they will continue to infect the practice of counseling and therapy.

The priority of this reckoning is those who are served by counselors and therapists. Clients should see and experience the assurance that they will receive authentically professional care. This care is validated by the profession through which it is expressed. Such care, generally speaking, must be characterized by integrity, competence, and cultural pluralism. While these qualities are necessary, clients are not likely to analyze their care toward understanding whether they see them in their caregivers. Instead of depending on clients to analyze and assess mental health care—although space for this should be provided—this is the conscience-constrained and standards-supported duty of all professional mental health care providers. Without a conscientious and persistent effort to discharge this duty and the delivery of such care, the profession tacitly commits to sustaining the very visible peril that threatens its existence.

Thus, based on a considerable volume of information about specifically religious orientations to counseling and therapy, as they are presented in this book and elsewhere, the needed reckoning begins with necessary and inevitable observations about counseling and therapy. Importantly, conclusions presented in this chapter require staking a justifiable claim for the integrity of counseling and therapy and the potential for clinical competence. The avoidance of staking such a claim has consequences. The avoidance is an acknowledgment of an illness, a disease, that predictably will get worse, without vigorous intervention. Further, such an avoidance leaves in place an enormous number of serious threats to counseling and therapy and acquiesces to the idea that counseling and therapy ought not to exist or, worse, that counseling and therapy can exist as almost anything that an individual therapist says it is, although its implementation may involve harm to clients. Necessary conclusions, therefore, arise, as difficult as they are to acknowledge and as daunting as they are to change. These conclusions constitute most of this chapter. Thus, this chapter contains two major parts. The first part discusses some of the major issues with which counseling and therapy are presently confronted, with an emphasis on religion-related issues. The second part provides a long list of more specific, grittier components of the major issues, with each one being an observation about counseling and therapy.

Major Issues

In a previous chapter, this discussion developed the observation that rampant and exaggerated individualism among counselors and therapists has skewed practice toward self-serving approaches to counseling and therapy and compromised client care. It indicated that a list of consequences of consequences of exaggerated individualism would be discussed, later. Now, the discussion turns to the following items.

Mindless disagreements that cannot be responsibly argued nor responsibly ended
Self-serving actions and attitudes.
Chaos disguised as healing.
Perpetuation of a delusional belief in being right.
Relating with clients without professional boundaries.
Obeisance to self-effacing impulses.
The debilitating paradox of diversity.
Suspension normative ethics.

Mindless Disagreements That Cannot Be Responsibly Argued Nor Responsibly Ended

From the beginning of the mental health movement, debates about many different issues have characterized the movement. While nascent psychoanalysis tip-toed toward finding a secure footing on which to stand, alternate approaches to therapy also began to search for a secure footing, igniting differences that persist to the present day. Among the many emerging beliefs about counseling and therapy, some held that the unconscious dominates psychological functions and consequent actions, while others held that the contingencies of reinforcement shaped behavior. Likely, most mental health care providers assume that these differences inhere in their world. And, likely, they feel no need or obligation to end them. After all, who has the better argument? Sigmund Freud or John Watson? Carl Rogers or Aaron Beck? Or, if almost any other pair of major influencers in mental health care are observed, conclusions about them are very similar. They disagree and this is the way it is and, maybe, the way it will always be.

However, the disagreements to which this discussion is concerned do not involve Freud, Watson, Rogers, Beck, or other major influencers. They involve tens of thousands of counselors and therapists who arbitrarily offer their respective therapies, as if they are truly therapies, without regard for evidence to support them, clinical judgment to clarify them, relevant client needs for which to offer them, or any plausible rationale for identifying them as therapies. They include Harp Therapy, Lady Warriors Counseling,

Sanctuary Counseling, Kuro Nitraguro Therapy, Labyrinth and Purpose-filled Living, and tens of thousands of others. Many of them are named in this book. Worse, not only are these aberrant approaches to therapy used, they are widely and openly advertised and practiced. Increasingly, the aberrant approaches to counseling and therapy define what counseling and therapy are. Largely, such approaches are the individualistic expressions of therapists. And, therapists who advertise and utilize these approaches meet virtually no scrutiny or concern from the profession of which they are members. Thus, lacking the effort to filter approaches into professional practice and efforts to filter them out of professional practice, disagreements about them cannot be responsibly argued or responsibly ended. For now and into the indefinite future, mental health care is stuck with ongoing decline, due to unrecognized and irreconcilable differences.

Self-Serving Actions and Attitudes

Self-service is not an entirely bad thing. In fact, self-service that is based on reasonable and proportionate self-interest may be a universally accepted value, among many widely accepted values. For example, the needs for food and shelter may be reasonably and responsibly met, when an individual, family, or other collection of individuals takes action to meet these needs in reasonable and socially conscious ways. After all, everyone needs food and shelter.

Those who provide counseling and therapy take important needs to their work, too. They need appropriate personal and professional status, degrees, licenses, certifications, and other indicators of endorsement from their respective states and from their peers. Also, as providers, they may place an important and proportionate value on success such as pursuing personal-professional growth and clinical effectiveness that ensues from such pursuits. Along with these kinds of needs, therapists hold important, personal values that they take to their professional work, with the understandable need to enact these values with integrity, including such values as honesty, service, and self-care.

However, the evidence is clear. A majority of counselors and therapists fail to consider and pursue the importance of maximizing effectiveness in the treatment of their clients. Instead of this, counselors and therapists oppose evidence-based approaches to their professional work, seek to maximize their ideology-driven self-satisfaction, and commonly exaggerate their clinical prowess and presumed, consequent effectiveness. Compatible with others' research, Walfish and his associates (2012, p. 641) reported, "Based on the data from the current sample of psychotherapists, all rated their effectiveness as above average when compared to other psychotherapists in the same discipline." An inflated view of therapists' self-importance may not be a problem, as suggestive as this may be. Sadly, though, this self-importance also translates into erroneous conclusions about their clients. As Lambert (2017, online), concludes, "the clinician's view of their own patients' outcome is much more positive than the measured outcome using self-report scales." Specifically, Lambert's report about 12 studies indicates that mental health clinicians believe that "85% of their clients recover or improve," but that "rates of improvement averages 35%, and deterioration varied from a low of 3.2% to a high of 14%." With regard to counselors' and therapists' effectiveness with children and adolescents, he adds, "The small body of outcome studies in community-based usual care settings yielded an overall mean effect size near zero." Confirming similar conclusions, Constantino et al. (2023) describe the over-confidence bias in counselors and therapists, adding that they are "poor prognosticators of their own problem-specific effectiveness" (p. 8), relying instead on self-perceptions of their clinical strengths. While these numbers may slightly rise and fall and conclusions lean in one direction or another, depending on the source from which they are drawn, the discrepancy between providers' self-assessment and their specific, measured results is extreme, strongly suggesting that their self-assessment is much more about serving their individual needs than serving the needs of their clients. (Refer also to Goldberg et al., 2016 and Spengler & Pilipis, 2015.)

Chaos Disguised as Healing

No doubt, concern about the massive proliferation of approaches to counseling and therapy continues to grow. Also, no doubt, it has received relatively little attention. In my earlier book, *Therapy Thieves: How To Save Mental Health Care from Its Providers* (Oxford University Press, 2020), this issue received major attention. Back then, the book included a chapter, "21,758: The Scariest Number in the Psychotherapy World." The number, 21,758, referred to the number of treatment orientations that I had located by the time the book was completed. Now, a few years later, the number of treatment orientation found on the websites of practicing counselors and therapists has grown to 38,373. [Refer to the Introduction for an account of "The Big List."] At least, the meaning of these numbers is that counseling and therapy have no agreed-upon treatments, no consensus about what counseling and therapy are, no effective way of monitoring the practice of counseling and therapy, and—critically important—no way to filter effective or ineffective treatments into the practice of counseling and therapy and no way to filter them out. The net impact of this is that chaos reigns. And, worse, chaos poses as counseling and therapy, largely omitting effectiveness and the possibility of effectiveness from its repertoire. The inevitable outcome, among others, is that clinical competence continues to decline.

Indeed, chaos is disguised as healing. The collective failure to establish useful professional boundaries in which counseling and therapy may be effectively delivered is the blurred, penumbral context in which random, individually initiated approaches to therapy proliferate. As demonstrated in this book, counseling and therapy may be anything that an individual therapist says that it is. For a list of therapies that easily illustrate how individuals claim that a therapy is whatever they as individuals say that it is, readers can refer to the Appendix. The partial list of religion-related therapies includes only 400 items. Alone, the list of religion-related therapies adds fuel to the fire that is consuming counseling and therapy.

While the sincerity of those who utilize unusual, if not harmful, approaches to counseling and therapy may be challenged, such a challenge is not likely to effect needed changes in the delivery of professional services. Possibly, when evidence is clear, relevant, and useful, instead of challenging the motivations of those who practice unusual approaches to counseling and therapy, the therapies themselves must be challenged. It is malpractice that must the eliminated, not individuals, assuming that those who stray from professionally accountable therapy are capable of regaining their professionalism.

Perpetuation of a Delusional Belief in Being Right

As stated elsewhere, the conclusion here is that a common view of tens of thousands of practicing counselors and therapists is "I believe what I believe and what I believe is right and because I am right about what I believe, I can practice what I believe." This view is what an unknown but very large number of preparation programs teach students. This strange phenomenon is described earlier in this book, with reference to several theological schools that advance extremely rigid ideologies that they incorporate into their presumed ideas about what counseling and therapy are. In addition, similar approaches are taken in many other preparation programs that give inordinate attention to the expectation that their students and prospective licensees will "choose a theory" by which they will conduct counseling and therapy. For example, a colleague recently stated, "Our [graduate] program was Adlerian all the way. We came out Adlerian. That's just the way it was." More broadly and generally, preparation programs establish the expectation among students and the licensees they become that they can and will create their own "unique" approach to counseling and therapy. While the adverse impact on clients is the most important outcome of this way of preparing students, it also leads to the massive proliferation of approaches to counseling and therapy. Indeed, if a therapist practices a unique approach to counseling and therapy, the approach is probably deficient and inappropriate. As noted elsewhere in this book, several research reports indicate very similar conclusions to those that appear in this paragraph.

To illustrate this delusional belief, new counselors and therapists were not likely taught or specifically led to believe that they should invent Running Therapy, Jedi Social Skills Therapy, Jewish Mysticism, Joyology, Karmic Release Therapy, Kita Peace Creating Sound Healing, Kiva Coaching, or thousands of others, but they did—because they believed they could and, maybe, should. They will continue to invent non-clinical, sometimes harmful, approaches to counseling and therapy because they can and they believe they are quite right to do so. To further illustrate this phenomenon, Chart 5.1 provides a list of unusual therapies.

The short list of odd therapies may not seem to be odd, given that it includes 100 items. Extracted from The Big List of 38,373, the short list provides a very limited indication of the much larger problem: the massive proliferation of approaches to counseling and therapy. More than proliferation—a phenomenon that could suggest growth—these approaches define an assault on counseling and therapy and perpetuate the highly individualistic, delusional thinking from which many of these approaches emerge. Framed differently and personally, if you are a practicing counselor/therapist who recognizes, say, only 20 of the approaches on the list of 100 approaches or, maybe, only five of them, are you really a member of the profession that utilizes these approaches? Or, do you recognize the profession of which you are a member? If you do not recognize most or maybe all of these approaches, may you conclude that your profession may not really exist? Many of the odd therapies in Chart 5.1 are either specifically religious or evoke religious thinking.

Relating with Clients Without Professional Boundaries

The list of approaches to counseling and therapy in Chart 5.1 does not explicitly demonstrate violations of professional boundaries in relating with clients. However, the probability is that when a counselor/therapist implements any one of the approaches in the list, the needs of the clients who are subjected to these treatments are not likely taken into account. Too obviously, the interests of the counselors and therapists who practice most of these approaches rise above the interests and needs of their clients. Insofar as this conclusion holds meaning for the present and future condition of counseling and therapy, it poses the unfortunate characterization of numerous counselors and therapists as being philopatric foragers, individuals who take their clients to a preferred sanctuary in which the therapist feels safely guarded within sacred walls where they can consume and dispose of client welfare, in deference to their own needs. With this characterization in view, a needed question is "What accounts for this kind or orientation to professional mental health care?" To be sure, the self-interest of the counselor/therapist is a factor. Beyond this, though, as

Chart 5.1 A Short List of Odd Therapies

Angelic Channeling	Buteyko Method
Esotherapy Natural Wisdom	Gemstone Therapy
Pray Therapy	Komichi Therapy
Shiatsu & Martial Arts	Sociotherapy
Usui Reiki Healing	Vedic Astrology
Yuen Method	Zanker Therapy
Young Living Oils—Thieves	HALO Light Therapy
Power Animal Retrieval	DeTUR Method
Divination	Plant Spirit Medicine
Universal Life Counseling	Advanced Past Life Therapy
Adyashanti Approach	An-Ra Energy Healing
Frum Therapy	God Designed Counseling
Rohun Purification Process	Capoeira
Biblical Christian Sex Therapy	Arno Temperament Profiling
Salt Cave Therapy	Holistic Money Coaching
Mud Therapy	Light Laser Therapy
Qabalistic Pathworking	Character Analytic Vegetotherapy
Chassidic Spirituality	Chinese & Ayurvedic Medicine
Orgone therapy	Wild Feminine Soul Psychotherapy
Neuro-Affective Touch (NAT)	Harmonic Medicine
Phage Therapy	Thermal Auricular Therapy
Christian ACT	Protector-Self Approach
Quantum Healing	Aromatouch (Massage)
Aura Therapy	Balametrics
Biblical Nauthetic Principle	Biofield Tuning
Mesotherapy	Immanuel Prayer Process
Scientology	Psychopomp Work
Time Traveling	Fundamental Scriptural Principles
GTD Methodology	Mental Feng Shui
Scriptural Principles Therapy	Psychosilence
Ichthyotherapy	The Nine Gamut Sequence (9G)
Shambhala Buddhist Approach	Life Between Life Spiritual Regression
Hyperbaric oxygen therapy	Metaphysics
Scriptural Values Counseling	Psychosynthesis Therapy
Wicca	Reincarnation therapy
Energetic Anatomy	John of God Crystal Healing Bed
Life SOULutions Therapy	Divine Integration Healing
Nondual Kabbalistic Healing	Maya Womb Healing
Pyramid Model	Secret Garden Healing
Holy Fire Karuna Reiki	Micro-Boundaries Therapy
Astral Soul Traveling	Eastern and Western Mystical Traditions
Astrocartograph	Cinemeducation
Eco-Somatic MFT	Luminous Body Integral Energy Medicine
Kunkel's We Psychology	Metaphors of Movement
Triathlon Training w/DBT	Provocative Changeworks
Satori Batterers Intervention	Subtle Energy Medicine
Neshama Counseling	Avron Method
Loss History Grapy Technique	Abundant Life Therapy
Alchemical Hypnotherapy	Akashic Record Readings
Alignment of Chakras	Ancestral Regression Therapy

previously noted, the profession of mental health care, more broadly, energetically advances individualism to such a degree that such individualism is devoid of minimal accountability to the profession or to the clients being served by it. Consequently, the positive potential of counseling and therapy exhibits major distress under individualism's burden.

Obeisance to Self-Effacing Impulses

In this book, previous discussions have given attention to rampant individualism. Almost all of this attention has referred to the extraordinarily large number of aberrant approaches to counseling and therapy. Surely, these approaches expose both goodwill and poor judgment, at least. However, in addition to aberrant approaches to counseling and therapy, individual counselors and therapists commit to other actions that betray their profession and themselves. Anecdotes cannot and should not be used to characterize an entire profession. When anecdotes are paired with carefully gathered data, they become somewhat more consequential in their importance. Considerable research is cited elsewhere in this book. For now, here are some anecdotes:

> An experienced, licensed therapist reported that she was upset and worried about her daughter who fell and fractured her femur. The therapist concluded that her "traumatized" daughter needed EMDR and that, because she was trained in EMDR, she would administer the needed treatment to her daughter.
>
> A presenter at a conference enthusiastically described her "walk and talk therapy." She stated that she met her clients for their hour of therapy at a large public park where "safety was pretty much assured because there were a lot of people there." She added that "one of the joys of going to the park is that she met some of her colleagues there" who were walking and talking with their clients. Does this situation hold violations of professional ethics?
>
> A student in a graduate program that prepared her for licensing as a mental health care provider asked to be considered for an internship where she was already receiving therapy. She was integrated into the clinical operations of the practice, while also being a client at the practice.
>
> The clinical director of a small group practice admired his client, an accountant. So, because his practice needed an accountant and his client needed a job, the director hired his client and continued to provide treatment for the new accountant.
>
> "My license renewal form came in the mail, but I really didn't think much about it. That was two years—and a few months—ago. It's not unethical for me to practice, is it?" This individual appeared to have little

or no awareness of the serious, potential consequences that could befall her clients, let alone the consequences for herself. For example, was she guilty of insurance fraud? Did her clients have legal privilege for two years during which she held no professional license? Was she committing ethical violations?

"All of my clients are my friends. They expect it. And, I give them my friendship as best I can. Most of them don't know how to be a friend. So, I can be friends with them and let them experience real friendship."

Each of these situations illustrates the frequent ease through which individual therapists succumb to self-effacing impulses. They not only serve themselves poorly but also serve their clients and their profession poorly.

The Debilitating Paradox of Diversity

On the one side, advocacy of diversity is an important professional value and, on the other side, diversity is tacit approval of almost any rationale for enacting aberrant therapies. The reality of this paradox is all too easily manifested in the extraordinarily large number of specifically religious approaches to counseling and therapy and the almost universal silence in addressing the obvious fact that many of them severely lack a reasonable connection to professionally accountable mental health care. If anyone, who openly and seriously speaks about whether Ancient Faith Healing should be a professional clinical service? Or, who speaks about Advanced Reiki Energy Healing? Or, African Healing Rituals? Or, Akoma Healing? Or, Alchemical Healing? Or, An-Ra Energy Healing? Along with many others, these six appear among those that begin with "A." Between "A" and "Z, tens of thousands of others appear. Among those that begin with "U," who, if anyone, openly and seriously speaks about whether Universal Healing Energy? Or, Universal White Time Healing? Or, Usui Natural Healing Methods? Or, Usui Tibetan Healing? Or, Usui Reiki/Crystal Healing/Matrix Energetics? Or, Usui Holy Fire Reiki? Or, near the end of the alphabet, how about Zapotec Healing Ceremonies? Any one of these indicators of the debilitating paradox of diversity is not much of a problem. One of them could easily and justifiably be ignored by the mental health care professional community. However, when the number of these aberrant approaches to therapy runs into the tens of thousands, the likely impact on mental health care services involves harmful compromises of the integrity of mental health care and elevates the likelihood of harming clients.

As important as this is, it should have more discussion than it receives here. The size of the discussion, though, should not diminish its importance. Clearly, diversity is an important professional value. Advocating for diversity has offered sanctuary for many individuals who would otherwise be outcasts from normative social functioning. Surely, these include LGBTQ+, trans individuals, victims of sexual assault, and many others. Similarly, within the professional community, advocating for diversity has helped to provide acceptance of alternate views on what therapy is and how it should be delivered, welcoming new ideas and approaches. However, as significant as diversity is and should be, can it survive the stress of carrying the burden of more than 5,000 specifically religious approaches to counseling and therapy, along with tens of thousands of other religion-related approaches, including Vedic Astrology-Soul Healing, Shamanic Energy Field Healing, or Biblical Evangelical Counseling?

Embodying and enacting diversity should continue because it is a fundamentally important and commonly supported value among counselors and therapists. Akin to enacting honesty, a virtue that almost never encompasses the venting of raw, unfiltered, and offensive expressions, including "raw" venting in the name of honesty. For example, a granddaughter of a terminally ill grandmother should not say, "My God, grandma, you look terrible; I'm not surprised that you're going to die. At least, I won't have to look at you any longer. Right now, you are damned ugly." The granddaughter's "honesty" may indeed be honest, but it also seriously lacks compassion, affection, discretion, and more. It is unnecessarily hurtful and harmful. Similarly, uncritical and thoughtless openness to welcoming anything different in the name of diversity betrays diversity and its magnificent potential for human understanding and enhanced well-being. So long as numerous, "diverse" approaches to counseling and therapy continue to proliferate, other basic values that inhere in counseling and therapy will be squelched and betrayed. Among the other values that are buried under the rubble of pre-scientific, anti-intellectual, and broadly unethical individualism, surely, client welfare, personal integrity, clinical competence, client autonomy, beneficence, and justice will be among them. All professionally accountable counselors and therapists must ask themselves why they persist in ignoring and, therefore, tacitly supporting the conspicuous abuse of diversity.

Suspension normative ethics

Along with the evidence from other researchers, the accrued evidence in this book requires the conclusion that, much too frequently, professional ethics have a marginal place in the practice of counseling and therapy. Some report that competence is declining among counselors and therapists (e.g., Goldberg et al., 2016 and Gonsalvez & Crowe, 2014). Some report that practicing counselors and therapists have exaggeratedly positive views of their performance (e.g., Constantino et al., 2023; Walfish et al., 2012). Others report that the most common cause for effective action against a licensee is the failure to attain continuing education hours (e.g., Grin, 2021; Wilkinson, Smith, & Wimberly, 2019). Others report that preparation programs increase prospective therapists' awareness of therapy-related issues, but does not increase their competence (e.g., Hill et al., 2015). Still, others report that "many psychotherapists incorporate religious beliefs and political ideologies in their "meta-theories" or their assumptive worlds by which they guide their practice" (Bilgrave and Deluty, 2002, p. 256). While none of these reports, taken separately, clearly establish the fact that religious or other ideologies seriously compromise the integrity and competence of counseling and therapy, taken together they raise serious concern about the likely deleterious impact of such ideologies and, therefore, the high potential for ethical violations.

Contributing to the growing body of information about this serious concern, this book provides considerable evidence about the suffusion of specifically religious approaches with counseling and therapy, the massive scale of this suffusion, and the attendant, poor judgment that accompanies this suffusion. It offers clear, widespread, and readily accessible evidence that confirms multiple ways such as religious organizations issuing licenses for so-called "counselors" and "therapists" that lack minimal credibility, that this suffusion very likely establishes punishing and abusive consequences for clients who need mental health care. Altogether, the consequence of the massive suffusion of specifically religious approaches with counseling and therapy is that normative professional ethics and accountability are suspended, if not consciously and conspicuously violated, by large numbers of both clearly "qualified" counselors and therapists who elect to provide services for which they are not qualified and clearly "underqualified" providers who presume to provide services for which they lack training and experience.

No doubt, a small number of the religious approaches to counseling and therapy contribute positively to the lives of clients. However, the general lack of relevant training among those who offer such approaches mitigates against positive contributions, along with those whose training is locked in pre-scientific, anti-intellectual, and/or pre-clinical views of being human. Also, when the lack of relevant training expresses itself in selecting approaches to clinical work that lack credibility, except in the mind of the therapist who practices them, the therapist, client, and the profession are likely harmed.

Further, those who practice any of the numerous aberrant approaches to counseling and therapy defraud themselves, insofar as they presume to immunize themselves from the necessary criticisms of their poor decision-making about what is clinical and what is not. Their indecent denial of their professional duties and accountability is likely accompanied by their denial of their humanity, too, often preferring to associate themselves with the absolutist view that they know as the inerrant word of God, among other such views. After all, if they are good enough to know the inerrant word of God when they see it and the rest of us lack this level of capability, from their perspective, they presume to have superior knowledge and, maybe, more suspiciously, superior connection with God. Instead of superiority, though, they illustrate how easily individuals may succumb to their inordinate desperation to separate themselves from others. Their indecency is that, by defining themselves this way, they claim to be superior to others. Worse, they hear such a critique and defend themselves by averring that it is God who is superior, not they. Thus, their immunization from criticism is sustained.

The idea that many counselors and therapists have suspended normative professional ethics requires more than writing the idea. The idea should have evidence that supports the idea. Without evidence, the idea, no matter how well it accommodates one's preferred conclusions, amounts to no more than whining.

Therefore, this brief exploration of professional ethics and religion comes as a necessary truncation, intended briefly to discuss the suspension of normative professional ethics. Much of this book provides evidence that supports the conclusion that numerous practicing counselors and therapists have suspended normative professional ethics. This is truly a sensitive matter, but the avoidance of it by those who perpetrate it and those who tacitly let it happen may contribute to the most common violation of professional ethics among counselors and therapists.

As documented in Chapter 7, therapists commit many microaggressions toward their clients. While the documentation refers to religion-related microaggressions, readers should reflect on the much larger variety of microaggressions that occur in their practices. Religion-related microaggressions constitute a substantive ethical issue that may be explored from the view of normative professional ethics. At least, they expose the potential for specifically religious approaches to suspend or reject the values that mental health care professionals have labored for decades to establish. While microaggressions are, by definition, relatively small and often hardly noticed by either clients or their therapists, their pervasiveness makes them a compelling and formidable challenge for all mental health care providers.

Among the major and by far the largest groups of mental health care providers, most are represented by the American Psychological Association (APA), the American Counseling Association (ACA), and the National Association of Social Workers. Each of these professional associations promotes ethical practice among its members. For example, similar to ACA and NASW, in its *Ethical Principles of Psychologists and Code of Conduct*, the American Psychological Association (American Psychological Association, 2016) lists its basic values or principles, as indicated below.

Principle A: Beneficence and Nonmaleficence
Principle B: Fidelity and Responsibility
Principle C: Integrity
Principle D: Justice Principle
Principle E: Respect for People's Rights and Dignity

More specifically, the ethical standards of the American Counseling Association says, "Counselors practice in specialty areas new to them only after appropriate education, training, and supervised experience. While developing skills in new specialty areas, counselors take steps to ensure the competence of their work and protect others from possible harm" (American Counseling Association, *Code of Ethics,* p. 8). Similarly, the National Association of Social Workers' Code of Ethics says, "Social workers should base practice on recognized knowledge, including empirically based knowledge, relevant to social work and social work ethics" (National Association of Social Workers Code of Ethics, 2023). Congruent with the ACA and NASW, the ethical standards of the American Psychological Association says, "Psychologists' work is based upon established scientific and professional knowledge of the discipline" (American Psychological Association, 2016, p. 5).

In contrast, the value orientation of the National Christian Counselors Association (NCCA) appears to be much less clearly committed to clients who receive services from the so-called "counselors" and "therapists" who get degrees and/or licenses from the Association. On the one side, in its *Code of Ethical Standards*, the NCCA says, "The *Code of Ethical Standards* herein expresses Christian and biblical distinctives. The primary focus of these ethical standards is to promote a therapeutic approach, according to the scope and limitations of a Pastoral Counselor's Ministry, designed for reconciliation, restoration and transformation, rather than being punitive in nature" (National Christian Counselors Association, 2021, online). On the other side, while ostensibly promoting "a therapeutic approach," NCCA repeatedly emphasizes its complete reliance on biblical principles, as indicated in "Article One: We believe the Bible is the inerrant, inspired Word of the Living God. The Bible is the final authority on all matters of life, faith and practice" (National Christian Counselors Association, 2021). The necessary question is whether the NCCA's claim of advancing "a therapeutic approach" is compatible with its avowed commitment to a document that it alleges is "the final authority on all matters of life, faith, and practice?" (Chapter 3 includes an analysis of NCCA-related therapists and their treatment orientations.]

At least, the priorities of these two kinds of association are different. While the American Psychological Association emphasizes its commitment to client, the National Christian Counselors Association emphatically avows its commitment to The Bible. One is professional and service-oriented and the other is idolatrous. One is open to wide differences of clinical views and the other is tightly iconophilic. One responsibly aspires to adapt to the needs of clients and the other aims to deliver an ideology to which clients are expected to adapt.

The NCCA ideologically aligns tightly with the academic institutions that are described above, along with others that are described in Chapter 8. And, it also ideologically aligns with several Christian, counseling-related associations. Adding to the usually tightly constructed ideologies of several Christian counseling associations, numerous individuals advertise specifically religious approaches to therapy or religion-related approaches. In this book alone, more than 1,100 of these approaches are named. Again, in contrast with genuinely professional associations, those who advocate for and practice these ideologies carry the burden for demonstrating that the presumed clinical treatments that emerge from these ideologies are effective. So far, they have failed to do this. Religion-related therapists have failed to demonstrate that practicing their faith as therapy has increased their effectiveness as professional mental health care providers. Until they do this, their presence in the professional community should be challenged, if not prohibited. By analogy, because of their Christian faith alone, without medical training, why would cardiac surgeons presume to meet the life-and-death needs of cardiac patients? Once their attempts to provide cardiac care are made, they would likely be arrested and tried for a crime.

The so-called "Biblical principles" or similar titles usually refer to Biblical mandates for some kinds of therapy and, of course, many specific behaviors. Several religion-based counseling associations definitively advocate for a view of The Bible as the inerrant Word of God. The kind of religion advertised by the NCCA is incompatible with counseling and therapy, just as a mandate to wear sandals, robes, and beards is incompatible with personal and intellectual freedom. Is this overstated? Maybe. Many of these largely entrepreneurial organizations may be challenged to explain several biblical mandates that refer specifically to apparel. One—1 Timothy 2:9-10 ESV—prohibits braided hair, wearing gold, pearls, or costly attire. This prohibition appears in several biblical statements. Another—Deuteronomy 22:5 ESV—says that "a woman shall not wear a man's garment." And, while there are many other biblical mandates that relate to apparel and jewelry, just one more may be instructive. Leviticus 19:28 ESV prohibits "any cuts on your body or tattoos." Given that everyone wears clothes and accessories, the NCCA would seem to have missed the biblical mandates to regulate their members and, possibly, everyone else's clothes and accessories. After all, the mandates are taken from "the inerrant Word of God."

Many who are not acquainted with the NCCA or several similar associations likely conclude that, because they are not acquainted with one or some of the others, they are relatively inconsequential organizations. This is a dangerous conclusion. While the "membership" numbers are not entirely precise, the American Association of Christian Counselors (AACC) boasts that it is the largest Christian counseling organization in the world. Its membership may be larger than the membership of the American Counseling Association, American Psychological Association, or the National Association of Social Workers. The Wikipedia page on the AACC says that its membership exceeds 50,000 (Wikipedia, 2022).

Typically, Christian counseling associations have taken a strong, oppositional view of sexual orientations that differ from a heterosexual orientation that is expressed only within marriage. Among other consequences of this view, so-called "conversion therapy" was widely practiced by these associations. However, public resistance to this practice has lowered its profile. In 2014, the AACC determined that it would remove conversion therapy from its code of ethics, due mainly to lawsuits that targeted some of its members. Prior to removing its long commitment to conversion therapy, AACC joined lawsuits to prohibit various states' attempts to eliminate conversion therapy (Merlan, 2013). A summary statement here is that the AACC has not been a friend to professionally accountable counselors and therapists, although it should be credited with serious gestures toward adapting its values to contemporary social realities.

According to the Movement Advancement Project (MAP), several states have banned conversion therapy. Specifically,

Twenty (20) states ban conversion therapy for minors
Five (5) states partially ban conversion therapy for minors
Twenty-two (22) states have no law or guiding policy
Three (3) states have unsettled lawsuits in which bans against conversion therapy are contested (Movement Advancement Project, 2022)

If the three legal contests are decided in favor of banning conversion therapy, the total number of states that prohibit or partially prohibit conversion therapy would be 28. Probably, the number of states that ban conversion therapy will rise, not fall. Regardless of individual counselors' and therapists' view of conversion therapy, all of them should ask about the condition of their profession, if professionally accountable clinical considerations are not a feature of treatment. Much more than clinical considerations that may have advanced conversion therapy, religious considerations have created and sought to establish conversion therapy as a feature of counseling and therapy.

The Grit and Grime of Crisis

This chapter stands on the conclusion that the profession of mental health care must be reformed. Some of the possible ways that reform is needed are discussed in Martin's *Therapy Thieves: How To Save Mental Health Care from Its Providers*, 2020). Later, this book adds to possible, needed reformative actions. The reforms discussed in this book emerge from evidence related to the place of religion in the practice of counseling and therapy. The need for reform, along with discussions around reform, is simple: Without reckoning with the massive and deleterious impact from the inappropriate suffusion of religion and therapy, the potential for a viable future for counseling and therapy will remain in serious doubt, if not forebode its inevitable demise. So long as the reckoning is avoided or postponed the condition of counseling and therapy will worsen. Vigorous intervention is needed.

In the context of huge volumes of evidence that call for reform in the practice of counseling and therapy, the need should be understood for what it is. More than a call for innovations or the creation of new forms of counseling and therapy, it is a simple and desperate need to recover and restore the integrity of professional practice and competence in the delivery of professional services. Among professionally accountable counselors and therapists, it is a mandate to affirm and practice within the boundaries of the best available evidence and competence. It is a mandate for every practicing counselor and therapist to embody in their professional practice the professional ethics that assign appropriate honor to their clients and to the profession of which they are members. Likewise, it is an equally strong mandate to deny the insidious incursion of tens of thousands of highly personal and many institutionalized ideologies that, by their very nature, reject evidence upon which mental health care can and should stand.

This chapter contains two major parts. Already presented, the first part discusses some of the major issues with which counseling and therapy are presently confronted. The second part provides a long list of more specific, grittier components of the major issues, with each one being an observation about counseling and therapy. Among the components, the following ones likely require consideration.

> Getting a license to practice counseling and psychotherapy is easy. It can be readily purchased, as reported in detail earlier in this book. Readily available licenses mean that, among other things, they may be easily acquired and advertised as if the holder of the license is capable of delivering a major health care service, when they clearly are not.
>
> Otherwise, if a license is not merely purchased, before entering the profession and confirming the broad decline in competence, an advanced degree and a state-issued license are required. However, appropriately

licensed counselors and therapists practice their religion, apparently believing that they are practicing counseling and therapy, despite the fact that almost 90% of them have no specific training that would qualify them to practice what they advertise.

Along with numerous other, often irrationally non-clinical approaches, religion has infiltrated the practice of counseling and therapy, with no recognized way to filter these approaches into practice or to filter them out of practice. For now, this conclusion is confirmed, by the fact that 3,908 titles of approaches to Christian counseling therapy have so far been located. No doubt, the number of these approaches among counselors and therapists is much larger than this.

Several sizeable organizations promote training and non-state licensing that is weak, at best, and likely harmful, to many of the clients they attempt to treat. Earlier chapters provide a detailed but partial accounts of this.

By adding a favored adjective, any approach to counseling and psychotherapy can be made into almost anything else. To illustrate, EMDR can be "Christian EMDR." Sex Therapy can be "Christian Sex Therapy." Jungian Therapy can be "Christian Jungian Therapy." Person-Centered Therapy can be "Christian Person-Centered Therapy." These adjectival inventions are very common. Such adjectival thinking appears to reveal much more about the personal needs and interests of large numbers of counselors and therapists than a minimally sufficient awareness of and commitment to professional accountability.

An approach to counseling and therapy can be "just made up." Such an approach needs no basis in anything appropriately related to counseling and therapy such as Kayaking Therapy, Power Animal Retrieval Therapy, DAFT (Depth & Freedom Therapy), Dance Ethnology and Mysticism, Keys of Enoch Counseling, Shamanic Extraction Cleansing and Healing, or Orgasmic Meditation. Another feature of many "just made up" models is that they appear to express marketing interests as much or more than clinical interests.

Among professional associations, little has been done to secure a useable future for counseling and psychotherapy, with regard to the relation of religious ideologies to the professional practice of counseling and therapy. Instead, through accrediting preparation programs, they have sometimes endorsed conspicuous anti-intellectualism, pre-scientific thinking, misogyny, and homophobia, among other adverse, discriminatory views and practices. (Refer to Chapter 8, for details about preparation programs.) While the explanations of this failure are currently lacking, it may stem from a misguided belief in diversity. Diversity is and should be an important value among counselors and therapists, but it may also leave them vulnerable to manipulation. Almost no one wants or intends to discriminate against others because of their religious views. A belief in diversity inadvertently encourages those who wish to take advantage of the goodness of the belief, by inserting inappropriate approaches to counseling and therapy, when their practice expresses hostility toward academic freedom, appropriate intellectual pursuits, women, or non-binary individuals. Then, religious views become harmful. And, when these views are practiced as counseling and therapy, all mental health care providers are compromised by them.

Many so-called "Christian" approaches to counseling and therapy take positions that betray counseling and therapy, including approaches that are homophobic and misogynist. Worse, they appear to meet little resistance among professionally accountable counselors and psychotherapists.

Personal ideology continues to triumph over professional accountability. Ideology-driven counseling and therapy is an incompatible concept. Authoritarianism in counseling and therapy has been an unwanted and poor clinical orientation, but has shown itself to have increasing appeal among providers.

Significantly, there are no standards for selecting and implementing approaches to counseling and therapy that are religious ideologies. An approach may be nicely and professionally integrated with, say, Cognitive Behavior Therapy or it may sternly and emphatically reject Cognitive Behavior Therapy. It may be affirming and welcoming of LGBTQ+ clients or condemning and punishing of them. It may involve Bible Study or hostility toward Bible Study. It may be conspicuously evangelical toward clients or highly resistant to such an approach. As an indicator of the extreme lack of standards, there are thousands of titles for some form of specifically religious approaches to counseling and therapy. The number of these approaches to counseling and therapy continues to rise, but the guiding authority for regulating them is lacking. Obviously, preparation programs lack capacity to filter into therapy or out of therapy approaches that may harm the profession for which they are preparing individuals. States do not generally approve of or disapprove of—filter in our filter out—approaches to therapy. Professional associations do not filter into practice or filter out of practice approaches that are "good" or "bad," respectively.

Almost any individual, anywhere, anytime can be licensed and/or certified to practice a stunningly large number of therapies. For example, Holden and Barker (2018) ask whether social workers should be engaged in certain practices. Their list of certifications among social workers includes Totem Pole Imagery Process Therapy, Cuddle Party Facilitator, Soul Entrainment, and Zero Balancing Practitioner, along with many others. Some organizations, such as the ones discussed earlier, sell licenses and certifications as religious activities. Others that are rigidly religious and anti-intellectual, along with other deficiencies, prepare individuals for "professional practice." The plain and obvious fact is that numerous individuals and organizations have usurped the rightful prerogatives of duly trained, licensed, and practicing counselors and therapists. This is usurpation that would not and should not be tolerated in any other area of health care such as pharmacy, ophthalmology, nurse practitioners, or imaging technologists. What may be the reaction to this: "Naturally, I am a pharmacist. I take pills, right! And I love them!" Or, this: "God tells me to love everyone, including women. And, I do. I love every one of them. And, the most loving thing I can do for women is to ensure that they are not stressed by the real world where men manage things for them. My job is to protect women. They're not equipped to handle life the way we are. It's my job, as a gynecologist. Right?"

Those who practice with little or no training and often without a license have become an acidic presence in the practice of counseling and therapy. Their presence demonstrates much more than a blatant lack personal or professional accountability. For example, as reported earlier in this book, 13 of 30 individuals who hold "licenses" issued by the National Christian Counselors Association have no degree of any kind, while advertising that they treat many of the personal problems with many of the same treatments provided by well-trained and state-licensed counselors and therapists.

The illogic of many so-called "Christian Counselors" or others who are dogmatically committed to utilizing their religion in therapy can be somewhat easily recognized and acknowledged, except by those who choose to live within the "like-minded" community of those who share their religious views. Within their pre-scientific, anti-intellectual confinement, they live in the proverbial "echo chamber." Their dedication to their echoed voices prevents openness to ideas and evidence in a manner that characterizes professional accountability.

Absolutism of many religious counselors and therapists appears to be common. As such, their work likely bespeaks their intolerance of ambiguity and, more largely, professional accountability.

As a large group of providers who presume to provide "clinical services," many religious counselors and therapists appear to have an unusually high interest in sex-related issues, although a preponderant majority of them have little or no training to treat sex-related issues. Nevertheless, they commonly advertise this as one of their specialties. Is their religion a means through which they suppress healthy sexuality?

The mental health movement has offered the promise of social justice. It has been a feature of those who advanced the movement, including "the father of the movement," Sigmund Freud. Freud expressed an accepting and possibly gracious view of homosexuality, for example. However, currently, social justice within the mental health movement has stalled and quite possibly has begun to fade. Numerous well-trained and state-licensed providers have committed to beliefs that betray social justice. They have advocated unreasoning and simple ideas such as using their "biblical principles" to defend their misogynist views and their rejection of LGBTQ+ individuals, among other things. Of course, those who observe this phenomenon should be as gracious toward misogynists as they would be toward any other person with whom they seriously disagree. Among professionally accountable mental health care providers, such an attitude comes hard. It requires them to acknowledge that the pre-scientific, anti-intellectual, client-compromising, and profession-harming attitudes and actions by many religion-driven counselors and therapists are harming them, too.

Another necessary observation is that harmful biases within specifically religious approaches to counseling and therapy are often hidden with expressed concern about the welfare of clients and/or prospective clients. The examples of this appear on the websites of counselors and therapists. "I am a Christian who asks Christ to guide my words in every session; but welcomes any belief system a client brings with them." Or, "as a Christian, I depend on Jesus Christ to lead my therapy, but everyone is welcome, whether they have faith or no faith." Or, "My goal is to help you to achieve the life that God has designed for you." As numerous as they are, these kinds of messages promote religion under the guise of concern for clients. They appear in every state and among all types of licensees. Individually and collectively, they appear to be too much like "I am a liberal Democrat, but welcome believers of all political views." Or, "I am virulently pro-life in my views of abortion, but I welcome your obviously inadequate pro-choice point of view."

The massive misuse of religion in counseling and therapy actively involves an intentional avoidance of clinically relevant facts. Instead of clinically relevant facts, personal preferences, especially religious ideologies, continue to squelch openness to facts, acceptance of differences, and the potential for delivering effective clinical services. Such avoidance, based largely on personal preferences, also involves magical thinking, with the inherent refusal to be duly impressed with evidence apart from their respective ideologies. This avoidance contradicts sound clinical judgment and promotes pseudo-therapies. As only one of tens of thousands of such examples, the following one represents large numbers of others. A graduate of Appalachian State University, with no other indications of training as a "Christian" therapist, posts this on her website:

As we partner together to find real-life solutions to real-world problems, we begin with the conviction that with God's help, we can find healing

> and restoration. As a Christian counselor with more than twenty years of experience, I have found that Christian counseling is not only unique, but also facilitates an excellent therapeutic outcome for the client. When applicable, we will apply Biblical principles during the process of counseling. When appropriate I will be blessed to pray for you during our session. Combined with sound therapeutic techniques, Christian counseling has proven to help people experience healing.
>
> I provide counseling to both children and adults. I utilize play therapy with younger children to facilitate the natural expression of feelings. Your child will love coming to therapy! For marriage counseling, I bring twenty-eight years of successful marital experience to the process of restoring and enhancing your relationship. Since 1992 I have worked successfully with thousands of individuals who were struggling with all sorts of personal challenges. Combining a strong Biblical worldview with evidence-based clinical techniques, I have been blessed to help individuals and families achieve successful treatment outcomes. I never forget that God's love triumphs! https://www.psychologytoday.com/us/therapists/lora-s-williams-garner-nc/161791

The absurdity of "combining a strong Biblical world view with evidence-based clinical techniques" is much too obvious. Such pronouncements are common and easily located. By analogy, if another health care provider—say, a physical therapist—advertised that she welcomed persons from all faith traditions and that healing of their specifically physical ailments comes because "God's love triumphs," she would very likely be censured by her licensing board and may lose her license. Her approach, though, may be reasonably extended to promote the idea that God will triumph over your pancreatic cancer. As uncomfortable as the analogy may be, it is a necessary one for serious consideration by mental health care providers, if they expect minimally appropriate acceptance and respect by other health care providers such as physical therapists, pharmacists, pediatricians, urologic surgeons, or psychiatrists.

Further, as indicated several times in this book, numerous so-called "Christian" counselors and therapists presume to advertise their "Christian" services merely because they want to. Except for wanting to advertise such services, they have no professional foundation for doing so. They reveal a kind of Christian imperialism—a readiness to occupy a profession that, except for merely wanting it, is not theirs to occupy. Whether it is labeled Christian imperialism, Christian supremacy, professional failure, or whatever, it should be further investigated. Among many issues that should be investigated is the question of whether those who advertise some form of Christian counseling contribute to racial bigotry, misogyny, or other beliefs and actions that betray the profession of which they claim to be members. Clearly and unfortunately, many of them practice misogyny and homophobia. In addition, from their study of Christian counselors and therapists, Perry and Whitehead (2019, p. 294) conclude that "being American with being Christian tends to activate a particular sector of society to constrain the boundaries of ethno-national group membership." Sadly, instead of an affirmation of cultural diversity and multicultural competence, Christian supremacy may be a defiance of these values, if not a conspicuous rejection of them.

Onofrio (2021) says that Christian supremacy is "that cooptation, that taking of Christianity and using it like a wolf in sheep's clothing—using its language, sacred texts, and traditions, to cause harm, to perpetuate domination, imperialism, racisms, sexism. That mixture, that marriage, that unholy union between power, systems of power, and religion ..." Allowing for all-encompassing scope of concern about the cooptation of Christian practices in Onofrio's comments, the idea is essentially correct. These observations are not new. For example, Burlein (2002) gives a detailed analysis of the convergence of "the Christian right" and "White supremacy." Referring specifically to the matter of race, Weir (2021, p. 401) gives a thoughtful, personal account of his work as a therapist, concluding, "I had not developed a relationship to myself as the white man in the room." And, tersely elaborated, "Because I had not suffered the consequences of a racialized identity, my white-ness remained invisible to me and left me naïve to the impact it had on [my client], who could see the white man in the room." How similar is Weir's thinking to the thinking of many "Christian" counselors and therapists? Clearly, within the profession of counseling and therapy, the cooptation of clinical and professional accountability is as widespread and obvious as it is crippling and unethical. This is the consequence of massive cooptation of counseling and therapy by Christian supremacists. Too often, in its application, Christian supremacy becomes gender supremacy, sexual supremacy, racial supremacy, moral supremacy, and probably economic supremacy. As such, it stands against the basic values of mental health care. And, moreover, it calls on professionally accountable counselors and therapists to work to ensure that the integrity of their profession is protected, with emphasis on providing competent services to clients.

Based on reviews of extensive research literature about our profession and the evidence that I have gathered, my conclusion may be simply stated:

> If religion is not removed from the practice of therapy, therapy should be removed from health care. With the presence of religion as it is currently practiced, counseling and therapy may no longer be professional and viable.

To be clear, religion has a place—an indispensable place—in the practice of counseling and therapy. The unfortunate reality is that religion has become a means of exploiting and harming professional counseling and therapy and the clients who are served by counseling and therapy.

The reasoning for removing religion from the practice of counseling and therapy leads to complicated explanations that involve multiple issues. This book carefully illustrates several of the issues, including the fact that it contains more than 1,100 religion-related approaches to counseling and therapy, with many of them showing that they are inappropriate approaches. This alone is only a deleterious and ongoing influence on the practice of counseling and therapy.

Another issue is that religious initiatives in counseling and therapy are sometimes much more entrepreneurial than clinical. It is profiteering. Another issue is that religious initiatives are sometimes aggressively evangelical, with the transparent aim of proselytizing clients. Another issue is that religion-based therapies exhibit clinical incompetence, along with a rejection of normative professional standards. Instead of promoting a welcoming environment within the professional community or for clients who are served by the professional community, religious initiatives much too conspicuously promote attitudes, values, and actions that betray the best interests of the professional community. Similar to the matters of incompetence and rejecting normative professional standards, religion in therapy has become a means through which agreed-upon and reliable evidence for effective practice has been opposed.

So long as mental health care is defined by specifically religious ideologies—or other ideologies—it is not mental health care. An Islam cardiac bypass surgery or Christian prostatectomy is no more credible, relevant and/or useful than Islam Emotion Focused Therapy, Christian Cognitive Behavior Therapy, or any of the tens of thousands of very similar approaches to therapy. When therapy is re-defined and re-issued as a religious activity, it is no longer therapy. And, when well-trained, licensed, practicing counselors, and therapists cannot recognize most of the treatment orientations that their peers advertise, it is no longer a profession.

In their comprehensive study of religious and spiritual abuse and trauma, Ellis, Hook, Zuniga, Hodge, Ford, Davis, and Van Tongeren (2022) examine and report about the empirical literature that has covered these issues. Among other conclusions, they state that the evidence suggests "a high prevalence rate" of religious/spiritual abuse and trauma (p. 223). The details of the studies about which they report are alarming. In one study, over 70% of participating adults felt manipulated at their current church and 84% felt manipulated at a prior church (p. 223). From another study, 95% of participating adults reported at least one instance of abuse in their Church of Christ, because of their sexual orientation (pp. 223–224).

Among their conclusions, they state, "Although" researchers highlighted variations in how R/S [religious/spiritual] abuse and trauma has been conceptualized and defined, three primary factors appear to be consistent across studies: (a) misuse of power, (b) psychological harm, and (c) spiritual harm (p. 228)." The relevance of this comprehensive report is that its authors conclude that the misuse of power accounts for widespread and extraordinary rates of abuse and trauma in religious settings. The question is whether the apparent proclivity for abusing others is also a feature of counseling and therapy that religion-based therapists provide, due to their misuse of power. Their conclusion likely traces the outline of multiple forms of abuse and trauma by religion-based therapies and therapists. Focusing more sharply on this issue and as only one of many expressions of the potential for harm around religious issues, the research reported by Trusty et al. (2021) in their article, "Religious Microaggressions in Psychotherapy: A Mixed Methods Examination of Client Perspectives," confirm the likelihood of potential harm to clients by their therapists when religion is an issue in therapy.

Moreover, insofar as these reports, along with others that are described in Chapter 7, are approximately close to the reality of likely potential harm from participating in religious organizations and receiving counseling and therapy from proponents of religion in clinical practices, the extremely heavy burden of proof, if such a thing is possible, of establishing the effectiveness of religion-based therapist falls on those who advocate and practice religion-related therapies.

A Disordered Profession

The question is "What is the place of religion in the practice of counseling and therapy?" At this time, a broadly agreed-upon answer(s) to this question is not available. Recognizing this, the more precisely stated attempt in this discussion is one of offering ideas about how the professional community may seek to answer this question. Toward achieving a workable consensus, built on a normative clinical understanding of professional accountability, Chapter 6 offers guidelines upon which courses of action may be pursued. The guidelines principles may be regarded as the outcomes of contemplating "career counseling for therapy" or, more accurately, career counseling for a disordered profession.

This—or any other—discussion of the place of religion in the practice of counseling and therapy may raise more questions than it answers. Insofar as it is an invitation to others to discuss their views, the approach in this book is to minimize any specific religious view so as to ensure that the discussion is a welcoming one. Recognizing that a widely accepted and agreed-upon understanding of the place of religion in the practice of counseling and therapy is not available at this time, the larger interest is to invite discussion.

A messaging aside: In whatever professional setting you work, please explore your views and practice of counseling and therapy, as they relate to the place of religion in them. As you explore your religious views and seek to advance your personal and professional accountability, I encourage you to utilize the material in this book, but in doing this, challenge the ideas here. Whether you utilize this book in your exploration or not, your exploration will likely provide benefits for our profession. Collectively, as all of us explore the question about the place of religion in our efforts to care for others, all of us will achieve gains from this. Moreover, as we take on other challenging questions—the hundreds of them that show up among us on a daily basis as we meet with clients—all of us gain from this, too, as we affirm our best intentions toward our clients and peers and attempt to express them in open and practical ways. So, while the story of our profession is to be determined, each of us and all of us hold the potential for shaping our profession as we have always shaped it—slowly, with intentionality, toward making it a cause and force for good. Surely, inherent in this cause is the necessity for an agreed-upon and enforceable compact within which the boundaries of professional accountability, integrity, competence, healthy pluralism, and a demonstrable commitment to effective self-governance and regulation can be established. Without reckoning with career and profession-altering issues, the necessity for such a compact and activating the standards that inhere in it, our collective future will remain in jeopardy.

A Professional Future

The Appendix contains 400 religion-related approaches to counseling and therapy. Some of them come from only one individual, while others come from hundreds or thousands. Whether the number of therapists who practice any of these approaches is one, a hundred, thousands, or some other number, the extraordinary variety of approaches merely offers hints about the number of approaches that are advertised by appropriately credentialed counselors and therapists. Given the currently accrued number (i.e., 38,373) of approaches that we have so far located, the general and necessary question for all of us is "What does this say about the current condition of counseling and therapy?" And, if the condition is truly deteriorating, "Who concludes this and what, if anything, should they do, once they have made such a determination?" If the determination is that mental health care is not healthy, what should they do?

The answers to these questions, along with others that could be raised, are complex. They involve the matter of whether preparation programs for counselors and therapists are minimally effective. They involve the question of whether counselors and therapists practice under minimally relevant regulations. They relate to the question of the relevance of professional ethics. And much more. Taken together, all of the concerns that may arise from these numbers and approaches to counseling and therapy necessitate an assessment of the current condition of counseling and therapy and judgment about whether they have a viable, truly professional future.

Framed in another way, each of us may want to ask, "If I am an active member of a health care profession in which I cannot recognize thousands of the treatments that my peers advertise, am I really a member of the profession?" Or, "Is my profession really a profession?" Or, asked another way, "How may aberrant and potentially harmful approaches to therapy be filtered out of clinical practice and how may productive and effective approaches be filtered in?"

Alternately and in addition, another way to inquire about the massive proliferation of religious approaches to counseling and therapy along with a demonstrable incapacity to regulate which approaches come into the practice of counseling and therapy is to ask, "If some aberrant, religious approaches to counseling and therapy are known to harm clients and the mental health care professions—or, at least, are known to be ineffective—what are the consequence of such tolerance?" Or, merely out of self-interest, "How may I protect my profession, including my income and clients, from those who persistently, and massively and compromise the integrity of my profession?"

Counseling and therapy cannot be everything that all counselors and therapists wish for them to be. Can they be both Qabbalistic Healing and Ancient Chinese Medicine? Can they be both Afterlife Mythology and Amma Therapy? Can they be both Contemplative Tibetan Buddhist Psychology and Inner Healing Prayer? Can they be both Applied Behavioral Analysis and Bible Study? Can they be both Sacred Geometry Practice and Stoic Philosophical Therapy (STOP)? To engage readers in considering such options, an exercise appears, below. It asks readers to review each item in column "A" and compare it with its mate in column "B" in Chart 5.2. Then, after their review of the options, readers are asked for their answer to a simple question, "Can counseling and therapy be both of them?" To readers, can you determine which therapy may be the more clinically relevant and viable therapy?

These "options" may fail to satisfy a reader's interest in examining strange approaches to counseling and therapy. In response to them, therapists' concern, if not alarm, should be aroused by the fact that all of these approaches to counseling and therapy are advertised by appropriately credentialed individuals. Then, if alarm is not aroused by this list of 100 items, added notice should be given to the fact that such lists could be

Chart 5.2 Therapists' Preferred Therapies

Column A		*Column B*
9 Rites of Munay-Ki	OR	Access Consciousness
After Death Communications	OR	Afterlife Mythology
Akashic Record Readings	OR	Alaska Wisdom Recovery
Alchemy	OR	Amma therapy
Anthroposophical Counseling	OR	Angel Therapy
Asian Inspiration	OR	Astrology
Astrotherapy	OR	Avesa Quantum Healing
Biofield Tuning Practice	OR	Bohemian Approach
Buddhist Jungian Psychology	OR	Celtic Healing
Chinese Herbal Medicine	OR	Clairvoyant Psychotherapy
Consegrity	OR	Core Shamanic Practices
Crystal Healing	OR	Dharmacharya
Diamond Approach	OR	Dianetics
Earth Sangha Meditation	OR	Earth-based Religious
Energetic Healing Modalities	OR	Energy Alchemy
Energy Psychology-Splanka	OR	Entheogenic Shamanism
Formational Prayer Counseling	OR	Eso-Phenomenological® Medicine
Goddess Psychology	OR	Havening Techniques
Healing Love Energy Direction	OR	Hermetic Philosophy
Ho'oponopono	OR	Hold Sacred Space
Huna Healing	OR	HypnoBirthing
Indian Saint Sri Kaleshwar	OR	Indigenous Healing Practices
Inner Healing Prayer	OR	Kalla Treatment
Light Energy Art Therapy	OR	Life Purpose/Maat-WellBalance(tm)
LSD psychotherapy	OR	Magical SOULutions
Marconic Soulful Healing	OR	Mayan Healing
Meridian Psychotherapy	OR	Morita therapy
MuZen Mindful Creative	OR	Mystic Aroma Therapy (MAT)
Nanj therapy	OR	Native Mesoamerican Healing
Oneness Blessing Giver	OR	Ontological Hermeneutics
Past Life Regression Therapy	OR	Personal Totem Pole Process
Pranic Healing	OR	Principles of Soul Healing Love
Psychic Medium	OR	Quantum Healing Hypnosis
Redemption Therapy	OR	Repentance Therapy
Ridhwan Approach	OR	Rituals & Rites of Passage
Sacred Card Readings	OR	Sacred Contracts
Sacred Role Play Therapy	OR	Secular Buddhism
Shamanic Energy Healing	OR	Shamanic Healing Practices
Sogyal Rinpoche	OR	Soteriological Counseling
Soto Zen Tradition Orientation	OR	Soul Entrainment
Soul Psychiatry [lpc]	OR	Soul Restoration
Soul Retrieval Therapy	OR	Soul Travel
Soul Wisdom Therapy	OR	Spiritual Divination
Spiritual Emergence Seekers	OR	Spiritual Healing Ceremonies
Spiritual Root System	OR	Spiritual Warriorship
Splankna (Christian based)	OR	Spiritually Fluent Psychotherapy
Splankna Energy Therapy	OR	Sufi Psychology
Ubuntu Philosophy	OR	T'ai Chi Chih
Taoist/Tantric Practices	OR	Tarot
Temperament Analysis Profile	OR	The Divine Mother Process

composed hundreds of more times. The number of similar items runs into the tens of thousands.

Also, readers should remember that, largely without the knowledge, let alone their consent, others in their profession created, adopted, and now practice these so-called "therapies." These therapies are "out there." They represent all counselors and therapists. As asked earlier, "Are you a member of a health care profession, if you cannot recognize most of the treatments that your peers in your profession advertise and practice." Or, "Does the profession really exist, if it can be so very many different things?"

The evidence that practicing counselors and therapists utilize evidence-based therapies is severely lacking. Moreover, the resources through which practicing clinicians can receive training in evidence-based therapies are lacking. In fact, numerous dubious substitutions for evidence-based training have effectively supplanted evidence-based training. Among other important implications of the evidence reported in this book and the analyses that accompany the evidence, practicing mental health care providers do not feel ambivalence about utilizing evidence-based therapies; they actively oppose evidence-based therapies.

Several evidence-based, research-validated approaches to mental health care for children have emerged during the past few decades. Which one is better than the others? Circle of Security (COS), Parent-Child Interaction Therapy (PCIT), Child-Parent Relationship Therapy (CPRT), Collaborative-Proactive Solutions (previously, Collaborative Problem Solving), Functional Family Therapy, or Trauma-Focused Cognitive Behavioral Therapy (TFCBT), to name only six of them? The short answer is "No." "No" does not answer the question about which of these approaches is better than the others. However, "No" is the best answer because, while these approaches are available, the evidence gathered from the websites of practicing counselors and therapists who treat children indicates that they almost never utilize these or other readily available evidence-based approaches. As noted earlier, practicing mental health care providers do not feel ambivalent about evidence for clinical work that is research-based; they oppose it.

Religion-related and other ideology-driven approaches to counseling and therapy receive far more support among practicing clinicians than evidence and research-based approaches Religion and ideology maintain the stagnation, if not promote decline in counseling and therapy, by their pre-scientific, anti-intellectual, and non-clinical orientation to clinical work. A widespread and obvious commitment to major theories, such as Adlerian Therapy, Person-centered Therapy, Solution Focused Therapy, or Psychoanalysis, augments this stagnation. Thus, whether the clinical approach is specifically religious or a more familiar "clinical" ideology, such as these, the clinician has likely refused to be impressed by, accept, and clinically utilize clinically relevant research and evidence. To frame the matter in a different way, how may therapists distinguish "Faith-based Therapy" from "Freud-based Therapy?" Or, how may therapists distinguish a "Humanistic Worldview" from a "Christian Worldview?" Or, how may "Torah Based Therapy" be a clinically and professionally accountable approach, compared with "Bible Based Theological Counseling?" More than evidence, ideology continues to ascend in clinical practice.

Counseling and therapy are not healthy. The material in this book may strongly imply that this observation/conclusion is justified, even while thoughtful individuals challenge it. Indeed, it ought to be scrutinized and challenged. Many others, though, have reached very similar conclusions. A detailed account of this appears in *Therapy Thieves: How To Save Mental Health Care from Its Providers* (Martin, 2020, pp. 30–47). Added confirmation appears in Chapters 8 and 9 in this book.

Authoritarianism in counseling and therapy has been an unwanted and poor clinical orientation, but has shown itself to have increasing appeal among providers. It appears mostly in the form of rapidly burgeoning, religious ideologies. The evidence cited in this book confirms this unfortunate reality and further indicates that the expanding influence of authoritarianism is very likely to continue into the indefinite future, accelerating the decline of counseling and therapy. Further, as Chapters 4 and 8 confirm, many preparation programs vigorously indoctrinate new counselors and therapists in tightly structured religious ideologies that pose obvious threats to a minimally healthy profession.

Having reached Chapter 6, much of the book remains to be read. It turns in a decidedly different direction. Chapter 6 answers the question, "How does religion relate to counseling and therapy?" and offers several guidelines for enacting this relationship. Chapter 7 examines clients' religious issues that appear in counseling and therapy. Then, with the clear aim of helping our profession to become much healthier, Chapters 8 and 9 offer practical recommendations for actions that may be taken by preparation programs, individuals, professional associations, licensing boards, state legislatures, and social service agencies. Finally, the book closes with an emphatic affirmation of our profession, by calling attention to those who persist in providing professionally accountable services for and with their clients.

References

American Counseling Association. (2014). *2014 Code of Ethics.* https://www.counseling.org/resources/aca-code-of-ethics.pdf

American Psychological Association. (2016). *Ethical principles of psychologists and code of conduct.* https://www.apa.org/ethics/code

Bilgrave, D. P., & Deluty, R. H. (2002). Religious beliefs and political ideologies as predictors of psychotherapeutic orientations of clinical and counseling psychologists. *Psychotherapy: Theory/Research/Practice/Training*, *39*(3), 245–260.

Burlein, A. (2002). *Lift high the cross: Where white supremacy and the Christian right converge*. Durham, North Carolina: Duke University Press.

Constantino, M. J., Boswell, J. F., Coyne, A. E., Muir, H. H., Gaines, A. N., & Kraus, D. R. (2023). Therapist perceptions of their own measurement-based, problem-specific effectiveness. *Journal of Consulting and Clinical Psychology, 91*(8), 474–484. 10.1037/ccp0000813

Ellis, H. M., Hook, J. N., Zunigal, S., Hodge, A. S., Ford, K. M., Davis, D. E., & Van Tongeeren. (2022). Religious/Spiritual abuse and trauma: A systematic review of the empirical literature. *Spirituality in Clinical Practice, 9*(4), 213–231. 10.1037/scp0000301

Goldberg, S. B., Miller, S. D., Nielsen, S. L., Rousmaniere, T., Whipple, J., Hoyt, W. T., & Wampold, B. E. (2016). Do psychotherapists improve with time and experience? A longitudinal analysis of outcomes in a clinical setting. *Journal of Counseling Psychology, 63*(1), 1–11.

Gonsalvez, C. J., & Crowe, T. P. (2014). Evaluation of psychology practitioner competence in clinical supervision. *American Journal of Psychotherapy, 68*(2), 177–193.

Grin, D. L. (2021). *Continuing education and predictors of self-reported professional competency among trauma counselors*. [Doctoral dissertation, Walden University]. https://scholarworks.waldenu.edu/cgi/viewcontent.cgi?article=12562&context=dissertations

Hill, C. E., Bauman, E., Shafran, N., Morrison, A., Rojas, A. E., & Gelso, C. J. (2015). Is Training Effective? A Study of Counseling Psychology Doctoral Trainees in a Psychodynamic/interpersonal Training Clinic. *Journal of Counseling Psychology, 62*(2), pp. 184–201. http://dx.doi.org/10.1037/cou0000053

Holden, G., & Barker, K. (2018). Should social workers be engaged in these practices? *Journal of Evidence-Informed Social Work, 15*(1), 1–13.

Lambert, M. J. (2017). Maximizing psychotherapy outcome beyond evidence-based medicine. *Psychotherapy and Psychosomatics, 86*(2), 80–89. doi:10.1159/000455170.

Martin, F. A. (2020). *Therapy thieves: How to save mental health care from its providers*. New York: Oxford University Press.

Merlan, A. (2013). *Dubious Christian "counseling" organizations sue New Jersey over Gay conversion therapy ban*. Retrieved from https://www.villagevoice.com/2013/08/27/dubious-christian-counseling-organizations-sue-new-jersey-over-gay-conversion-therapy-ban/

Movement Advancement Project. (2022). *Conversion "therapy" laws*. https://www.lgbtmap.org/equality-maps/conversion_therapy

National Association of Social Workers (2023). *Code of ethics*. Retrieved from https://www.socialworkers.org/About/Ethics/Code-of-Ethics/Code-of-Ethics-English/Social-Workers-Ethical-Responsibilities-to-Clients

National Christian Counselors Association. (2021). *Code of ethical standards*. Retrieved from https://docs.google.com/document/d/1OZuiUJftOr592arU8GRieUMoUXuzeWJke5VDYz1i4O preview

Onofrio, A. (2021). *Christian supremacy is a front for power.* https://www.opendemocracy.net/en/5050/christian-supremacy-is-a-front-for-power-reverend-alba-onofrio-explains/
Perry, S. L., & Whitehead, A. L. (2019). Christian America in black and white: Racial identity, religious-national group boundaries, and explanations for racial inequality. *Sociology of Religion: A Quarterly Review, 80*(3), 277–298. doi: 10.1093/socrel/sry046
Spengler, P. M., & Pilipis, L. A. (2015). A comprehensive meta-reanalysis of the robustness of the experience-accuracy effect in clinical judgment. *Journal of Counseling Psychology, 62*(3), 360–378. 10.1037/cou0000065
Trusty, W. T., Swift, J. K., Black, S. W., Dimmick, A. A., & Penix, E. A. (2021). Religious microaggressions in psychotherapy: A mixed methods examination of client perspectives. *Psychotherapy, 59*(3), 351–362. doi: 10.1037/pst0000408.
Walfish, S., McAllister, B., O'Donnell, P. & Lambert, M. J. (2012). An investigation of self-assessment bias in mental health providers. *Psychological Reports, 110*(2), 639–644.
Weir, D. (2021). The white man in the room: Finding my position as a white therapist. *British Journal of Psychotherapy, 37*(3), 390–403. doi: 10.1111/bjp.12650
Wikipedia. (2022). *American Association of Christian Counselors.* Retrieved from https://en.wikipedia.org/wiki/American_Association_of_Christian_Counselors
Wilkinson, T., Smith, D., & Wimberly R. (2019). Trends in ethical complaints leading to professional counseling licensing boards disciplinary actions. *Journal of Counseling and Development, 97*(1), 98–104.

6 How to Relate Religion with Therapy

Guiding Principles

Religion has a role in the practice of counseling and therapy. The presence of religion in the practice of counseling and therapy is indisputable and considerably larger than most counselors and therapists likely recognize. No doubt, as plentiful and valuable research has demonstrated, clients receive both very good mental health care and very bad mental health care because of the presence of religion in the practice of counseling and therapy. No doubt, much of the very bad mental health care comes from counselors and therapists who implement their religion in providing care for their clients, instead of placing pre-eminent priority on the clinically relevant needs of their clients. As noted, this book includes more than 1,100 religion-related approaches to counseling and therapy, confirming that countless numbers of counselors and therapists probably deliver their religionist, alloplastic aggression toward their clients and reveal their marginal awareness of, if not indifference to, the needs of their clients. Such aggression includes numerous forms of overt actions such as Christian evangelism, but also numerous forms of real, serious microaggressions. At least, in response to this, incumbent on practicing counselors and therapists is the obligation to ask, "What may be the clinically appropriate understanding and utilization of religion in mental health care?" Albeit a partial one, the answer to this formidable question and as a way to offer assistance to those who wish to answer the question, this chapter recommends several guiding principles for relating religion with mental health care.

At the risk of speeding over important events and persons and fast-forwarding to the current time, what are some useful, productive ways to think about personal religious commitments and counseling? While numerous factors may influence and produce answers to this question, the approach here relies on principles to which most practicing, professional counselors and therapists are likely to agree. The principles stand on a simple assumption. It is that counselors and therapists are clinicians, broadly defined. This is not a bold assumption. It merely confirms what almost everyone knows to be factual. More than this fact alone, however, it

DOI: 10.4324/9781003472469-7

strongly implies that most of our thinking about clinical work is, well, clinical thinking. Thus, if we try to identify useful, productive ways to think about personal religious commitments among counselors and therapists, what are some guiding principles and how may they manifest clinical thinking? Some guiding principles are discussed below.

Think and Act Clinically

The umbrella principle is this: *Think and act clinically.* "Thinking and acting clinically" refers to a commitment that virtually all counselors have or should have. It is that they provide professional services in response to clients' clinically relevant needs. As such, except for rare circumstances, they do not provide services in response to clients' non-clinically relevant needs. For example, they do not provide shelter for clients. They do not provide entertainment for their clients. They do not provide employment for their clients. And, as ethics and law require, they do not provide intimate relationships for their clients. While there are numerous other things that they do not provide, they do think clinically and provide clinical services. This is essential for counseling and therapy, although they are obviously more complex and demanding that a single sentence can capture. Naturally, the emphasis on thinking clinically evokes the question, "What is clinical thinking?" Or, how may clinical thinking be recognized?

Clinical Thinking Places the Needs of Clients at a Much Higher Level of Priority Than One's Own Needs

This way of thinking may complement or defy the therapist's religious commitments. It suggests that a therapist's personal, tightly held religious views should not obviate the needs of clients. This is poignantly critical when a client's personal, tightly held religious views are significantly different from the therapist's or when they reject the therapist's views. As evidence from research about the place of religion in the practice of counseling and therapy shows, the religious commitments of the counselor/therapist often lead to micro-aggressions by the therapist and other potentially adverse events. Some of this research is covered in Chapter 7.

Placing a high priority on the needs of clients appears to be a commitment that numerous counselors and therapists do not make. Instead, usually with a religious rationale for doing so, they avow that their views about the roles of men and women, the proper composition of marriage (i.e., one man and one woman), sexual orientation, abortion, and/or the absolute necessity of marriage as the only setting for sexual partnering have a higher status than the views of their clients about these and other deeply personal issues and values. Clearly, the abrogation of clients' needs fails to comply with minimal professional standards. Also, it expresses an anti-intellectual, anti-scientific, and pre-scientific attitude. In any kind of health care, this is a dangerous attitude.

Clinical Thinking Intentionally and Self-Consciously Addresses Client Needs

More elaborately, clinical thinking receives the client's needs and assesses them as well as possible and enacts clinically appropriate and professionally accountable services, as responses to these needs.

Clinical thinking draws from the accrued wisdom and established evidence for good clinical work, regardless of the therapist's personal feelings about the client. For example, this means that a therapist treats a mother with good clinical skills and an accepting attitude, although the therapist's feeling of disgust may be a genuine response to the mother's confessions about repeatedly and intentionally burning her child with steaming hot coffee. Further, no matter how genuine the response to a mother's disgusting behavior may be, it is not a sufficient basis for attempting to conduct therapy. The necessary caveat here is that several research reports indicate that almost all practicing counselors and therapists lack evidentiary bases for their clinical activities and interventions. In various ways, others conclude that the gap between science and practice continues to widen (e.g., Bilgrave & Deluty, 2002; Constantino et al., 2023; Dozios, 2013; Dufort et al., 2021; and, Vannatta & Steen, 2019). Utilizing the best evidence for clinical decision-making and active interventions would seem to be self-evidently desirable and necessary among counselors and therapists, but this is apparently not self-evident (e.g., Crowe, Collie, Johnson, & Wiltsey, 2020). Instead, religion in counseling and therapy has too often become a serrated ideology that cuts through clinical evidence, personal and professional ethics, client welfare, and the integrity of counseling and therapy. This is to say that, in other words, when large numbers of practicing counselors and therapists avoid examining the sentimentalizing of therapy by mixing it with religion, their avoidance compromises the integrity and effectiveness of the profession to which they belong. Obviously, this mitigates against evidence-based, research-validated approaches to clinical practice. The unfortunate consequence is that they give tacit approval to the widening gap between science and practice.

This view, notwithstanding, others conclude that the burden for narrowing the gap falls much more heavily on the shoulders of researchers than on practicing counselors and therapists (e.g., Lyon et al., 2018). In response to this latter group, practicing clinicians who wish to succumb to sentimentalism will find limited comfort and reassurance.

Clinical thinking expresses genuine interest in and curiosity about clients, instead of reacting to the client's presentation. While there is no universally acceptable response to some client's intentional or unintentional attempts to provoke reactivity in therapists, becoming reactive is generally not clinical nor productive. When a client states, "You don't care. You're in it for the money. You don't really give a damn about me," clinical thinking understands that the client is usually not commenting about the therapist, but is revealing himself, instead. So, maybe, a reasonably good response would be, "Is it hard to accept that I might genuinely care for you, even if you pay me?" Likewise, a not-so-good response may be "Oh, I really do care. I'm sorry I have to charge you a fee." Obviously, the tone of such a response matters. As an important professional asset, curiosity is addressed, later.

With the necessary recognition of the critical importance of intentional and persistent professional accountability, *clinical thinking demonstrates itself in a wide array of measurable and commonly accepted clinical skills.* A casual search for these skills will likely be productive because they are ubiquitous. Surely, for example, Allen Ivey (Ivey, Ivey, & Zalaquett, 2022) and his associates have identified many of these skills. And, in their book on clinical supervision, Martin and Turner (2020) describe many of the essential skills, too. Locating, defining, and understanding commonly recognized skills are easily achieved tasks. Implementing them so that therapists' clinical effectiveness increases is another, very different challenge, but a necessary one. It is one to which practicing therapists should commit.

Clinical thinking necessarily involves the ability to appropriately examine, assess, and address clinically relevant client needs that arise in practicing counseling and therapy. This ability may be expressed in numerous ways, although the most common by far is the clinical interview. Embedded in the clinical interview, critical thinking becomes a necessary adjunct to thinking and acting clinically.

Think Critically

Critical thinking is a necessary adjunct to clinical thinking. Thus, clinical thinking is also *critical* thinking, a disciplined focus on facilitating client change toward solving specific problems and living an improved, if not ideal, life. *Critical* thinking refers to an increasing ability to analyze clinical data and to integrate professionally accountable clinical interventions into the therapeutic relationship. To frame this idea in another way, *critical* thinking in the practice of counseling and psychotherapy answers the question, "Can you, the therapist, describe your client's needs and your clinically appropriate responses to these needs in ways that almost all of your professional peers would accept what you say as professionally accountable, even if they disagree with you?" Allowing for a variety of clinically relevant perspectives, the premise of critical thinking is that counselors and therapists seek to deliver a professionally accountable service to their clients. This rightly presumes that counselors and therapists maintain accountability not only to their clients but also to the profession in which they are members.

With regard to religious and spiritual interests of clients, mental health care providers frequently demonstrate sensitivity to the cultural and social dimensions of their clients. They recognize this as a necessity if they provide clinically appropriate care. Critical thinking, then, is not only a clinical imperative but also an ethical one. (Refer to the discussion of diversity, later in this chapter.)

Seek and Rely on the Best Evidence

Currently, the standards of accountability among counselors and therapists are, at best, sketchily defined and loosely applied to clinical work. Recognizing this, Martin and Turner (2020) sought to clarify the concept of professional accountability.

> Along with the idea that psychotherapy is professionally accountable, the idea necessitates the question, "To what or two whom should therapists be accountable?" While the evidence leads to the conclusion that many practicing therapists lack professional accountability, many practicing therapists demonstrate the opposite of this. Such accountability may be seen in several ways.
>
> 1 Professionally accountable therapists utilize approaches to therapy that their profession endorses.
> 2 They seek to comply with identified standards of competence.
> 3 They place the needs of their clients above their own needs, when providing clinical services.
> 4 They maintain currency with their clinical skills, specialized clinical services, relevant research, evolving ethical standards, evolving legal issues, and other indicators of commitment to professionalism.
> 5 They seek to maintain and enhance the viability of the profession of which they are members, supporting it in specific ways.
> 6 They monitor and seek to improve their personal well-being and their clinical effectiveness.
> 7 They place positive value on diversity among their peers and their clients, recognizing that potentially harmful biases should be recognized and neutralized.
> 8 They demonstrate that they affirm positive values, such as trustworthiness, honesty, integrity, curiosity, accurate self-awareness, service, tolerance, collaboration, democracy, justice, adaptability, grace, generosity, altruism, benevolence, and so on. (pp. 22–23)

This conceptualization should be placed in the context of a somewhat more sharply focused emphasis on evidence in and for clinical practice. Probably, the reference to evidence evokes thoughts of dreadfully dull research reports, for many practicing counselors and therapists. As unfortunate as this is, it also suggests that preparation programs and ongoing practice have not allowed practicing clinicians to value their expertise with regard to evidence for their work. Thus, as Martin and Turner (2020) ask, "How may clinicians conceptualize the evidentiary basis of their practice?" Their thoughts about evidence need not be limited to research reports. Instead, practicing clinicians may conceptualize evidence differently. Martin and Turner (2020) offer a polarized conceptualization of evidence, with one pole having the highest level of reliability and the other pole having the lowest level of reliability (p. 54).

Highest level of reliability

- Blended evidence from other levels, except highly individualized judgment
- Meta-analyses of randomized and controlled studies
- Randomized and controlled studies
- Non-randomized and controlled studies
- Informal, non-randomized studies
- Supervision and consultant-based evidence
- Clinical experience and judgment
- Highly individualized judgment

Lowest level of reliability

Every practicing counselor and therapist readily recognizes the limitations of published research reports. Although they may consume and attempt to utilize such material, their experience as clinicians requires them to integrate it with their knowledge of their individual competencies and the clinically relevant information that they gather from a client. Integration of this kind confirms the importance of research and the necessary and fundamental significance of clinical experience. Further, for counselors and therapists who aspire to be highly effective, these sources of evidence become critically important ones in relating religion to therapy.

Endorse, Affirm, and Practice Diversity

While diversity is defined in a variety of ways in clinical mental health care, those who are therapists should be committed to it. Obviously, among counselors and therapists, those who are Mormons and Muslims, Atheists and Agnostics, Baptists and Buddhists, and many other variations of personal religious commitments, along with many who have a comfortable indifference about religion, may be easily located. In addition, there are multiple variations of diversity with which counselors and therapists should become knowledgeable.

Obviously, these variations are seen in our clients, too. In addition, our clients demand a steady and clear affirmation of diversity, just because of who they are. Among many things, they are

Suicidal	Seniors.	Young children
Rapists	Bigots.	Overly emotional
Self-loathing	Rape victims	Intellectualizers
Shame-burdened	Perfectionists	Substance abusers
Religious fanatics	Shy introverts	Excessively anxious
Irrationally hostile	Painfully lonely	Terminally ill
Menopausal	Abundantly sweet	Perpetually confused
Strangely avoidant	Unkempt	Healthily generous

They are members of huge families. Some live entirely alone. They are political zealots. They are welcoming. They are adventuresome. They are …, well, just about any problem, ethnicity, sexuality, location, income level, and so on, that may describe human beings. Practicing counselors and therapists cannot avoid diversity. Instead, in response to it, they must individually decide what they believe about it and how they want to manage it.

One of those sometimes overt and challenging, but also alternately subtle tests of therapists' belief in diversity comes with others whose religious views and commitments are different from theirs. Each of them/us should ask, "How well can I affirm the religious view of the other person, whether the other person is a colleague or a client?" Or, "How well do I, say, as a somewhat liberal Congregationalist, affirm my client whose religion is conspicuously a Southern Baptist fundamentalist?" Or, "If my religion is Muslim, how well do I affirm my Christian client's religion?" Or, "If my view of religion is that of a skeptic or atheist, how well do I relate with a devout Hindu client?" Or, "If my personal history has left me angry, or even bitter, toward religion, how well do I relate with a client who speaks about her sincere, fulfilling personal faith?" This kind of test of a therapist's attitude toward diversity is quite common. Religious/spiritual diversity describes the professional mental health care community. No doubt, the professional community includes all of those to whom this paragraph refers, along with many who are not mentioned.

The dimensions of diversity among counselors and therapists are almost impossible to measure. However, the list of approaches to counseling and therapy in the Appendix provides a snapshot of such diversity. Possibly, it is a picture of diversity that is more extreme than most therapists could have imagined. Readers may scan the list and possibly locate their respective approach on it.

The necessary tasks of endorsing, affirming, and practicing diversity generally hold great appeal for practicing counselors and therapists. The idea of affirming others who are "different invites others to be affirming of one's self. Also, the idea reminds us of the importance of "doing the right thing." However, our commitment to diversity also beckons us to examine our not-so-affirming attitudes toward individually selected others. Thus, we may ask, "Who are the others for me?" Are they atheists? Or, Jews? Or … To encourage therapists to consider their challenges in managing their responses to diversity, the following questions may be useful: Who makes me uncomfortable? In response to whom do I feel fear? Or anger? Or exaggerated attraction? Are there others whose views solicit my deeply felt resistance?" Each counselor or therapist reacts differently, say, to clients who are attorneys, preachers, child abusers, overly emotional, intellectually low functioning, ugly in appearance or gorgeous, convicted criminals, or any of numerous others. If diversity is practiced well, individual counselors and therapists will adapt to their own vulnerabilities, with regard to their clients who evoke reactions from them, and come to appropriate comfortableness in relating with others who are different or even repugnant.

Practicing diversity is compelling. It is good. It may also be daunting or even unwanted, at times, when differences between therapists and clients may be confusing, threatening, or lead to incompatibility. Nevertheless, practicing counselors and therapists should account for their compliance or non-compliance with their professional ethics. Duty to clients is a pre-eminent ethical commitment.

In addition, virtually all of the major codes of ethics require that providers avoid discriminatory attitudes and practices with regard to the religion of their clients. The codes of ethics of the National Association of Social Workers and the American Counseling Association exemplify the importance of such attitudes and practices. Among other related ethical standards, the National Association of Social Workers includes these in its code of ethics.

> Social workers should demonstrate knowledge that guides practice with clients of various cultures and be able to demonstrate skills in the provision of culturally informed services that empower marginalized individuals and groups. Social workers must take action against oppression, racism, discrimination, and inequities, and acknowledge personal privilege.
>
> Social workers should obtain education about and demonstrate understanding of the nature of social diversity and oppression with respect to race, ethnicity, national origin, color, sex, sexual orientation,

gender identity or expression, age, marital status, political belief, religion, immigration status, and mental or physical ability. (National Association of Social Workers, 2023)

Similar to the standards in NASW's code of ethics, the American Counseling Association *Code of Ethics* includes these.

A.4.b. Personal Values: Counselors are aware of—and avoid imposing—their own values, attitudes, beliefs, and behaviors. Counselors respect the diversity of clients, trainees, and research participants and seek training in areas in which they are at risk of imposing their values onto clients, especially when the counselor's values are inconsistent with the client's goals or are discriminatory in nature. (American Counseling Association, 2014, p. 5)

C.5. Nondiscrimination: Counselors do not condone or engage in discrimination against prospective or current clients, students, employees, supervisees, or research participants based on age, culture, disability, ethnicity, race, religion/spirituality, gender, gender identity, sexual orientation, marital/partnership status, language preference, socioeconomic status, immigration status, or any basis proscribed by law. (American Counseling Association, 2014, p. 9)

Surely, in providing a professional service in which personal issues and personalities register as highly significant, openness to the experience of others usually comes somewhat naturally, with training and professional development, of course. For many therapists, encountering those whose experience is different from theirs, even significantly different, becomes a satisfying adventure. More than tolerating differences, the adventure of conducting therapy offers the possibility of new forms of professional fulfillment.

In contrast, some therapists—any one of them on any given day—encounter the client, a substance abuser who tried to operate his pickup truck, crashed into a car, killed a child, and critically injured another child and their mother. More likely than not, he intended to harm no one. However, when he meets with you, his therapist, he explains, "I came to see you because my lawyer thought it would be a good idea. He told me it would help me with my defense. I have to find a way to get out of this. This whole thing has brought me back to God, you know what I mean?. I'm just human, but now I've got God. In my heart. I don't think I did anything wrong. I can forgive myself and I think they ought to, too." Conceivably, this client or another one may justify dangerous, threatening, or abusive behavior as an expression of their religion or as non-relevant because of their religion.

During the most recent three decades, the professional mental health community has been far more supportive of integrating religion and therapy than invested in opposing religion in therapy. Probably, those who have welcomed expressions of religion from their clients have been disappointed at times. Independent of those who welcome expressions of religion from their clients, most counselors and therapists have met clients who justify their behavior with their misuse of religion. Alternately, they have assisted clients whose mental anguish came from abuse that was perpetrated on them because their perpetrators believed "God led me to do this." As reported by a therapist:

> I remember all too well the woman who came to therapy because her husband and teenage children demanded it. They had grown weary of their wife and mother being completely controlled by her church. They felt frustration and anger because she gave her total income to her church, received directions from the church about how she and her husband should raise their children, including which school they should attend, took instructions about when and how to have intimate contact with her husband, and demanded changes in her employment because of directions from her church. The woman's husband and children had decided that they should help her or separate from her, if she refused to get help. Reluctantly, she came to therapy. Initially, she was overwhelmed with guilt about the possibility of separating from her church. Eventually, she separated from her church and, through conjoint therapy with her husband and children, comfortably integrated into her family.

Through considerable anguish, the woman escaped from the complete control of her church. Experiences of religion such as hers challenge therapists in more than one way. Obviously, the woman and others like her challenge therapists' clinical abilities. However, they may also challenge therapists' well-being with their own religion, insofar as they have personal religion.

Insofar as therapists are religious, they should be, at least, comfortable with their personal, lived experience of being religious. For many of them, the positive features of this experience come readily to mind. They include opportunities for sharing important values, such as generosity, interpersonal honesty and support, learning and growth, and many others, not to mention the importance of gaining a personal philosophy that helps them to make sense of themselves and their world. Importantly, many of them experience the inspired and needed experience of worship. And, often, their personal religion teaches them about acceptance and inclusion and provides them with ways to express such teachings. In short, many therapists experience their religion as good, including their readiness to affirm cultural pluralism.

As individuals, therapists or not, countless individuals acquire a personal and positive acquaintance with religious life. However, as therapists, they also come to understand that religion is sometimes expressed in conspicuously harmful ways. An exploration of "sick religion" would take this discussion far beyond its intentions. Suffice it to say that almost every evil perpetrated by human beings has had a religious rationale to support it. Easily, the exploitation of women comes to mind, along with human slavery and multiple wars. Similarly and easily, shame-saturated or guilt-suffused religion comes to mind, too. The recognition of these things challenges an easy endorsement of diversity, with particular reference to religion. Counselors and therapists recognize that religion holds great positive potential and great negative potential. Often, then, they reject an easy endorsement of religion because such an endorsement defies the clinical interests and the needs of their clients. In short, they can think clinically about religion and their clients' experience of religion and, simultaneously, welcome their clients with a genuine openness to and practice of diversity.

Attempt to Make Ideologically Neutral Clinical Judgments

For many counselors and therapists, making ideologically neutral clinical judgments may be more of a challenge than it appears to be. Usually, they take assurance from their ability or presumed ability to maintain objectivity in their service to their client. Objective judgments, though, are not easily, let alone perfectly, provided or measured. In addition, clinically sophisticated and effective counselors and therapists correctly understand that their judgments are frequently and appropriately informed by subjectivity. For example, when a counselor hears from a young widow about the tragic murder of her husband—including details about how his body was brutalized and mutilated—and that she discovered him in their garage, simple objectivity and neutrality are not likely responses. Hearing her story evokes many different responses, including empathy, sympathy, assessment of her clinically relevant needs, but also a sense of the horror of seeing the mutilated body of one of her husbands. And, if a counselor hears, say, four other similar stories, the level of objectivity could easily decline and become supplanted by personal, understandable skepticism about others and strong views about victimization of others, critical life-changing and tragic events, crimes and desired consequences, and criminal prosecution, among other emergent opinions. Such skepticism is not inevitable, but its potential arises from our humanity—for good or ill.

Research reports have concluded that an ideology-driven approach to counseling and psychotherapy is not effective. Generally, such reports say that the more ideology-driven an approach is the less effective it is, with the strong implication that ideology cannot supplant clinical judgment.

Apparently, in many clinical situations, sound clinical judgment cannot bear the burden of a superordinate ideology. Regardless of the ideology, the more strongly it is advocated by a therapist, the less likely the therapist achieves desirable clinical goals. For example, as a result of their study of counseling and clinical psychologists, Bilgrave and Deluty (2002) conclude,

> In this study, we found that different amalgams of religious beliefs and political ideologies predicted different psychotherapeutic orientations. In addition, it found that the majority of the participating psychologists asserted that their religious beliefs influenced their practice of therapy and almost half claimed that their political beliefs influenced their practice. Finally, it found that the majority of therapists disagreed with the assertion that science provides the only truths about the world. Together, these findings challenge the ideal of the therapist as a scientist–practitioner. (p. 256)

They add that the increasingly clear departure from science is a cause for concern, insofar as it transitions the practice of counseling and therapy toward losing one of its primary strengths and sources of credibility, its reliance on science and evidence. Their view, though, is far from being a commonly accepted one. In contrast with theirs, Carere-Comes argues, "[I]t is difficult to understand how a critical science can avoid being conditioned by all sorts of preconceptions that a theory-driven scientist does not know how, or does not want to, bracket off" (p. 346). In addition to Belgrave and Deluty, a small sampling of similar reports includes the following ones: Campbell & Kay, 2014; Choma, Hanoch, Gummerum, & Hodson, 2013; Haavind, H, 2003; Hansen, 2007; Hodson, 2014; LaMarre, Smoliak, Cool, Kinavey, & Hardt, 2019; Michaels & Datta, 2016; Parker, 2014; and, Silander, Geczy, Marks, & Mather 2020. If nothing else, these clinicians and scholars express an easily viewed phenomenon: the profession of counseling and therapy contains numerous and often contradictory ideologies, as almost everyone in the profession readily recognizes.

Significantly, ideology-driven counseling and psychotherapy is not necessarily religious. It may be specifically clinical. For example, a therapist who is strongly committed to, say, Eye Movement Desensitization and Reprocessing (EMDR), and attempts to utilize it with almost all clients, is not likely an effective therapist. In short, the ideology becomes more important than the needs of clients. This is somewhat sadly demonstrated in a study by Noble and Rizq (2019). They studied individuals who were committed—maybe, over-committed—to Cognitive Behavioral Therapy and concluded, in the words of one of the study's participants, "It's led me astray." Studies of other major orientations to counseling and psychotherapy have reached similar conclusions (e.g., Barlow & Brown, 2020; Keng et al., 2017). Translated in a summary fashion, when a therapist declares, "I am a Gestalt therapist" or another ideology, the therapist is likely also declaring a commitment to ineffective therapy. While clear and consistent interpretations of this phenomenon may not be available at this time, its deleterious impact on counseling and therapy is clear and consistent.

Ineffective or compromised clinical judgment may also come from an over-commitment to a religious ideology. When counselors and therapists are strongly committed to, say, Christian Discipleship as a clinical orientation, they are likely ineffective therapists. While their faith may be entirely wholesome, it does not necessarily translate into a plausible clinical approach. For example, a licensed counselor (Counselor, 2022) who completed her graduate studies at state-sponsored university advertises,

> "For God so loved the world that He gave His one and only Son, that whoever believes in Him shall not perish but have eternal life." Together let's find out what love means for you and your relationship with Jesus. His love is the key to all successful relationships! His love heals the broken core, find out how!

The clinical meaning, if any, of this invitation to counseling and therapy may be somewhat mysterious for those whose views do not align with it, while they also respect the counselor's religion. This counselor's invitation prompts many, no doubt, to wonder whether she could be effective in providing clinical services. Can she or other counselors and therapists who promote approaches like this fulfill their promise of exposing clients to divine healing love? Is the promise of divine healing love an appropriate expectation from counseling and therapy? More generally, can personal faith be compatible with professionally accountable clinical judgment? As important and obvious as this question is, it has received attention from many researchers. For example, Anderson and McGuire addressed the topic, "Personal faith and professional ethics: Best Practice with the Families of Sexual and Gender Minority Youth." Similar investigations have been reported by Bidell (2014); Greenberg, Pievsky, and McGrath (2015); and, McGeorge, Carlson, and Toomey (2015).

More than this should be said. To frame the discussion in a slightly different manner, counseling and therapy are not specifically religious activities. They are clinical activities. As such, generally, they do not include specific religious activities such as worship, evangelism, prayer, or others. Also, research has consistently shown that ideology-driven approaches to counseling and therapy are not effective, insofar as such approaches too often compromise clinical thinking and clinical judgment. As this discussion has already reported, several studies have shown that counselors and therapists who strongly commit to their respective clinical orientation demonstrate relatively poor clinical judgment. Clearly, this kind of over-commitment sometimes appears among those who seek to implement a specifically religious approach to counseling and therapy.

In personal correspondence, a professional peer wrote,

> "They [religion-oriented therapists] cannot inspire confidence in their professional judgment. Instead, they refuse to do so, as they hide their humanity. More than contributing to friendship, community good, or most other needed relational resources, they actively construct the conditions of severance and alienation. Their plumage of security in the moment conceals their dread of a future without hope—a nice suit on a corpse. Their close-hearted authoritarianism (e.g., "The Bible is the inerrant Word of God. Therefore, I know how you ought to live and how to run your life.") They promote cultural and intellectual snobbery."

Among counselors and therapists, ideologies that oppose religion have been prominent, too. Maybe, no one represents the anti-religion ideology among counselors and therapists more than Albert Ellis. In his typically acerbic but well-informed manner, Ellis made his argument in *The Case Against Religion* (1985) where he expressed his views, most famously. However, as non-typical as Ellis was within the community of counselors and therapists, he represented his views many times. Somewhat succinctly, in 2004 in an interview with George Halasz, one of the questions gave Ellis another opportunity. In the interview, Ellis stated that he is "a probabilistic atheist." He explained, "… a probabilistic atheist is not a dogmatic atheist who says that there is no God and that there can't be. He says that in all probability there is none and therefore, since the probability of there being a God is 0.00001, I will assume there isn't any deity. If there is, and if he ever comes and talks to me, I'll ask him to prove that he really is God" (p. 327). Then, Halasz asked, "Has that happened yet?" Ellis answered, "No, he hasn't appeared to me and I've lived very well without his help" (p. 327).

By definition, ideologies can be neither proven nor disproven. No matter what the ideology is, it invites some level of speculation, non-factual faith, cultural affirmations, almost inevitable disputations, and much more. And, whatever the ideology may be, attempts to utilize it as a foundation for conducting counseling and therapy almost inevitably compromise clinical judgment and its potential effectiveness. Whether the ideology is 99 Divine Principles, Christian Biblical Principles, Kingdom Leadership Therapy, Apostolic Counseling, Cognitive Behavior Therapy, or Solution-Focused Therapy, ideology-driven therapy serves the interests of therapists more than the interests and needs of clients.

Maintain a Professional Perspective

In ordinary discourse, conclusions are far more easily reached than reasonably defended. The ease of reaching conclusions or impulsively grabbing them depends to a large measure on the person who views any particular conclusion. Members of couples know this all too well. They know that "evidence" may not support any particular conclusion. If they have been a couple for, say, eight years, they have likely learned that their hopefully infrequent arguments often represent misunderstanding and hastily drawn conclusions. He needs something he didn't get and, because of this, becomes pouty and somewhat distant. Already suffering with an annoying toothache, his partner also withdraws, leaving both of them feeling lonely and distracted by uncomfortable feelings toward the other person. From the view of each member of this couple, the other one is "wrong." And, as sometimes happens, when each member of the couple reveals thoughts and feelings to the other member of the couple, the skewed and incorrect conclusions are easily seen.

Counselors and therapists should avoid such easy conclusions. However, among them, conclusions and misunderstanding them come much too easily. One may be devoted to Dialectical Behavioral Therapy, while the other one despises it. One may skillfully utilize play therapy, while the other one views it as mere sophisticated pandering. Psychodynamic therapists may have little patience with their peers who boldly advocate for Gestalt Therapy or Behavior Therapy. One may view Person-Centered Therapy as the all-encompassing and singularly appropriate approach to therapy, while another views it as a passive and negligent approach. The point is that disagreements and easy conclusions commonly appear in the professional clinical mental health community. Indeed, just as it does with everyone else, the humanity of mental health care providers makes them vulnerable to having points of view that have come much too easily and that may be enacted awkwardly, if not inappropriately, in their clinical work.

Because of this, each counselor and therapist should give serious attention to maintaining a professional perspective and, likewise, avoiding personal and professional mythologies. Very likely, in the clinical environment, human beings who are therapists relate with human beings who are clients. This holds great promise of change toward increased health for clients and usually a small risk of harm. Maintaining the viability of the promise is obviously important, while minimizing the risk of harm is also important. It is this latter potential that most therapists do not acknowledge, insofar as it may characterize their individual clinical service. As many researchers have confirmed (e.g., Constantino et al., 2023; Walfish et al., 2012), therapists generally hold positive views of the therapeutic alliance and its outcomes that do not comply with the evidence.

The clinical relevance of the therapeutic alliance, as it is commonly called, may be appropriately affirmed by therapists. Obviously, a positive, clinically relevant, and useful relationship with clients has been broadly recognized as important and confirmed by a considerable body of research. However, therapists' ready affirmation of the importance of the therapeutic alliance may mitigate against their recognition of their clients' view of the alliance. For example, Bedia and Duff acknowledge that "… we still know very little about how clients understand and experience the alliance and its formation independent of the lens of practitioners and researchers" (p. 1). Depending on the clients' experience of the therapeutic alliance, regardless of the level of clinical skill that therapists display, their respective clients may or may not gain from such skill. Therapists need to assess the therapeutic alliance with careful accounting for clinical outcomes stands quite apart from therapists' genuine goodwill toward their clients. Thus, caution is needed, as therapists rightly reflect on their clinical effectiveness and consider the therapeutic alliance from the view of their clients.

Such reflection and consideration may confirm the fundamental importance of the therapeutic alliance, as Cirasola, Midgley, Fonagy, IMPACT Consortium, and Martin (2022) report, "The results of the present study provide some evidence for the existence of differences in the mean alliance strength across three therapy types, which were shown to be equally effective for treating adolescent depression in the clinical trial from which this data was taken" (p. 338). A somewhat more moderate confirmation of the therapeutic alliance is offered by Bartholomew, Kang, Joy, Robbins, and Maldonado-Aguiñiga (2022). They conclude, "The alliance developed in psychotherapy between clients and therapists is a profoundly critical component of change in psychotherapy. However, the concept of change has long been operationalized as a reduction of symptoms rather than a simultaneous increase in positive characteristics" (p. 321). However, rating of the therapeutic alliance raises concerns about it. As Lokhorst and Reich (2022) state, "[W]hen objective and observable relational events are held constant, alliance ratings are nonetheless biased by perceptions of therapeutic success or failure. This finding underscores the global evaluative nature of alliance ratings. In theory, adopting descriptive measures that involve coding for the presence or absence of concrete and objective behaviors, rather than ratings of subjective quality, may ameliorate this threat to our science" (p. 305). The importance of these and other reports—each one a serious attempt to study what therapists do and how well they do it—is that, at least, they challenge practicing counselors and therapists to examine their work with clients and to maintain a professional perspective, in contrast with a personal perspective or assumptions about their professional work that may not be entirely correct. Also, significantly, to highlight the theme of this book, such reflection and consideration strengthen integrity and competence in clinical practice.

Another common myth is that the longer therapists practice, the more effective they become. The evidence indicates that the opposite is correct. Among a majority of practicing therapists, competence declines over time (e.g., Goldberg et al., 2016; Spengler & Pilipis, 2015; Spengler et al., 2009).

Among many details that may be associated with maintaining a professional perspective, each therapist should understand and account for her/his ordinary limitations and assets, including specifically religious commitments. This feature of a professional perspective supports the therapist's obligation to give preeminence to the client's welfare. Among other implications of this feature, therapy ought not to be seen as an opportunity for making disciples of the therapist's religion, evangelizing clients, or otherwise persuading clients to accept the therapist's religious point of view.

On the other side of limitations, though, therapists have professional assets that can be appropriately integrated into a professional perspective. While they may easily be taken for granted, some of the important assets are a considerable body of professional knowledge, specific clinical experience, say, with eating disordered clients, a useful and reliable network of referral sources, skillful peers who are available for consultation, and many others. In addition, a therapist's personal religion may be another asset, so long as a therapist demonstrates respect for the inherent power imbalance in the therapist–client relationship and maintains a clear and enduring focus on the welfare of clients. The importance of such respect is that it inhibits the common microaggressions from religion-based practices in counseling and psychotherapy (Trusty et al., 2021). Likewise, the commensurate importance of such respect is that the therapist's religious experience, theological perspectives, and related commitments may provide reassurance and comfort for clients whose needs include confirmation of their religious experience.

Therapists maintain a professional perspective by carefully and self-consciously integrating their alignment with their profession into their clinical practice and, with high predictability, enhance their integrity and competence. This is to say that they demonstrate their professional accountability to the profession of which they are members. In application and in the context of a discussion of the place of religion in the practice of counseling and therapy, this means that those who hold a professional perspective understand that their attempts to insert their religion or any other ideology into their clinical practice imply that their peers endorse such insertions. Similarly, when a therapist goes badly rogue and injures a client, say, through developing a harmful duality as therapist and as close friend (e.g., sharing picnics, vacations, and hobbies), their actions imply that this is normative among counselors and therapists. In short, the actions of one therapist have implications for all therapists, for good or ill.

Integrate Clients' Religion into Clinical Decision-Making

In treating clients, counselors and psychotherapists should integrate clients' religion as a feature of clinical decision-making, but not as a religious pursuit. When clients' religion is viewed as a clinical feature of the therapeutic experience, it may be comparable to clients' experience and understanding of, say, parenting, sex, marriage, self-discipline, friendship, or other features of their personal views of themselves and others. As such, clients' religion becomes a demystified and somewhat utilitarian feature of their clinical picture. In other words, the religious experience and theological views of a client are not as important as the specifically clinical needs that the client presents. Swift, Callahan, Cooper, and Parkin (2018) and Barnett and Johnson (2011) provide clinically relevant and practical recommendations about how clients' religion can be integrated into clinical decision-making. Their work is discussed later in this book. For now, integrating clients' religion as a feature of clinical decision-making should be recognized as the complex reality that it is. Serious and competent counselors and therapists understand that clients are truly complex and that a client's religion may be more an expression of mental-emotional distortion and disorder than genuinely religious.

Complete Relevant Training

If therapists wish to integrate religion and/or spirituality into their clinical work, they should seek training prior to attempting to do so. Having a religious and/or spiritual perspective without training should not be tolerated among counselors and psychotherapists, particularly when training is commonly available. No matter how sincerely therapists hold their respective, personal religious beliefs and faith orientation, such beliefs and orientations alone, without professional training, are inadequate bases on which to provide counseling and psychotherapy. Research indicates that a small minority of those who advertise that they provide "Christian Counseling" or other specifically approaches to counseling and psychotherapy have any training for such counseling (Martin, 2020). As an aside, a majority of those who advertise play therapy and sex therapy also usually have no training for either of these therapies. Among providers, the lack of training for their advertised approaches is fairly common. With regard to religion, training may be acquired through several means, including the ones discussed next.

One, while it is insufficient alone, subscribing to and studying a relevant professional journal(s) can contribute to professional development, with regard to providing counseling and psychotherapy related to religion and/ or spirituality. Numerous journals are available. Here is a very short list of some of them:

Journal for the Scientific Study of Religion
Journal of Religion and Health
Journal of Religion and Spirituality in Social Work
Mental Health, Religion & Culture
The International Journal for the Psychology of Religion
The Journal of Psychology and Christianity
The Journal of Spirituality in Mental Health

Two, seek regular and probably long-term consultation with peers who are experts in integrating counseling and therapy with religion and spirituality. This may be accomplished in many different ways. The consultation may be one-to-one discussions. Another way is to organize and participate in a discussion group with other counselors and therapists. In such a group, individuals can gain from others' experience of providing professional services, with regard to whatever members of the group need. For example, consulting about clinical cases is almost always beneficial. Another focus of consultation could easily be the place of religion in the practice of counseling and therapy. Generally, highly effective therapists seek consultation with their professional peers.

Three, attend relevant professional development events. Usually, these events may be easily located. As a beginning of such a search, a review of several commonly recognized national professional associations and their respective state chapters is likely to lead to events that give attention to the place of religion in counseling and therapy. Along with their state chapters, these associations include "the big three:" American Psychological Association (APA), the American Counseling Association (ACA), and the National Association of Social Workers (NASW), along with their respective state chapters.

Four, a therapist may seek therapy with a provider who can assist with understanding and personal growth toward a healthy integration of the therapist's personal religion and the delivery of professional services.

Five, practicing therapists can enroll in academic courses that can expand understanding and professional practice, with regard to the place of religion in counseling and therapy. In consideration of this possibility, therapists may want to define the questions that they wish to answer. For example, a question may be "What is a theological understanding of anxiety or of relationships?" Or, a question may be "How does my faith orientation relate with the faith orientation of client whose religious views are different from mine, in such a case, for example, where my faith is Muslim and my client's faith is Christian?"

Six, therapists may want to pursue ways to gain understanding and meaningful expression of their religious interests and commitments, insofar as they have these interests and commitments. This may come in a variety of ways. In anticipation of such a pursuit, they may wish to formulate the questions that they need to answer for themselves. This would be an exercise that assists them in refining their personal views of religion and, therefore, increased clarity about what perspectives on religion they take to their clients. As a visible influencer among counselors and therapists, this seems to be Gerald Corey's (no date) emphasis, when he asked, "At this point, what do you think is the heart of your spirituality or religion?" Then, he suggests that his readers "reflect on the [several] questions about your religion or your spirituality to determine whether it is a constructive force in your life?" For consideration, here are only three of his questions:

Is the way that I live my life congruent with my religion or spirituality?
Does my religion or spirituality encourage me to put my beliefs into action?
Does my religion or spirituality encourage me to question life and keep myself open to new learning?

Given that presumably all therapists have a clear and positive commitment to their profession, they likely have questions to add to Corey's. What useful questions may be added? More narrowly, readers may ask, "What are my questions about the place of religion in counseling and therapy that will help me to with my professional and, maybe, personal development?" Raising your own questions may be more formidable than it first appears. For example, asking, "Should religion be connected with counseling and therapy?" is easy. It is primarily the substance of an intellectual exercise. Personalizing the questions is harder, such as asking and answering the following questions.

Which religious points of view do I hold that may interfere with my practice of counseling and therapy?
How welcoming or intolerant am I toward religious orientations that oppose mine?
Are there features in the story of my religious history that should alert me to the need to show diligence in how I regard the story of others' religious history?
How likely am I to visit a religious worship service at a church, synagogue, or mosque, to gain insight into my clinical work?

Which features of religion, including mine or others, as I understand it truly annoy or frustrate me?
In what specific ways may my religious views and attitudes harm my clients?

Among other concerns, these questions remind therapists of the importance and sometimes difficulties of personal growth. Also, they invite therapists to affirm the "good" and the "bad" of their humanity.

Seven, read articles and books that can assist with understanding religion and spirituality, particularly ones that may expand the scope of therapists' comfort in treating religion-relating clients. The list of such articles and books in itself could occupy multiple volumes. Later, in Chapter 7, ten articles are discussed in detail. To add to a short list of resources to read, here are two recommended books. Yaden and Newberg's (2022) *The Varieties of Spiritual Experience: 21st Century Research and Perspective* offers numerous and valuable insights into the extraordinary variety of spiritual and religious experiences, with a strong foundation of research-based evidence. In contrast, Dowd and Nielson's (2006) *The Psychologies in Religion: Working With the Religious Client* takes readers inside the feelings, attitudes, and beliefs of clients and proposes ways to assist them in counseling and therapy.

Demonstrate Support for Religious Freedom

Quite apart from their role as mental health care providers, counselors and therapists work in a large and complex social environment in which multiple varieties of religious expressions are easily located. Among the many expressions of religion, some embody the practice of openness to alternate religious expressions. Obviously, some do not. Likewise, among counselors and therapists, a range of closed-mindedness and openness will be found, too. Nevertheless, professionally accountable counselors and therapists should seek to maintain their individual openness to alternate expressions of religion. They should demonstrate their support of religious freedom, just as they expect their respective personal expression of religion to be respected and supported by others.

As it has evolved in America, freedom of religion has been an ever-present right. The right should be respected. This right for individuals who are counselors and therapists should be protected and respected, too. Among other sensitive and mostly unanswered questions is how this right may be included in or excluded from the practice of professionally accountable counseling and therapy. In the Appendix, a representative sample of collected approaches to counseling and therapy demonstrates the larger observation that counselors and therapists in large numbers express their personal religion through their conduct of therapy, including more than 1,100 titles of religion-related approaches in this book. The very large number of specifically religious approaches to counseling and therapy necessitates questions: Can counseling and therapy sustain the proliferation of tens of thousands of religious approaches within the practice of counseling and therapy? In other words, within the profession of counseling and therapy, how may freedom of religion be balanced with professional accountability that encompasses integrity and competence?

Adapt to the Limitations of Faith and Religion

Just as all other human beings, counselors and therapists live with limitations. Whether the category of human experience is time, energy, money, affection, information, empathy, dedication to a cause, or others, they adapt to the reality of limitations. As much as their dreams and aspirations may cause them to imagine immense and positive possibilities for themselves and their clients, they are limited. This is an ordinary human reality. More than a reality with which they must reckon, adaptation to this reality is rich with potential. Indeed, it is this adaptability that is associated with clinical effectiveness, according to several researchers (Martin & Turner, 2020, pp. 61–64). In this context, countless numbers of counselors and therapists find life-enhancing and life-sustaining meaning in their faith and religion. This potential can be and usually is affirmed by counselors and therapists, for themselves and for their clients.

Because of personal faith and religion and sometimes in spite of it, both mental health care providers and those who receive their care adapt to disturbing or otherwise compelling facts. Without mindlessly accommodating facts, such as parental abandonment, terminal illness of a spouse, accidental death of a young child, or whatever the specific tragedy is, pursuing life-affirming adaptations always arises as a desirable goal. Other courses of action, such as denial, substance abuse, attempts to avoid struggle, or other means of denying the facts and life itself, subordinate the best of what clients—or their therapists—can be. Similarly, therapists who promote therapy-denying approaches to therapy, including religious ones, frustrate the healthy expression of faith and religion. Worse, these therapists deny—or sometimes actively prevent—their client's growth toward health, not to mention that they deny their own growth, when they enact their religious views as therapy. Many such approaches are included in the list of therapies in the Appendix.

Along with others, counselors and therapists sometimes hold sincere faith in God and other aspects of their personal religion. And, in some cases, such faith takes the character of absolutism. Apart from life-denying absolutism, though, and regardless of the belief that God is almighty, omniscient, and much more, the fact is that faith also expresses the humanity of the believer. It is this fact that invites counselors and therapists to adapt to the limitations of faith and religion. At the core of faith and religion is a simple statement: I chose to believe. The decision-making of the believer expresses humanity, much more than it defines God, the purity of a holy book, or other commonly sanctified features of faith and religion. Thus, no matter how strong and meaningful their faith may be, counselors and therapists also reckon with the human limitations of living their lives and conducting therapy.

Affirm Highly Effective Therapists

The profession is perpetually and, maybe, forever unfinished. Instead of finishing its development, therapists often promote changes in it. A broad view of its current status and functioning shows clearly that the profession is not what it was, say, 30 years ago, let alone 100 years ago when it had achieved nascent momentum toward becoming a profession. Compared with most of its history, one of the current emphases is that, instead of a preoccupation with theoretical orientations or a cluster of techniques, it is trying to clarify what makes therapy work well by recognizing that individual therapists provide therapy, not theories or techniques. Thus, with increasing clarity, the profession continues to define who highly effective therapists are.

While a brief list of some of the important characteristics of highly effective therapists may be provided, the personal and professional reality of living these characteristics is far more complex than they may indicate. Adding to this complexity and as a feature of their clinical mastery, therapists must also seek to accommodate their clients' religion. This sometimes poses extraordinary demands on counselors and therapists, particularly those whose personal religious views stand in contrast or opposition to the religious views of their clients. Borrowing from the work of Martin and Turner (2020, pp. 61–64), the following discussion of the characteristics of highly effective therapists is intended to ease some of this demand. Drawn from multiple sources (e.g., Ablon & Jones, 1998; Blatt, Sanislow, Zuroff, & Pilkonis, 1996; Delgadillo et al., 2022; Eells, 1999; Fox, 2023; Goldfried, Raue, & Castonguay, 1998; Huhra, Yamokoski-Maynhart, & Prieto, 2008; Jennings & Skovholt, 1999; Lafferty, Beutler, & Crago, 1989; Liszewski, 2022; Martin & Turner, 2020; Owen et al., 2019; Skovholt & Jennings, 2004; Vaz & Sousa, 2021; and, Wampold & Owen, 2021), these characteristics include the following.

Proclivity for intellectual complexity

The importance of this quality may be understood as necessary for effective mental health care because clients are almost always immensely complex.

Or, to state the matter negatively, simple answers to complex human problems and linear thinking lack the cognitive assets that effective mental health care requires. At least, this characteristic of highly effective therapists facilitates the process of listening alertly to what clients say, but also hearing the meaning of what they say. Also, it helps counselors and therapists to engage with confounding, inherently contradictory, and disturbed relationships among clients such as couples, families, or groups. This calls for maintaining attunement to the frequently recognized, unspoken intentions and feelings that clients present and that they often have difficulty claiming and voicing.

The nature of religion is that it is complex. Obviously, religion may be expressed by innocent, young children whose knowledge of and presentation of their religion are understandably and predictably simple. However, it may also be expressed with intellectual muscularity, through such individuals as Jim Wallis—referred to earlier in this book—professional ministers, priests, mullahs, and rabbis, not to mention their intellectual leaders or historic figures such as Dietrich Bonhoeffer, Martin Luther King, Jr., or Augustine of Hippo. Thus, as a practical and clinical matter, a proclivity for intellectual complexity is a positive and necessary feature of highly effective therapists.

Indefatigable Curiosity

Likely, one of the signs of depleted curiosity among counselors and therapists appears in the form of a compulsion to advance an ideology. In the context of conducting counseling and therapy, the unfortunate outcome of such a compulsion is that clients become targets of the ideology. And, whether the ideology is a specifically clinical one or a specifically religious one, the potential for effective decision-making and clinical interventions is impaired. Additionally, a truism about conducting mental health care is that clients usually contain more clinically relevant information than clinicians seek from them. Thus, pursuing clinically relevant questions with clients is almost always superior to giving information or directions to clients. Such a pursuit calls for the authentic exercise of high curiosity. Well-exercised curiosity may solicit easy agreement until it is tested. Toward testing genuine curiosity, Maurer (no date) offers a challenging exercise.

> Let me propose a way for you to test your skills in this area. First, consider your position on a specific social issue and find someone who has the opposite opinion. Then, ask that person ten open-ended, non-judgmental questions designed so you can truly understand their point of view … the whole time giving them no indication whatsoever that you do not agree. You will know if you are succeeding if they are becoming

animated and verbal as they talk with you, a curious listener. If you find this task nearly impossible (and most people do), then you have your answer ... curiosity may be a challenge for you!

No doubt, clients present to their therapists a countless variety of thoughts and behaviors with which therapists disagree, or even vehemently reject. And, when therapists function well as therapists, including being curious, they provide services to those with whom they disagree, "giving them no indication whatsoever that you do not agree."

High Tolerance for Ambiguity

Human beings are highly ambiguous. In response to this, mental health care providers should expect and welcome ambiguity, instead of attempting to pose solutions that defy ambiguity. Most individuals feel stressed by ambiguity, particularly when it arises in a critically important situation such as when a loved person is terminally ill or when a client is imminently suicidal. In such familiar but daunting situations, counselors and therapists not only discover the limits of their tolerance of ambiguity but also develop their internal and external skills in demonstrating their increasing tolerance. Among many other sources of stimulation toward developing in this way, clients who present specifically religious problems—another complex layer of ambiguity—pose the demand for such development.

Emotional Attunement

Mental health care providers who demonstrate emotional attunement, with special emphasis on their internal coherence and authenticity, function with more effectiveness than those who are out of sync with their emotions. They feel their feelings with an acuity that allows them to utilize these feelings on behalf of their clients and themselves. Based on such internal awareness, therapists increase the likelihood of being accurately attuned to their clients' emotions. This is important when uncomfortable emotions are deeply felt. It is such emotions that evoke doubt about one's clinical prowess. Nevertheless, uncomfortable emotions usually hold the potential of being used on behalf of clients with whom such emotions arise. While the confirmatory research about accurate empathic awareness has been in place for decades, no doubt, therapists almost always recognize the truth of its importance in their effectiveness.

Strong Relational Skills

The degree to which experienced clinicians demonstrate strong relational skills is the degree to which they are effective mental health care providers.

Further, these skills protect the welfare of the clients whom they serve. Highly effective counselors and therapists recognize the importance of these skills and conscientiously seek to pursue their ongoing development. Many of these skills are discussed in detail in Martin & Turner, 2020, pp. 136–159).

Intentional and Sustained Self-Care

Studies confirm that intentional and sustained self-care is correlated with effectiveness in providing mental health care. While caring for oneself may be expressed in many different ways, these studies indicate that superior self-care pervades several basic aspects of human functioning, including nourishment, rest, recreation, scheduling, exercise, and others. Healthy and sustaining religion may be added to this list.

Important Relationships/Social Support

Effective therapists pursue ways to meet their relational needs. They find ways to care for others and to meet their need for care from others. Conversely, they are not usually loners or inclined to avoid others. And, they do not depend on their clients for relational support or most other relational needs.

As research continues to define who highly effective therapists are, a necessary and almost inevitable outcome of this is that theories, techniques, models, orientations, and approaches—by whatever title they may be known—become subordinated to individual counselors and therapists who possess the needed qualities for practicing highly effective therapy. This has real potential implications. For example, over time, it may mean that we have fewer and fewer discussions of and references to historically significant theoretical orientations, even individually preferred ones. It may mean that preparation programs give far more attention to individual-personal growth and development than to academic achievement. It may mean that discussions about the place of religion in counseling and therapy become somewhat less needed and relevant. It may mean that mental health care can restore its professionalism, including its providers' belief in the integrity of their profession. It may mean that individually and collectively, therapists can fulfill their promise to our clients to provide them with clinically effective services, carefully and predictably demonstrating clinical competence. No doubt, there are other implications from the emerging emphasis on highly effective therapists, not the least of which is that, when therapists can justifiably identify themselves as one of them, they like themselves better.

Trends That Matter

When questioning the relation of religion to counseling and therapy, the context matters. If the context is military combat, immersing in questioning is impractical and likely inappropriate. However, absent such extraordinary circumstances, the flow of history creates a context that must be taken into account. Currently, one of the visible trends in counseling and therapy has been the steadily rising visibility and utilization of tactical orientations to therapy. While each of them may have theoretical flavors, practicality is their essential character. Among many, they include Compassion Focused Therapy, Parent-Child Interaction Therapy, Emotion Focused Therapy, Solution-Focused Therapy, and Trauma-Focused Cognitive Behavioral Therapy. In addition to these somewhat broadly scoped approaches to therapy, others, are tactical, including various mindfulness-oriented techniques, contemplative therapy, and anti-anxiety relaxation techniques. Along with other developments, this one helps to contextualize the place of religion in the practice of counseling and therapy as a clinical issue.

Another set of trends involves neuroscience. Some of the practical expressions of this kind of approach to counseling and therapy include Brainspotting and Eye Movement Desensitization and Reprocessing. These are familiar approaches that utilize neuroscience, but the range of possible interventions is much broader than this. For example, Duenyan and Luke (2019) discuss some of them in their article, "Neuroscience for Counselors: Recommendations for Developing and Teaching a Graduate Course." Similarly, in their prescient composition, Ivey, Ivey, Zalaquett, and Quirk (2009) nicely forecast the importance of neuroscience in the practice of counseling and therapy, from their view of it in 2009. Along with many others, including Presti (2015, 2018), these authors confirm a trend that has likely moved from a trend in counseling and therapy to an established orientation. Goss (2016) reports about neuroscience in counseling and therapy, as if it is, indeed, an established orientation.

Another trend takes counseling and therapy toward complex and demanding challenges. It is the expanding lack of access to mental health care. Numerous reports conclude that the lack of access to mental health care services perpetuates a crisis (e.g., American Association of Medical Colleges, 2023; National Council for Mental Well-being, 2023; National Alliance on Mental Illness, 2023). The lack of access to counseling and therapy, along with other critically important demands for competent services, exposes weakness in current delivery potential and threats from it.

Additional trends in the practice of counseling and therapy could easily be included here, but the significance of these trends is not so much that the list of them is complete but that important changes in professional practice continue to evolve and, by virtue of their research-based quality and clinical efficacy, invite, if not required, practicing counselors and therapists to integrate them into their clinical work.

References

Ablon, J. S., & Jones, E. E. (1998). How expert clinicians' prototypes of an ideal treatment correlate with outcomes in psychodynamic and cognitive-behavioral therapy. *Psychotherapy Research*, *8*, 71–83. 10.1093/ptr/8.1.7

American Counseling Association. (2014). 2014 Code of Ethics. https://www.counseling.org/resources/aca-code-of-ethics.pdf

American Association of Medical Colleges. (2023). Exploring barriers to mental health care in The U.S. https://www.aamc.org/advocacy-policy/aamc-research-and-action-institute/barriers-mental-health-care

Barlow, I., & Brown, R. J. (2020). A systematic review of measures of therapist competence in psychodynamic, interpersonal, and/or relational models. *Psychology and Psychotherapy: Theory, Research, and Practice*, *93*, 408–427.

Barnett, J. E., & Johnson, W. B. (2011, March). Integrating spirituality and religion into psychotherapy: Persistent dilemmas, ethical Issues, and a proposed decision-making process. *Ethics and Behavior*, *21*(2), 147–164. 10.1080/10508422.2011.551471

Bartholomew, T. T., Kang, E., Joy, E. E., Robbins, K. A., & Maldonado-Aguiñiga, S. (2022). Clients' perceptions of the working alliance as a predictor of increases in positive affect. *Journal of Psychotherapy Integration*, *32*(3), 310–325. 10.1037/int0000265

Bedia, R. P., & Duff, C. T. (2014). Client as expert: A Delphi poll of clients' subjective experience of therapeutic alliance formation variables. *Counselling Psychology Quarterly*, *27*(1), 1–18. 10.1080/09515070.2013.857295

Bidell, M. P. (2014). Personal and professional discord: Examining religious conservatism and lesbian-, gay-, and bisexual-affirmative counselor competence. *Journal of Counseling and Development*, *92*, 170–179.

Bilgrave, D. P., & Deluty, R. H. (2002). Religious beliefs and political ideologies as predictors of psychotherapeutic orientations of clinical and counseling psychologists. *Psychotherapy: Theory/Research/Practice/Training*, *39*(3), 245–260.

Blatt, S. J., Sanislow, C. A., Zuroff, D. C., & Pilkonis, P. A. (1996). Characteristics of effective therapists: Further analyses of data from the National Institute of Mental Health Treatment of Depression Collaborative Research Program. *Journal of Consulting and Clinical Psychology*, *64*(6), 1276–1284.

Campbell, T. H., & Kay, A. C. (2014). Solution aversion: On the relation between ideology and motivated disbelief. *Journal of Personality and Social Psychology*, *107*, 809–824.

Carere-Comes, T. (2015). Process-driven psychotherapy does not need empirical research. *Journal of Psychotherapy Research*, *25*(4), 346–352.

Choma, B. L., Hanoch, Y., Gummerum, M., & Hodson, G. (2013). Relations between risk perceptions and socio-political ideology are domain- and ideology-dependent. *Personality and Individual Differences*, *54*, 29–34.

Cirasola, A., Midgley, N., Fonagy, P., IMPACT Consortium, & Martin, P. (2022). The therapeutic alliance in psychotherapy for adolescent depression: Differences between treatment types and change over time. *Journal of Psychotherapy Integration*, *32*(3), 326–341. 10.1037/int0000264

Constantino, M. J., Boswell, J. F., Coyne, A. E., Muir, H. H., Gaines, A. N., & Kraus, D. R. (2023). Therapist perceptions of their own measurement-based, problem-specific effectiveness. *Journal of Consulting and Clinical Psychology*, *91*(8), 474–484. 10.1037/ccp0000813

Corey, G. (n.d.). Integrating spirituality in counseling practice. VISTAS Online. https://www.counseling.org/docs/default-source/vistas/integrating-spirituality-in-counseling-practice.pdf?sfvrsn=7ddd7e2c_10

Counselor. (2022). [no title]. https://www.psychologytoday.com/us/therapists/wendy-leann-centralia-il/455506

Crowe, C., Collie, C., Johnson, C., & Wiltsey, S. S. (2020). An intervention mapping process to increase evidence-based psychotherapy within a complex healthcare system. *American Psychologist*, *75*(8), 1116–1129.

Delgadillo, J., Deisenhofer, A.-K., Probst, T., Shimokawa, K., Lambert, M. J., & Kleinstäuber, M. (2022). Progress feedback narrows the gap between more and less effective therapists: A therapist effects meta-analysis of clinical trials. *Journal of Consulting and Clinical Psychology*, *90*(7), 559–567. 10.1037/ccp0000747

Duenyan, D. L., & Luke, C. (2019). Neuroscience for counselors: Recommendations for developing and teaching a graduate course. *The Professional Counselor*, *9*(4), 369–380. https://tpcjournal.nbcc.org/neuroscience-for-counselors-recommendations-for-developing-and-teaching-a-graduate-course/

Dowd, E. T., & Nielson, S. L. (Eds). (2006). *The psychologies in religion: Working with the religious client.* New York: Springer.

Dozios, D. J. A. (2013). Psychological treatments: Putting evidence into practice and practice into evidence. *Canadian Psychology/Psychologie Canadienne*, *54*(1), 1–11.

Dufort, V. M., Bernardy, N., Maguen, S., Hoyt, J. E., Litt, E. R., Patterson, O. V., Leonard, C. E., & Shiner, B. (2021). Geographic variation in initiation of evidence-based psychotherapy among veterans with PTSD. *Military Medicine*, *186*(9-10), e858–e866. 10.1093/milmed/usaa389

Eells, T. D. (1999). What do we know about master therapists? *Journal of Psychotherapy Practice Research*, *8*, 314–317.

Ellis, A. (1985). *The Case Against Religion: A Psychotherapist's View and the Case Against Religiosity.* Cranford, NJ: American Atheist Press.

Fox, S. (2023). Therapist perceptions on factors differentiating the most from least effective therapists. [Doctoral dissertation]. Indiana University of Pennsylvania.

Goldberg, S. B., Miller, S. D., Nielsen, S. L., Rousmaniere, T., Whipple, J., Hoyt, W. T., & Wampold, B. E. (2016). Do psychotherapists improve with time and experience? A longitudinal analysis of outcomes in a clinical setting. *Journal of Counseling Psychology*, *63*(1), 1–11.

Goldfried, M. R., Raue, P. J., & Castonguay, L. G. (1998). The therapeutic focus in significant sessions of master therapists: A comparison of cognitive-behavioral and psychodynamic-interpersonal interventions. *Journal of Consulting and Clinical Psychology*, *66*, 803–810.

Goss, D. (2016). Integrating neuroscience into counseling psychology: A systematic review of current literature. *The Counseling Psychologist*, *44*(6), 895–920.

Greenberg, M. J., Pievsky, M. A., & McGrath, R. E. (2015). Navigation of ethical conflicts among religious psychotherapists treating lesbian and gay patients. *Spirituality in Clinical Practice*, *2*(2), 134–144.

Haavind, H. (2003). Pro-feminist and non-psychoanalytic and other pros and cons of psychotherapy. *European Journal of Psychotherapy, Counselling & Health*, *6*(1), 35–50.

Halasz, G. (2004). In conversation with Albert Ellis. *Australian Psychiatry*, *121*(4), 325–333.

Hansen, J. (2007). Should counseling be considered a health care profession? Critical thoughts on the transition to a health care ideology. *Journal of Counseling and Development*, *85*, 286–293.

Hodson, G. (2014). Ideology matters (Too much): Does super-sizing ideology make ideology a risk to society? Psychology Today. https://www.psychologytoday.com/us/blog/without-prejudice/201511/ideology-matters-too-much

Huhra, R. L., Yamokoski-Maynhart, C. A., & Prieto, L. R. (2008). Reviewing videotapes in supervision: A developmental approach. *Journal of Counseling and Development*, *86*(4), 412–418.

Ivey, A. E., Ivey, M. B., Zalaquett, C., & Quirk, K. (2009). Counseling and neuroscience: The cutting edge of the coming decade. Counseling Today. https://ct.counseling.org/2009/12/reader-viewpoint-counseling-and-neuroscience-the-cutting-edge-of-the-coming-decade/

Ivey, A. E., Ivey, M. B., & Zalaquett, C. P. (2022). *Intentional interviewing and counseling: Facilitating client development in a multicultural society* (10th ed.). Belmont, CA: Cengage.

Jennings, L., & Skovholt, T. M. (1999). The cognitive, emotional, and relational characteristics of master therapists. *Journal of Counseling Psychology*, *46*, 3–11.

Keng, S-L., Waddington, E., Lin, X. B., Tan, M. S. Q., Henn-Haase, C., & Kanter, J. W. (2017). Effects of functional analytic psychotherapy therapist training on therapist factors among therapist trainees in Singapore: A randomized controlled trial. *Clinical Psychology and Psychotherapy*, *24*, 1014–1027.

Lafferty, P., Beutler, L. E., & Crago, M. (1989). Differences between more and less effective psychotherapists: A study of select therapist variables. *Journal of Consulting and Clinical Psychology*, *57*(1), 76–80.

LaMarre, A., Smoliak, O., Cool, C., Kinavey, H., & Hardt, L. (2019). The normal, improving, and productive self: Unpacking neoliberal governmentality in therapeutic interactions. *Journal of Constructivist Psychology*, *32*(3), 236–253.

Liszewski, K. (2022). The qualities and characteristics that distinguish most effective therapists: A survey of clinical supervisors and directors. [Doctoral dissertation, Indiana University of Pennsylvania]. http://gateway.proquest.com/openurl?url_ver=Z39.88-2004&rft_val_fmt=info:ofi/fmt:kev:mtx:dissertation&res_dat=xri:pqm&rft_dat=xri:pqdiss:28860875

Lokhorst, S. L., & Reich, C. M. (2022). The alliance-outcome correlation: Is there a halo effect? *Journal of Psychotherapy Integration*, *32*(3), 301–309. ISSN: 1573-3696. 10.1037/int0000285

Lyon, A. R., Stanick, C., & Pullman, M. D. (2018). Toward high-fidelity treatment as usual: Evidence-based intervention structures to improve usual care psychotherapy. *Clinical Psychology: Science and Practice*. 25:e12265. Pp.1–15.

Martin, F. A., & Turner, J. P. (2020). *Clinical supervision in the real world: A practical guide to ethics, legal issues, and personal development*. New York: Routledge.

Maurer, R. J. (2017). The power of curiosity. Psychology Today. https://www.psychologytoday.com/us/blog/the-traits-excellence/201704/the-power-curiosity

McGeorge, C. R., Carlson, T. S., & Toomey, R. B. (2015). An exploration of family therapists' beliefs about the ethics of conversion therapy: The influence of negative beliefs and clinical competence with lesbian, gay, and bisexual clients. *Journal of Marital and Family Therapy*, *41*(1) 42–56.

Michaels, T. M., & Datta, V. (2016). Evidence, not ideology, should guide the use of psychotherapy. *The British Journal of Psychiatry: The Journal of Mental Science*, *209*(2), 171.

National Alliance on Mental Illness. (2023). The doctor is out. https://www.nami.org/Support-Education/Publications-Reports/Public-Policy-Reports/The-Doctor-is-Out

National Association of Social Workers. (2023). Code of ethics. https://www.socialworkers.org/About/Ethics/Code-of-Ethics/Code-of-Ethics-English/Social-Workers-Ethical-Responsibilities-to-Clients

National Council for Mental Well-being. (2023). Study reveals lack of access as root cause for mental health crisis in America. https://www.thenationalcouncil.org/news/lack-of-access-root-cause-mental-health-crisis-in-america/

Noble, A., & Rizq, R. (2019). "It's led me astray": How cognitive behavioral therapists experience personal therapy in clinical practice. *Counseling and Psychotherapy Research*, *20*, 29–38.

Owen, J., Kivlighan III, M., Kopta, M., Drinane, J. M., Miller, S., & Imel, Z. (2019). Are high-performing therapists both effective and consistent? A test of therapist expertise. *Journal of Consulting and Clinical Psychology*, *87*(12), 1149–1156. 10.1037/ccp0000437

Parker, I. (2014). Psychotherapy under capitalism: The production, circulation and management of value and subjectivity. *Psychotherapy and Politics International*, *12*(3), 166–175.

Presti, D. (2015). *The foundational concepts in neuroscience: A brain-mind odyssey*. New York: W. W. Norton.

Presti, D. (2018). *Mind beyond brain*. New York: Columbia University Press.

Silander, N. C., Geczy Jr., B., Marks, O. & Mather, R. D. (2020). Implications of ideological bias in social psychology on clinical practice. *Clinical Psychology: Science and Practice*, *27*, 1–14.

Skovholt, T. M., & Jennings, L. (2004). *Master therapists: Exploring expertise in therapy and counseling*. Boston, MA: Allyn and Bacon.

Spengler, P. M., White, M. J., Ægisdóttir, S., Maugherman, A. S., Anderson, L. A., Cook, R. S., & Rush, J. D. (2009). The meta-analysis of clinical judgment project: Effects of experience on judgment accuracy. *The Counseling Psychologist*, *37*(3), 350–399.

Spengler, P. M., & Pilipis, L. A. (2015) A comprehensive meta-reanalysis of the robustness of the experience-accuracy effect in clinical judgment. *Journal of Counseling Psychology, 62*(3), 360–378. 10.1037/cou0000065

Swift, J. K., Callahan, J. L., Cooper, M., & Parkin, S. R. (2018). The impact of accommodating client preference in psychotherapy: A meta-analysis. *Journal of Clinical Psychology, 74*, 1924–1937.

Trusty, W. T., Swift, J. K., Black, S. W., Dimmick, A. A., & Penix, E. A. (2021) Religious microaggressions in psychotherapy: A mixed methods examination of client perspectives. *Psychotherapy, 59*(3), pp. 351–362. doi: 10.1037/pst0000408

Vannatta, R., & Steen, S. (2019) Pedagogical practices in CACREP accredited group counseling courses: A content analysis. *The Journal for Specialists in Group Work, 44*(2), 138–150. 10.1080/01933922.2019.1599477

Vaz, A., & Sousa, D. (2021). Persuasiveness: An underappreciated characteristic of effective therapists. *Psychology of Consciousness: Theory, Research, and Practice.* 1–16. Advance Online Publication, November 2021. 10.1037/cns0000309

Walfish, S., McAllister, B., O'Donnell, P. & Lambert, M. J. (2012). An investigation of self-assessment bias in mental health providers. *Psychological Reports, 110*(2), 639–644.

Wampold, B. E., & Owen, J. (2021). Therapist effects: History, methods, magnitude, and characteristics of effective therapists. In M. Barkham, W. Lutz, & L. G. Castonguay (Eds.), *Bergin and Garfield's handbook of psychotherapy and behavior change: 50th anniversary edition* (pp. 297–326). New York: John Wiley & Sons.

Yaden, D. B., & Newberg, A. B. (2022). *The varieties of spiritual experience: 21st Century research and perspective.* New York: Oxford University Press.

7 Clients' Religion in Therapy

Countless individuals, families, and communities experience their religion as desirable and good. They find that their experience of religion brings them closer to those whom they love, offers assurance about their understanding of life, provides a community in which they experience belonging, opens doors of opportunity for service to others, and much more. In short, their experience of religion is mentally and emotionally healthy. And, with regard to counseling and therapy, these are the ones who seldom present their religion in therapy as a source of pain or struggle.

Healthy religion poses little or no challenge for counselors and therapists. Unless they are members of such a religion, they may seldom, if ever, see it. It is the absence of healthy religion that may skew their view of religion, just as any clinical population may evoke in counselors and therapists a jaundiced view of others. At least, recognizing this may offer modest reassurance for practicing counselors and therapists. As noted already in the previous chapter, practicing counselors and therapists should acknowledge their limitations and, while maintaining their internal credibility and integrity, provide services within the boundaries of their competence, just as professional ethics and standards prescribe. To state this view in another way, the fact is that individual counselors and therapists cannot and should not claim expertise in all or nearly all areas of work in their profession. A therapist who specializes in treating clients who suffer with eating disorders may not hold much expertise in treating over-anxious young children or elderly persons who are terminally ill, for example. And, none of these areas of expertise necessarily relate to providing treatment that requires expertise in religion or religion-related problems that clients bring to therapy.

No doubt, counselors and therapists, along with numerous others, have reasons to be skeptical of religion and religious experience. With little or no effort, they can refer to The People's Temple, David Koresh, Hale-Bop Comet, the conspicuous politicization of religion in recent years, religious justifications for racist, homophobic—even harmfully aggressive—attitudes,

DOI: 10.4324/9781003472469-8

and so on, not to mention what they see in clinical consultations with their clients or their personal experience of religion. However, just as they understandably have reasons for being skeptical of many personal and family behaviors, such as parenting, marriages, misuse of substances, and so on, but accept clients who reveal their problems in these areas of life, they owe to their clients a commitment to suspend such skepticism with regard to clients' religion.

More than suspending skepticism, counselors and therapists either accept the religious experience of their clients and demonstrate a clinically appropriate level of empathic awareness or they decline to treat such clients. This is what professionally accountable counselors and therapists do with clients, while clearly also refusing to endorse unhealthy attitudes and behaviors. For example, a therapist can be accepting, empathic, and encouraging of parents whose parenting is demonstrably deficient, even when such parenting is rationalized with specifically religious ideation. Such an approach does not require approval of deficient parenting or the parents' rationalizations. At the core of this kind of thinking about clients' religion is the expectation that counselors and therapists will show respect for clients and their religion. Writing from an apparently Christian and conservative outlook, Shaler (2019) nicely and competently frames an appeal for counselors and therapists to respect the religion of both clients and their peers. She reflects on therapists' common temptation to be skeptical of their clients' religious beliefs. Also, she includes specific recommendations for expressing such respect, the first one of which is this:

> Listen: As the saying goes, listen to hear rather than to respond. If your first instinct is to prepare a rebuttal, that is a clear indication that you need to take a step back. Understand first, respond second. This is true not only in the counseling room with our clients, but also in communication with our fellow counselors. We should be willing to hear from those who are not like us without making assumptions or jumping to conclusions. (Shaler, 2019)

This chapter gives attention to three topics related to clients' religion in therapy. The first is "The Conversation about Religion in Therapy." This is a brief presentation of several research reports about clients' religion in therapy. The second is "Anticipating Treatment of Clients with Religious Concerns." This is a discussion of some of the major models of ways to integrate clients' religion into the process of therapy. And, the third is "Clients' Presentation of Religion-related Issues." This is a brief account of 18 specifically religion-related problems that clients bring to therapy.

The Conversation about Religion in Therapy

Respecting clients' religion may come somewhat easily for counselors and therapists. A larger challenge than showing respect is integrating clients' experience into the process of providing services. As a foundation for achieving clinically relevant integration of clients' religion into the process of helping them, counselors and therapists should gather information that may help to inform them about the possibilities for such integration. In this discussion, some of this information will be provided in brief annotations of ten selected articles. The articles are intended to suggest, at least, that there is a vigorous intellectual, research-based, and clinically relevant conversation about religion in counseling and therapy. The discussion also reveals how very complex religion in therapy is. For ease of tracking, the articles are numbered.

One: Captari et al. (2018) through a comprehensive meta-analysis, aimed to analyze 97 outcomes studies and offer direction for integrating clients' religion and spirituality into psychotherapy. Pursuing this daunting task, Captari and her associates reached several conclusions about how therapists can understand clients' religion and spirituality and integrate them into therapy. The details of their analysis add professional muscularity to their conclusions; this discussion includes only their conclusions (Captari et al., 2018, pp. 1949–1950).

> Treat religion and spirituality as a potentially important aspect of the client's identity. Express curiosity about each client's lived experience. Explore R/S [religious/spiritual] history, values, and commitment as part of the intake process, and consider intersectionality with other dimensions of diversity.
>
> Incorporate a patient's R/S values and worldview in psychotherapy as requested and when clinically indicated. Research shows that accommodative psychotherapies are at least as effective as secular approaches in reducing psychological symptoms, and can be provided by therapists regardless of their personal R/S background.
>
> Consider R/S adaptations in psychotherapy for their unique benefits to clients' spiritual lives, including greater spiritual well-being and increased connection with the sacred. When a client's treatment goals include not only symptom remission, but also spiritual development, integration of R/S within psychotherapy is a treatment of choice.
>
> Tailor treatment especially when working with patients whose R/S is an influential force in their day-to-day life. Preliminary findings suggest that accommodative psychotherapies may result in the greatest symptom reduction among clients with a high level of R/S commitment.
>
> Follow the client's lead when incorporating R/S beliefs and practices into psychotherapy. Avoid making assumptions based on

religious identification, and instead, explore their unique desires, needs, and expectations.

Practice respect and cultural humility when discussing patients' religious worldviews and practices. Be especially sensitive to one's own potential biases about organized religion and to clients' experiences of the sacred.

Two: Coburn and McGeorge (2019) asked a simple question, "What do Christian Clergy Say?" and discussed "Advice from Christian Pastors to Family Therapists about Working with LGB Clients.' They address a common "test" issue for those who seek to relate religion with homonormative sexual identities and behaviors. In their qualitative study, they interviewed 21 Christian pastors whose organizational affiliations include several mainline Christian denominations. Among their observations, they report, "These pastors clearly articulated that identifying as LGB and Christian is not only possible but supported in some Christian faith traditions and religious communities" (p. 242). This view from pastors in this study expanded into positions that likely offer comfort to LGBTQ+ individuals. Specifically, the pastors "highlighted the importance of religious communities engaging in active challenging of traditional heteronormative assumptions that would contribute to the exclusion of those with marginalized sexual orientations" (p. 242). The authors add, "These pastors also expressed a belief that religious faith and involvement in religious communities can be beneficial to LGB individuals, relationships, and families" (p. 242). Further, Coburn and McGeorge offer clinical implications of their study. "First, participants suggested that it is important that family therapists explore their own religious and spiritual beliefs about LGB individuals, relationships, and families" (p. 243). The second clinical implication "focuses on the need for family therapists to receive more training on how to appropriately utilize the spiritual and religious beliefs of their clients in order to support therapeutic change" (p. 243).

Finally, the last clinical implication "... is that family therapists could enhance their practices and better serve their LGB clients by actively enlisting religious leaders within their communities as a support network" (p. 244). Toward developing such a network, the clergy in this study emphasized that "family therapists can offer added assistance, through the help of clergy, to clients who have questions about spiritual issues or the teachings of their faith community" (p. 244).

Also, in their attempt to offer practical help, Coburn and McGeorge (2019) provide an excellent set of questions for self-reflection about the issues that they address. The set is too large for inclusion here. Suffice it to include only two of their reflection questions. One, "What types of people do I believe are involved in religious or spiritual communities? Who do I expect to see in churches? What experiences have I had that led me to hold these beliefs?" (p. 244). Two, "If applicable, what did my religious or spiritual community(ies) teach me about marginalized sexual orientations and LGB relationships? If my religious or spiritual community did not talk about LGB identities and relationships, what did that silence communicate?" (p. 244).

Three: Paine, Sandage, Ruffing, and Hill (2018) titled their publication, "Religious and Spiritual Salience, Well-Being, and Psychosocial Functioning Among Psychotherapy Clients: Moderator Effects for Humility'. Paine and his colleagues sought to "investigate dispositional humility as a potential moderator in the relationship between religious and spiritual salience and (1) well-being and (2) psychosocial functioning outcomes in a clinical sample" (p. 2398). What is the relevance of dispositional humility—a commonly identified virtue among religious and spiritual devotees—and social functioning, life functioning, and well-being? Following apparently sound research protocols, the authors' answer to this question is relatively simple. One, their hypothesis "of a positive association between religious and spiritual salience and psychosocial functioning" was supported (p. 2409). Moreover, "Those whose religious beliefs are important to them seem to exhibit fewer problems in well-being and life functioning than their counterparts. This finding supplements the growing body of evidence for a positive correlation between religion and spirituality and adaptive psychological outcomes" (p. 2409). From their data, the authors also conclude that "persons lacking humility may find it difficult to draw on religious and spiritual resources for support in times of struggle. In fact, religion and its associated moral precepts may be a source of distress for those lacking in humility" (p. 2409).

Four: In his article, Friedson (2015) addressed a challenge that has confronted countless therapists: "Psychotherapy and the Fundamentalist Client: The Aims and Challenges of Treating Jehovah's Witnesses." Apparently, Friedson has developed a comprehensive, compassionate, and empathic understanding of fundamentalist clients. Associated with the Derner Institute of Advanced Psychological Studies at Adelphi University, Friedson has successfully attempted to bring readers, particularly mental health clinicians, into this understanding. As noted, "This paper focuses specifically on the issues that may arise in the psychotherapeutic treatment of Jehovah's Witnesses" (p. 693). Allowing for the disparate ideologies of Jehovah's Witnesses and much of psychotherapeutic thinking, Friedson skillfully discusses transference and countertransference issues that may arise when therapy includes these ideologies. For counselors and therapists who find themselves in such clinical situations, the cautions and encouragements in this article can easily become a valuable resource for providing services for Jehovah's Witnesses, along with other individuals from fundamentalist communities, and individuals who come from non-religious, authoritarian families and communities, too. Friedson concludes, "There is clearly a need for culturally sensitive psychotherapeutic interventions for former and current Jehovah's Witnesses and other fundamentalist populations who are experiencing psychological distress" (p. 711). As a resource for practicing counselors and therapists, this article can be a practical guide for those who treat clients to whom Friedson gives attention and, based on this guidance, treat them with increased effectiveness.

Five: Cragun and Frielander (2012) investigated "Experiences of Christian Clients in Secular Psychotherapy: A Mixed-Methods Investigation." The small sample of Christians, an acknowledged limitation, who received secular psychotherapy makes Cragun and Frielander's report somewhat difficult to generalize. However, their careful study of the population provides insights and practices that many mental health clinicians will find helpful. Their primary findings indicate that clients for whom religion is important felt hesitant to discuss their religion, but that they experienced their therapists as open to such discussions. At odds with this view, "Dissatisfied clients reported that their therapists expressed opposing religious views or avoided discussing religious or spiritual issues" (p. 379).

The generalizations in this article are informatively augmented with narratives from interviews with the subjects in this research. The narratives give a level of livingness to the report that discloses the rich and detailed thinking of individuals who identify as Christian and who seek therapy from non-Christian therapists. For example, a "participant, who told her therapist directly that talking about her faith would be important, reported that the therapist often did not understand her religious beliefs but asked about them respectfully:"

> She treaded very gently. She did what most therapists do—which is, you know, let the patient do the talking and let the patient teach you. She would ask me questions like … I believe in speaking in tongues, and at one point it came up, I don't know how, and I told her what that means. And one thing that came up over and over again was going up to the altar at church and praying. And she didn't understand that at all, so I had to break it down for her and tell her why that was important and why that was emotional for me. (p. 385)

The lesson from Cragun and Frielander appears to be that, when Christians seek help from secular therapists, therapists who welcome them as they would other clients show respect for clients' religious experience, seek to understand the personal relevance of clients' religious experience, and, therefore, relate with clients in a manner that is clinically helpful, the therapeutic alliance more likely becomes effective. Or, because clients seek needed help, some Christians "intentionally seek out secular therapists because they prefer a less biased perspective and want to control how much to incorporate their faith into treatment" (p. 388).

Six: Trusty, Swift, Black, Dimmick, and Penix (2021, November 22) likely raise apprehension among counselors and therapists, as they report about "Religious Microaggressions in Psychotherapy: A Mixed Methods Examination of Client Perspectives." In response to the thought of religious microaggressions, therapists may understandably wonder, "Are religious microaggressions really committed by counselors and therapists?" Albeit sophisticated research, the insightful and practical answer from Trusty et al. is clearly "Yes." More than a simple "yes," though, their work aptly and ably describes several microaggressions committed by counselors and therapists. A review of the microaggressions should alert counselors and therapists to their potential for imposing them on their clients.

At 35.6%, "the most commonly reported category of religious microaggressions was avoiding religion in sessions" (p. 7). When clients wish to discuss a matter of importance to them and their therapist refuses or avoids such discussions, the therapeutic alliance is weakened. For example, a client affiliated with The Church of Jesus Christ of Latter-Day Saints (LDS) stated,

> I brought up my religion and how I was struggling with some questions about my life and how I felt alone and that God was not listening to me. My counselor just avoided talking about religion and told me that it's normal and okay to feel lost and confused at this time in my life and that I should focus on the things I do know and that matter to me. (p. 8)

If related to other features of a client's presentation how may this microaggression be understood? What may be the impact on the therapeutic alliance, if a therapist avoids depression, anger, sex, emotional intensity, or other uncomfortable and/or unpleasant features of a client's presentation?

"The second most common type of microaggressions was related to therapists making stereotypical comments about clients based on their religion … . This included verbalizing assumptions about clients' beliefs, practices, struggles, or abilities based on their religious identity" (p. 8).

The third category of concern involved therapists who indicated that "clients' religious beliefs were harmful" and expressed "disapproval of clients' beliefs" (p. 8). For example, a Jewish client shared: "In the first session, [my therapist] asked if I was religious. When I said that I am Jewish, her attitude completely changed. She just had a rude look on her face and she was much shorter with me when I was speaking … . She kept mentioning that we need to have short sessions because I'm a "'penny pincher'" (p. 8).

Other microaggressions included: "Therapists offering suggestions or discussing topics that clients felt were unhelpful or uncomfortable because of their religion" (p. 8); "therapists pressuring clients to live in line with their religion or to become more religious" (p. 8); "therapists incorporating their own religion, rather than the client's, into therapy" (p. 9); and, "therapists displaying a lack of knowledge or competence in addressing religious issues in therapy" (p. 9). According to Trusty et al., approximately 39% of clients in this study experienced microaggressions from their therapists (p. 9). They conclude that the marginalization of clients whose religion is important to them aligns the clients' experience with the experience of other marginalized clients such as racial minorities and sexual minorities.

Probably, an important takeaway from Trusty et al. is the necessary question, "Toward which clients am I likely to commit microaggressions?" Are they religious clients? Are they a different gender or sexual orientation? Are they a different race? Economic class? Height? Substance abusers? Attitude? Age?

Seven: Sunderania and Moodley (2020) explore "Therapists' perceptions of their use of self-disclosure (and nondisclosure) during cross-cultural exchanges." Among other cross-cultural factors that Sunderania and Moodley include in their research, religion emerges as an important one. They place these cross-cultural factors in the context of identifying therapists' judgment about self-disclosure and non-disclosure of their personal experience and points of view about these factors. They assess that the decision about disclosing or not "can become a complex and confounding process" that involves processes that are both conscious and unconscious, and that the major issues of disclosure do not occur "in the context of the Big 7 (race, gender, class, sexual orientation, disability, age and religion)" (Sunderania & Moodley, 2020, p. 751). While the research itself poses considerable challenges for those who conduct it and for those who wish to benefit from it, Sunderania and Moodley deliver specific implications of their research that ease the complexity and confounding nature of such challenging tasks and relief for those who wish to benefit from their research. Their implications are:

> Practitioners can strive to be mindful of whether what they reveal about themselves positively impacts the client or that it may also elicit and/or trigger a negative internal experience within the client.
>
> Practitioners [should] be cognizant of the nonverbal channels through which personal information is communicated (e.g., wearing a wedding ring, family photographs, office décor).

> Practitioners may develop a greater awareness of how their accent, skin color, can communicate cultural information about themselves to the client (also see Litjmaer et al., 2013).
>
> Practitioners may recognize that clients will enter the counselling room with pre-existing ideas about the therapist because of the limited amount of personal information they have to go on (e.g., from a professional website, name of therapist on a business card), thereby potentially stirring up culturally-based projections and culturally-based transference reactions.
>
> Practitioners may also be aware of the ways in which clients' cultural transference reactions could stimulate their own cultural-countertransference counter reaction.
>
> Practitioners can also be aware that hesitations to disclose, albeit a prudent choice, stifle excellence and creativity within their work with their clients. (p. 753)

Eight: In his report, Kizilhan (2014) offers compelling reasons for giving it serious attention. In his report, "Religious and cultural aspects of psychotherapy in Muslim patients from tradition-oriented societies," Kizilhan offers compelling reasons for giving it serious consideration. Quite possibly, the reasons for studying this article are the same reasons for thinking about avoiding it. This is to say that, for those whose consciousness of their world usually excludes Muslim clients, this article may be viewed as a necessity for study, after it has been read. Kizilhan has gathered evidence, to be sure, but has also effectively communicated layers of subtlety about understanding and relating with clients whose culture, with emphasis on their religion, is different from the culture of the therapist. The careful articulation of concepts of psychotherapy, Muslim belief and cultural expressions, and case studies make Kizilhan's work important, recognizing that briefly reporting the insightful subtleties inherent in the issues is truly difficult. Nevertheless, perhaps, a question for those who read this book will encourage them to learn more about their assumptions about how their own culture works and possibly locate Kazilhan's article to help with this. Thus, what may be the meaning of this: "A 58 year-old man from Turkey first noticed the influence of black magic in 1980 when he discovered a pile of soil at the entrance to his flat" (p. 338). Apparently, Muslim clients know what this may mean. Similarly, during the initial stages of treatment, are Muslim clients more or less likely to place an emphasis on the body or the soul? Kizilhan expertly addresses this matter.

Nine: Oxhandler and Parrish (2017) may provoke consternation among therapists, as they report their evidence in their article, "Integrating clients' religion/spirituality in clinical practice: A comparison among social workers, psychologists, counselors, marriage and family therapists, and nurses.' This research article emerged from Oxhandler and Parrish's survey of 550 therapists, using the Religious/Spiritually Integrated Practice Assessment Scale and background questions. As they indicate, "The purpose of the current study is to better understand how five helping professions, who often work together to alleviate mental and behavioral health issues, assess and address this area of clients' lives in clinical practice" (p. 684).

In their discussion of their findings, Oxhandler and Parrish state, "This study resulted in several noteworthy observations. Within our sample, LMFTs [Licensed Marriage and Family Therapists] are the most confident and perceive the least number of barriers with regard to integrating clients' RS [religion/spirituality] in practice" (p. 688). Their discussion does not indicate an awareness of the fact that LMFTs are more likely to have completed their training in religion-oriented programs than the other types of licensees in this study. However, allowing for this, they also state, "All five professions held very positive attitudes toward all aspects of integrating RS" (p. 688) into counseling and therapy. While this observation appears to be encouraging, with regard to mental health care professional's attitudes toward religion and spirituality in counseling and therapy, there are differences among the five types, too. As Oxhandler and Parrish write, "The behavior items involving assessment and engagement with clients on integrating of RS into practice were more encouraging for LCSWs, LPCs, and LMFTs" (p. 689) and less encouraging for psychologists. "Given that that many of the empirically supported interventions have emerged from psychology, it was interesting that psychologists reported the lowest frequency of using such interventions" (p. 690). "However, it is concerning that less than half of all licensed professions are conducting a biopsychosocial-spiritual assessment" (p. 690). This article helps counselors and therapists to gain awareness of both their professional assets and, as the authors suggest, aspects of their work that need attention.

Ten: Harris, Sisemore, Pargament, and Brown (2014) offer largely affirmative insights about religion in therapy, in their report, "The Relationship of Decline in Spiritual Struggles to Psychotherapy Outcomes: Evidence from a Large Scale Survey of Psychotherapy Clients." Observing that "the majority of research has shown that spiritual struggles are often linked with negative psychological functioning, such as increased depression, anxiety, and PTSD symptoms," (p. 40), Harris and colleagues hypothesized that a dramatically different outcome to spiritual struggles may occur with clients. They hypothesized "that there would be a positive relationship between decreasing spiritual struggles and improved psychotherapy outcomes" (p. 40). As identified Christian researchers who published their articles in a Christian journal, curiosity about whether these researchers may have discovered what they sought to find should be acknowledged. However, as necessary as such curiosity may be, the essential rationale of these researchers nicely accommodates a common rationale for engaging clients in their various struggles. Namely, as clients actively engage in their struggles, they likely experience improvement. Obviously, this generalization has its exceptions. Harris and colleagues concluded, though, "This study supported the hypothesis that as a person's spiritual struggles decrease during the course of therapy, his or her psychological functioning is most likely to improve" (p. 46). An implication of their study is that counselors and therapists may want to welcome religious and spiritual struggles of their clients so that clients may actively engage with such struggles and, therefore, achieve improved mental-emotional functioning.

As a whole, this collection of articles raises ideas and practices that may enlarge the perspectives that counselors and therapists take to their work. For example, as good-hearted, empathic, resourceful, relationally oriented, and clinically savvy individuals, counselors and therapists may need to give attention to the potential that they may commit microaggressions as they provide therapy for their clients. Or, they may need to consider the positive potential that comes from actively engaging clients in their religious struggles, with the idea that such struggles can lead to improved relationships and mental-emotional well-being. Or, they may need to engage in serious reflection about their personal experience of religion-related features of their personal lives.

Anticipating Treatment of Clients with Religious Concerns

Inevitably, counselors and therapists meet clients who present many different kinds of issues related to their religion. Acknowledging this, Leighton offers a sagacious insight. "It is not realistic to assume that a counselor can possibly assimilate both the quantity and quality of theological information about religious systems to hold court with their clients all the time" (Leighton, 2014, p. 297). If nothing else, the ten articles presented above confirm Leighton's view. Indeed, almost all clients present complexity, whether the specific category of concern is their religion, prolonged depression, marriage, overwhelming fears, parenting, excessive anxiety, or any thousands of other concerns or combination of concerns. With the need to focus on religion-related concerns, though, a good beginning question is how counselors and therapists may think about and anticipate the specifically religious concerns with which come to therapy. Toward developing a clinically appropriate orientation to focusing on religion-related concerns in therapy, help is available, as this discussion shows.

A useful and relatively simple entré into therapy with clients who present religion-related concerns is the "FICA" approach. Cotton, Grossoehme, and Tsevat (2007, p. 149) recommend this approach as a screening tool through which clients' concerns may become the focus of treatment. In short, their approach raises four questions, as follows.

> F (faith): What is your faith tradition?
> I (important): How important is your faith to you?
> C (church): What is your church or community faith?
> A (address): How would you like me to address these issues in your healthcare?

Another, more detailed, screening approach to addressing religion-related concerns in counseling and therapy is BRAIDS. Developed by Leighton (2014), the acronym, BRAIDS, stands for beliefs, relational, application, integration, diagnostic, and self. The aim is to engage clients in relevant mental-emotional change as it relates to religious beliefs, while maintaining clients' comfort with their religion, as needed. Leighton's brief description of the BRAIDS Screening Tool may be helpful. "As a catchment tool for therapists providing services to devoutly religious clients, the following is designed to establish, build and maintain therapeutic rapport while exploring the interface between psychological methods and strong religious beliefs."

In their article, "Integrating Spirituality and Religion Into Psychotherapy: Persistent Dilemmas, Ethical Issues, and a Proposed Decision-Making Process," Barnett and Johnson (2011) offer a somewhat more comprehensive approach to addressing specifically religious concerns in counseling and therapy. Their approach includes nine stages. The first one (p. 159) is titled, "Respectfully Assess the Client's Religious or Spiritual Beliefs and Preferences." They add recommendations that partially explain this stage.

> When feasible and appropriate to the psychotherapy context, consider employing established assessment tools and techniques which are valid for assessing religious or spiritual beliefs and practices. (Griffith & Griffith, 2002; Hall & Edwards, 2002; Hathaway & Ripley, 2009; Hill & Pargament, 2003)
>
> Accord respect and dignity in all matters but especially when assessing religious or spiritual beliefs that are unfamiliar or to which you have a negative personal reaction. (Beit-Hallahmi, 1975; McLemore & Court, 1977)
>
> As one component of the informed consent process offer a clear rationale for asking questions about religion and spirituality.
>
> Tailor the level or intensity of religious/spiritual assessment to the individual client, the psychotherapy context, and the client's own preference for consideration of these issues.

Without the explanatory details included in their article, Barnett and Johnson's title the other stages in the following manner.

Stage 2: Carefully Assess Any Connection Between the Presenting Problem and Religious or Spiritual Beliefs and Commitments
Stage 3: Weave Results of This Assessment Into the Informed Consent Process
Stage 4: Honestly Consider Your Countertransference to the Client's Religiousness
Stage 5: Honestly Evaluate Your Competence in This Case
Stage 6: Consult With Experts in the Area of Religion and Psychotherapy
State 7: If Appropriate, Clinically Indicated, and Client Gives Consent, Consult With Client's Own Clergy or Other Religious Professional
Stage 8: Make a Decision About Treating the Client or Making a Referral
Stage 9: Assess Outcomes and Adjust Plan Accordingly

The three approaches presented above have much to offer. Each one has positive value in working with clients who bring specifically religious concerns to counseling and therapy, but also has gaps and weakness. For example, one of the visible strengths of Leighton's BRAIDS Screening Tool is that it includes an emphasis on relationships. Barnett and Johnson include an emphasis on the need for counselors and therapists to assess their competence to treat clients whose concerns are specifically religious.

A good example of the current emphasis on how religion may be clinically and ethically understood in the conduct of counseling and therapy is Rosenfeld's "Contributions from Ethics and Research that Guide Integrating Religion into Psychotherapy." Somewhat presciently, Rosenfeld (2011) states, "The emerging integration of religion into traditionally secular psychotherapy can be seen as a reconciliation of the clash between those who believed religion was a cause of pathology and a defense against treatment and those who advocated that psychotherapy should teach the values and adopt the healing practices found in religion" (p. 197). While incomplete—probably, in perpetuity—this reconciliation is presumed here to be the place of religion in counseling and therapy, despite obvious reasons discussed earlier in this book in detail for increasing scrutiny of religion-related approaches to counseling and therapy.

Clients' Presentation of Religion-Related Issues

This discussion of client's presentation of religion-related issues refers to the complaints and problems that clients identify during the process of receiving treatment. While these complaints and problems arise and should be the focus of treatment, they are not in themselves an assessment of religion. Similarly, an individual may bring complaints about, say, his family. Such complaints should be taken seriously, but are not in themselves an assessment of families. By analogy, a patient who visits her physician and complains about her sore and painful shoulder from lifting a heavy object to an overhead shelf in her closet does not require her physician to assess bodies. The physician would and should address the patient's problem with a painful shoulder. This understanding of addressing specifically religious concerns is reflected in the client-presented complaints and problems discussed below.

Religion as a Failed Source of Strength and Meaning

Following the loss of his wife to death as a result of breast cancer, a widower says, "I guess I figured that somehow God would come through for us. You know, something would happen that would save her." The death of his spouse brings enormous consequences for this individual, but also for anyone who endures such an experience. Similarly, following the murder of a brother, life is not as it was before the brother's death. "I just feel like I got up one day and found that God had disappeared. Nothing made sense anymore." For counselors and therapists, the clinical demand is to relate with the client in such ways that confidence in life can be restored and sustained. The inherent demand for such a relationship may be tested when, for example, a seriously diseased and terminally ill, older man tells the therapist that he is "bitter toward God" because of his illness.

Desperate Search for Positive Meaning

Ever since Viktor Frankl's book, *Man's Search for Meaning*, appeared in 1946, mental health care providers have given heightened attention to their clients' sometimes desperate search for meaning. Instead of having experienced religion as a failed source of strength and meaning, clients also bring a void of meaning that emerges from failure, betrayal, loss, injury, or other insults to life that cause them to search for meaning or, sometimes from abundance, as suggested by a client.

> It's been really hard. I've been kicked pretty hard, but not nearly as hard as most people I know. I've actually had it pretty good. I have a job I love to go to. My family loves me. My health is pretty good. I just feel like I should have something in my life that I'm lacking, you know? I should be doing something with my life, but I have no idea what it is. I'm just lost, you know? I don't know what it would be like, but I somehow want to connect with God, you know?

The anguished absence of meaning is not unique to clients who seek therapy. Indeed, very likely, almost everyone is acquainted with questions of personal meaning across a wide spectrum of intensity. As obtuse as the concept of meaning may be, substantially good help for therapists is available for those clients who present their desperate need for meaning. For example, Dieser (2023) practices meaning-centered therapy through therapeutic recreation and Armstrong (2009) takes meaning-based therapy to sex-related problems.

Hurt, Embarrassed, or Betrayed by One's Faith Community

Many faithful Catholics have been harmed individually and embarrassed generally by the multiple revelations of the sexual abuse of children by their priests. Despite this, most of them have remained faithful Catholics. The harm to them was not uniquely personal, except of course to the individuals and families who were abused. When the damage is uniquely personal, remaining faithful becomes exponentially difficult. Here is what a client reported:

> We just feel so deeply hurt. It all started when my younger sister, Katie, had problems with drugs. Back then, I remember bringing my concern to our church, asking for prayer for my sister. Everyone there was so very supportive. We loved being a part of the church. We weren't married at that church, but we began to go there shortly after we were married. Until recently, this was the only church that our kids ever knew. It's always been like home to them. Our oldest is Serra—eighteen. She will go to college this fall. Of course, they visited other churches sometimes with their friends, but this was always home for them—their church home. We loved our church.
>
> Anyway, Katie's drug problems got worse. And, for several months, we lost all contact with her. It wasn't until we got a call from the jail, the county jail, to let us know that she had been arrested and sent to jail for several crimes. For us, though, the turning point—the thing that changed our lives—was that Katie was pregnant. The only reason the sheriff's office contacted us was to see whether we could take care of the baby when it was born. Of course, we said that we would. Anyway, Katie had her baby.
>
> Now, if you look at us, you can tell that we are white, as pale as people can get. Katie's baby was not white. She was very dark skinned. We don't know anything about who the father is. We tried to find out, but nothing came of it. Anyway, we took our new baby to church. She is now officially our daughter. We adopted her. We had not done that when we first took her to church. When we got to church the first time, we were

told by several people that we could not come into the building with a 'nigger.' We were so confused, at first. Then, thinking that we must have misunderstood what happened, we went back. The anger at us was overwhelming. I can still see the face of one of our 'friends' yelling at us. "We don't allow no goddamn niggers here." And they yelled a lot more. We left and have not been back. We do not want to go back. We were so devastated by what they did. Even now, I can't imagine how so many of them could be Christian and treat others like they treated us.

Religion Integrated into Mental-Emotional Distortions and Disorders

This problem is not really about religion; it is about religion becoming a feature of a mental illness. In the long history of mental illness, observers have noted that paranoid individuals, for example, sometimes integrate Satan into their personal problems, referring to being "filled with the Devil," for example. This is sometimes a way to account for inexplicable behavior and, at other times, a way to make sense of the individual's internal and stormy distortions. When religion manifests itself in this way, it should be understood, first, as a sign of mental illness and not as a specifically religious problem. Understanding that an individual may be suffering with a major mental disorder also somewhat simplifies the complexity of making sense of other distortions such as those that involve race, sex, religious beliefs, and others. The disorder itself explains the distortions.

Moral Dilemmas That Stem from Faith Commitments

Individuals who seek to fulfill the moral imperatives of their respective faith commitments sometimes find themselves in opposition to the position that their faith and faith communities have taken. "Well, back then, that's not what women did." The frail, tinny, and sometimes squeaky voice is that of an elderly woman. She continued. "No. Having been a member of my church from the earliest days I can remember, I blended in real well. What my church believed, I believed, too. That's just the way it was. Not only that, I could read, too. And, my reading of Scripture told me that a woman's place is not one of leadership in her church. That's what I believed. As a young woman, though, I knew I wanted to lead a church as a senior minister. So, I was in conflict, whether anyone else knew it or not. It wasn't really something I could talk about back then. My conscience was torn. Do I support myself and do what I believe I should do—lead my church—or do I support my church and do what I believe I should do? How in the hell do you solve something like that?"

Moral dilemmas that stem from religion often appear in mental health care. They are sometimes expressed as parenting problems: "We aren't sure what to do. Our son is dating a girl we can't quite approve of. She comes from a pretty rough family. They're not Christians." They may arise as marital conflict forces uncomfortable questions: "Our marriage just is not working, but we feel like we must make it work. We didn't get married so that we could get a divorce. Divorce has never been an acceptable thought for us. Our faith just doesn't permit it. Yet, here we are. Divorce seems like the only thing to do, at this time." More broadly than parenting problems and marital conflict, moral dilemmas that stem from religion result from ordinary and extreme religious views, because almost by definition religion holds its adherents to high standards of behavior and beckons them to be better than they are.

Beyond this somewhat personal and ordinary array of moral dilemmas, some moral dilemmas become ominous or pose deadly consequences. For example, an individual may strongly disapprove of sexual orientations that are not his own, but refuses to consider violent actions toward others. Unfortunately, as his views incorporate themselves in various groups of which he may be a member, including his religious group, his strong disapproval may prompt others to take violent actions. For some individuals and the groups in which they hold membership, expressions of violence or intended violence pose an intense and critical moral dilemma.

Conflict between a Client's Beliefs and Behaviors

Incongruence is common. Surely, in counseling and therapy, clinicians are readily and constantly aware of clients whose values and behaviors are conflicted. They recognize that some of their clients have pledged their affection to a partner in marriage, but also seek affection with partners outside of marriage. They accept the fact that many clients report that their individual lives should be good because they have all they need, but obsess with the idea that they wish to die. They understand, too, that some of their clients present similar conflicts around their religious beliefs and commitments. The young man is handsome, smart, married, successful, and a stalwart Christian. "As a dad, I do great. I love my two kids—a boy and a girl—and would do anything for them. I get a lot of rewards from being their dad. It's exciting to see them grow and become their own persons. It's amazing to watch them and be a part of their growth. My kids are not my problem. And my wife is not really a problem. She's a good mom and a good wife. I have no complaints about her. And we could talk about our marriage and how it has developed over these eleven or so years. There's not really a problem there. I am the problem. It's me, not her or the kids. I have a kind of secret life going. And it goes against everything I believe is right. As a Christ follower, I'm doing things that I know explode all that I say I believe. I don't really want to talk about it, but if I don't I will go crazy. My secret life involves partners. Romantic, sexual partners. The guilt and frustration with all of this is taking over my life."

Political Divisions and Alienation from Religion

Those who have immersed in the literature of the American Civil War have sometimes discovered letters and other documents that tell the stories of divided families. Some members of families supported the North and others supported the South. And, in some cases, their support took them to battlefields where a brother fought for one side and another brother fought for the other side. Reconciliation between them, during or after the war, seemed to be mostly impossible. Recently, the client says, "Our family is in trouble. I'm on Trump's side. My brother is a die-hard Democrat. We don't speak anymore. It's that simple. Neither of us is going to change sides. We used to go everywhere together. My wife and I went on several vacations with my brother and his wife. That has not happened for a couple of years. It doesn't look like it will ever happen again. We always went to church together, too. But that doesn't happen anymore, either. I believe that Trump is God's man for the hour, but my brother thinks differently. Probably, the nail in the coffin of our relationship came when our pastor publicly spoke about her political preferences. Up to that time, my brother and I pretty much kept our differences out of sight. But, when she publicly advocated for Donald Trump, that triggered his anger. He told me to go to hell and said he would not be attending our church after that. We haven't spoken since then. He hasn't been back at church. Who would have thought that two brothers would be separated by politics and church—especially feeling so much bitterness. I know that I feel it, just like he does. Both of us can't be right."

Controlling, Manipulative Religion

Eventually, if news reports are followed, a story of extreme control and manipulation by a church or another religious group will appear. Some of the stories will endure almost indefinitely because of their intensely dramatic character. For decades, those who heard the story of The People's Temple, led by Jim Jones, remember the story. Apparently, a paranoid and charismatic minister, Jones founded The People's Temple in the 1950s in Indianapolis, moved it to California, and eventually moved it again to the jungle in Guyana in 1974 (Britannica, 2022). In relocating his congregation to Guyana, Jones' apparent aim was to isolate his followers from the contaminating influences of the world. When family members and government officials lost contact with many of Jones' followers, a small number of family members and a United States Congressman went to

Jones' compound—Jonestown, Guyana—to investigate. The Congressman was killed by Jones' guards. And, the horror that perpetuated this story in memory was that almost 1,000 individuals died as a result of a massive murder-suicide on November 18, 1978 (Britannica, 2022). Most control and manipulation by a religious group are far less dramatic and known than the story of The People's Temple. More commonly, they involve perfectionistic standards of behavior, excessive demands for financial support, or coercion toward believing specific religious dogmas. Much closer to everyday living than the story of Jonestown, controlling and manipulative religion arises everywhere, allowing for the fact that most religious groups are not and should not be characterized this way.

With regard to over-controlling and manipulative religion, the story of "Andie" is somewhat extreme, but in attitude is not unusual. Andrea—or "Andie"—is a 23-year-old, self-identified "very attractive woman." Indeed, as her therapist notes, "Andrea presents in a confident, poised manner, almost oblivious to her stunning and beautiful appearance." Dressed impeccably, "Andie" presents in a manner that defies her appearance. She is miserable. She refers to herself with terms like "disgust," "immoral," "ashamed," and "guilty." Andie tells a story of the "purity culture" in which she was raised. She reports numerous events that confirmed her view of her personal history.

> My mom and dad sent me to a Pure Love Camp. I was just twelve or, maybe, thirteen. And, all they talked about was sex. I remember the leader, a frumpy middle-aged woman, holding a tea cup out and passing it around the group. Then, she explained that this is your sex. Then, she dropped the tea cup so it broke into a thousand pieces. She made her point. "If you have sex outside of marriage, you are no good. No one who is decent will ever want you. You are broken." Of course, everything there required prayer. Purity is Christian, you know?

Somewhat wryly, Andie added, "She wasted a lot of tea cups."

> You won't believe this, but about a year later in another Christian purity camp, another teacher told us we would have a competition to see who could drink a glass of water the quickest. So, she filled two glasses and asked for volunteers. I did not volunteer. My friend did. And another girl volunteered, too. Then, this woman took out a bag of dog shit—except she said "dog poop." She explained that she would put the poop in the glasses and ask the girls to drink it. Of course, she was saying that no one would want water contaminated with dog poop. Her point was much too clear. If you contaminate your body with sex, no one will want you. The sick thing was that one of the girls didn't

> believe that the poop was really poop. And she drank some of it. She got really sick. She wretched like crazy. She may have been hospitalized—I'm not sure about that.

Andie describes herself as a "sex magnet." "I can have sex anytime, anywhere. If I go to the mall, I can have a guy in a dressing room in fifteen minutes. I've done it. Several times. It's easy. I go to the beach and attract guys. And I know that in minutes we will be in his room or mine. We may have a little wine to loosen us up, but it doesn't matter. We are going to have sex. Then, I feel so ashamed. I can't sleep. I remember those awful lessons from back then, especially from my mom." Tormented by her internal conflicts, Andie adds, "My mom and dad won't even speak to me, now. They still think that a girl's only purpose is to save herself for the man she marries and to serve his sexual needs. That' it. That's her reason for being alive—marry, have sex, serve your husband." Andie reports that she did not have sex until she was almost 22 years of age, but that once she had it, she constantly craved it. From her own point of view, Andie migrated from purity to debauchery. When she discusses her sex-related behavior, she talks about how disgusted she is with herself. She adds that she feels bad about herself all of the time. "I don't know who I am, anymore. I just don't know. I'm in a cage called 'religion' and I can't get out." Andie is the outcome of over-controlling religion.

Disturbed Parenting

Karyn lives with her parents and two younger brothers and a younger sister. Her father is a minister and her mother a homemaker who is active in the church as the minister's wife. Karyn's mother is a quiet, unassuming woman. She has devoted her life to serving others. She spends several evenings a week with church-related activities. Kathy's father cares for the children these evenings, unless he too has church-related obligations. Karyn then has the responsibility of caring for the other children. When Karyn was 12, her father began finding excuses to come into the bathroom when she was bathing and watch her out of the corner of his eye. Karyn would ask him to leave, but he repeatedly told her there was nothing wrong with his being there; after all, he was her father, and he'd seen her naked all her life. About six months later he began going into her bedroom at night. He began by fondling her, moved to finger penetration, and finally began intercourse when Karyn was 14. Her father told her that God thought the human body was beautiful, and that the relationship between parents and children was the most sacred of all human relationships. However, he said, other people who weren't as close to God wouldn't understand, and if she ever said anything to anyone about their "special relationship," he would be banned from the church, and they would lose their home and the family would break apart.

Disturbed parents who violate their children are not likely to harm their children in the devastating way that Karyn's father harmed her. More likely than such devastation, disturbed parenting will induce guilt, impose unrealistic standards, demean the self-image of their children, neglect the emotional well-being of their children, and impair their children's social skills. However, thoughtful concern about the children of overtly religious parents should also account for the positive contributions that these parents make to their children. The work of Bornstein et al., 2017 stands as a reminder to account for such contributions. Their careful integration of a large volume of information about religion-related practices among parents confirms, in their language, "the mixed blessings" of such practices. In contrast, counselors and therapists are not likely to provide treatment for parents and children whose religion-related parenting practices lead to mental health and general well-being.

Godly or Godless Squabbles

In polite, cultural exchanges that almost inevitably occur in most communities, differences in faith orientations are taken for granted. Few conflicts of significance arise because of these differences. Some of the less consequential differences occur when a woman becomes the administrative superior in an organization where she will oversee the work of men or when an African-American will oversee the work of a mostly white workforce. However, serious differences in religion sometimes occur when two individuals "fall in love," try to anticipate how their religious differences will shape their future, and agonize about how to introduce their relationship to their respective families. From 2010 to 2015, interfaith marriages rose by 39% (Murphy, 2015). With the ongoing rise in the number of interfaith marriages, the frequency of conflict around religious issues has also risen.

Janeé and Cris, wife and husband, come from different faith traditions. Janeé describes her family of origin as "conservative Baptists" with whom she largely agrees. Cris describes his family as Mormons. He, too, indicates that he is loyal to his family and his church. Prior to their marriage, Janeé says that she decided to join Cris and become Mormon. Much to her disappointment, she reports that her mother and father expressed shock and anger about her decision, vowing never to see her again. She says that her parents' reaction seemed to be extremely out of character for them, because "they have always been supportive of my decision making and independence." She reports that her parents refused to attend her wedding or to offer any other kind of endorsement of her marriage. Now, almost five years later, Janeé says that she would love to reconcile with her parents, emphasizing that she wants her children—Allie and Jared, four and two, respectively—to know their grandparents. Following phone calls and email messages to her parents, Janeé cries, as she confirms that their only condition for accepting their grandchildren is that Janeé convert back to being "Christian." Her parents' demand has caused tensions between Janeé and Cris.

Abandonment of Family and Religious Traditions

While poor parenting by those who exhibit high religiosity may lead to adverse consequences for their children, their children may struggle with additional suffering when they seek to overcome the effects of poor parenting. Many experienced counselors and therapists have likely provided professional care for the client who says, "I can't talk to my mom or dad any more. They will want to talk about religion. I know I can't go there with them. I will have to leave or a fight will break out." Usually, this kind of message is accompanied by the client's conclusion that the faith commitments of their parents are no longer acceptable. Such a conclusion evokes ambivalence about whether abandoning the family's religious traditions and practices is better or worse than squirming with the recognition that an acceptable, let alone desirable, alternate does not seem to be available.

Anxious Exploration of Alternate Religions

Feeling suspended between a family history that makes sense and a future that makes no sense poses an awkward and sometimes insurmountable dilemma. Common statements that reflect this suspension are "I just don't know what to believe," "I used to be able to recite my religious beliefs, but now it's all a mass of confusion for me," or "I'm kind of lost, hoping that somehow I will see something that helps me to accept some sort of faith." Recalling such a client, a counselor reported that his client, a young woman, pursued several different faith orientations. He indicated that she relinquished her connection with a conservative Presbyterian family and experimented with the Church of Latter Day Saints, Buddhism, Oriental mysticism, and the Episcopal Church, among others. According to the counselor, his client expressed her need for personal religious faith, with a clear preference for something Christian, but also felt extraordinary apprehension about committing to it. Finally, the counselor observed, "Once she caught on to the idea that exploration might be a good idea, she began to relax. After venting a lot of frustration with her lack of answers about personal faith, she turned in the direction of welcoming the adventure of exploring many alternative ways of being religious, without having to persist with the empty idea that faith required her to live in an ideological box—or cell. So, for her, the freedom of exploring became more important that the discovery. It's an old story."

Abuse by Religious Persons

Due to widespread news reports about sexual victimization by church leaders, information about it no longer comes as a surprise. Sadly, it is not news; it is a reminder of a large class of victims. Often, because it received massive coverage, the perpetration of sexual abuse by officials in the Roman Catholic Church is presumed to be most of the story of such abuse. This is understandable. As Claudia Lauer and Meghan Hoyer (Lauer & Hoyer, 2019) reported,

> Nearly 1,700 priests and other clergy members that the Roman Catholic Church considers credibly accused of child sexual abuse are living under the radar with little to no oversight from religious authorities or law enforcement, decades after the first wave of the church abuse scandal roiled U.S. dioceses, an Associated Press investigation has found.

As dramatic as this report is, it is far from complete. Globally, abuse by Catholic leaders likely includes hundreds of thousands of victims. But, as immensely significant as this obviously is, sexual abuse by Catholic leaders may distract attention from leaders in other church organizations that perpetrate sexual victimization. For example, for an extended period of time, sexual abuse by leaders among clergy in the Southern Baptist Convention (SBC) has been reported through various news media. Because the SBC is headquartered in Nashville, Tennessee, the city's newspaper, *The Tennessean,* has delivered frequent and detailed coverage of this abuse. Liam Adams, a religion reporter for *The Tennessean*, has published many detailed reports about sex abuse perpetrated by Southern Baptist ministers. Adams has documented abuse of individual congregants and accounts of their perpetrators. His reports are easily located online. Recently, he reported about the current response of the SBC's Executive Committee, titled, "Firm named to create Southern Baptist Convention database of ministers accused of abuse" (Adams, 2023). From the time, clergy abuse of their congregants to the present time, the response has been mostly denial and avoidance of the abuse. According to National Public Radio's Terry Gross, the SBC "kept a secret list of over 700 offenders. The list was even kept secret from most of the church's leaders" (Gross, 2022).

No doubt, sexual abuse by religious leaders pervasively and forever changes the lives of victims. Whatever specific character changes the victim may have, the widespread silencing of their voices adds to the intensity of their betrayal and their deep emotional injury and trauma. In their study of child victims of sexual abuse by religious leaders, Tener, Katz, Marmor, & Lusky-Weisrose (2020) observed, "The participants responded to the abuse mostly with fear. Some tried to actively resist, and we wonder how many of them have been prepared to react that way. All displayed understanding that what happened to them was forbidden by God … ." This is not a complete picture of the experience of child sexual victimization by religious leaders, but it provides important clues about the consequences of such victimization and the issues that these victims often present to counselors and therapists.

In this discussion, the importance of these brief comments about sexual abuse by religious leaders is that the consequences of the abuse appear in individuals and families who seek counseling and therapy. An analysis of the specific clinical needs of these clients lies beyond the scope of this book. Suffice it to observe that they may receive any of several relevant diagnoses such as Post Traumatic Stress Disorder (PTSD) or Major Depression. More experientially, they may be characterized as suffering "moral injury," "shattered faith," or, as Shooter (2016), says, "traumatic wounding." Whatever the specific diagnosis or characterization may be, victims' view of their personal religion has been radically altered as a result of their sexual abuse. In the context of providing clinical services, counselors and therapists must seek to be aware of their personal religious views so as to protect clients from them. For example, a secure attachment by a therapist to personal religious beliefs and experiences may be affronted by an injured client's deep skepticism, cynicism, or hostility toward such beliefs and experiences. Abuse by religious leaders may erupt from other matters, too, such as sexual orientation. Among many other considerations, this requires that conscientious, professionally accountable counselors and therapists persist in their own growth and remain open and adaptable to the endless variety of challenges that appear before them, as they seek to ease the suffering of their clients and facilitate health and well-being.

Harmful Discrimination

Among the many valuable assets that most mental health care providers bring to their work is a belief in and readiness to embody diversity. In providing professional care for clients, embodying diversity may or may not be conspicuously significant. After all, this is what counselors and therapist do somewhat routinely and naturally. Their embodiment and practice of diversity may lower their awareness of how truly significant such embodiment and practice are for the clients whom they seek to help. A therapist reported that she was somewhat surprised to hear her client reflect on the importance of diversity. The client said, "Dr. Bradford, you get me, you know? Do you know how hard it is for an old Black lady to talk openly with a young White doctor? I'm so glad to have found you." The therapist's report about this client indicated that the client had very likely received harmful discrimination because of the client's race, but that, more than race as the issue of concern, the client indicated that she had been ridiculed at her place of employment because of her religion. "Just like Cassius Clay changed his name to Mohammed Ali, I changed my name, too. That was before I went to work at my current job. So, they hired me knowing that I was Muslim, not Christian. Not everyone there who is Christian has been rude or insulting, but the ones who have been this way remind me in a lot of ways that I should 'get over that stupid stuff.' Somebody put little cross stickers on my desk. I can still see the outline of where the crosses had been stuck to the desk. I've been angry about what they have done to me. I have had that evil thought, 'I hate Christians,' but I refuse to let them win. Still, I have to go there and take it. I cannot let them win. I should say that the owner of the company, a fine lady, has said that she will fire anyone who is caught doing these things. So, my job is secure."

Compromising Transference-Related Challenges

Along with many others, Abernethy and Lancia (1998, p. 281) agree with the thought that "the examination of transference and countertransference is an essential and challenging dimension of psychotherapy." Understanding this means that when clients request or demand a therapist who shares their religion, astute therapists will be alert to the possibility of compromise of their clinical professionalism. On the one side, a client may be seeking comfort and compatibility that come with knowing that their religious commitments will be safe and free of adverse reactions from their therapist. On the other side, a client may be preparing a prospective therapist for a compromise of clinical professionalism. A simple question, such as "Are you a Christian?," may be loaded with unspoken expectations of a therapist that a client anticipates will be actualized.

Such expectations may take the form of specific religious beliefs. When this is the situation, the reality of these expectations generally evolves to a time when the expectant client poses a belief, as if the therapist ought to agree with it. "Jesus is the Son of God and the only one who can give us happiness and/or mental health, right?" Or, "My problems may be serious, but the only solution for them is to pray. Don't you think so?" Of course, when a therapist fails to display sufficient agreement with the expectant client, the client's response is likely—either overtly or covertly—one of concluding that the therapist is not really the believer whom she claimed to me. Therefore, the client dismisses therapy and the therapist as likely hostile or rejecting toward the client's religion.

Alternately, expectations may take the form of social-cultural or familial beliefs and behaviors. When this is the situation, the expectant client may, for example, assign to the therapist a level of compliance with the client's view of a personal or family situation. This may also be a condition for receiving therapy. Speaking to their therapist, a husband described a situation toward which he expected agreement from the therapist.

> We've been pretty stressed out with each other lately. We've already told you a lot of the story. Usually, I think Cherry does not respect me and my way of looking at things. The thing that came up since we last met happened just last night. We went to a concert. She told me about the concert and wanted to get tickets. I said, "Sure. Sounds good to me." And she bought the tickets. So, I went to the concert with the idea that we would enjoy some good entertainment. It was sort of entertaining, but mostly it was kind of vulgar. I wasn't embarrassed by crude language, but I was confused about why she would want to go to hear the trashy stuff we heard. It wasn't the music. It was the stupid comments. This band talked about women's body parts in pretty explicit terms and politics. Their comments were disgusting. You may not believe in the Bible, but I do. And I know and believe that the Bible is right when it talks about how we must be modest in our dress and speech. It's what's in our hearts that matter. I mean, that's just the way it is.

This client expects their therapist to comply with his point of view. He believes that his view is nearly absolutely defensible because he can reference the Bible. Too often, the issues with which clients expect their therapist to comply involve sexual behavior (e.g., "We tell our daughter that God expects her to abstain from sex until she gets married."), abortion, sex roles, and, political issues. While the presentation of these issues can be subtle and disarmingly sincere, they can be no less coercive because of their subtly and sincerity. Significantly, on the therapist's side of such dialogues, no matter what the religion-related issue may be, counselors and therapists must show caution about presuming that their religious views and expressions of their views will likely receive ready acceptance by their clients. Instead of acceptance, the religious views and expressions of their views may seriously exacerbate the problems with which clients are seeking help, insofar as the socialization, including its internal security, that sometimes accompanies religion means that changing a religious commitment, even when the commitment is clearly self-defeating, becomes much too formidable for clients. Surely, in the health care crucible of the consulting room, clinical decision-making requires neither an obligation nor professional accountability to protect the therapist's religion from insult by clients nor to advocate clients for a religion. While this view may be entirely understandable or even desirable, it is likely to remain a nagging, challenging feature of clinical work with some clients. At least, on occasion, clinical work will immerse therapists in the thick mixture of their personal and strongly held beliefs, conscience about what is right and wrong, awareness of the necessary boundaries that inhere in clinical work, and normatively acceptable behavior, with the equivalent and incompatible presentations by their clients.

Religious Beliefs as Accelerants of Personal Problems

While religious beliefs cannot be regarded as predictors of personal problems, the reality of such consequences of religious beliefs has been confirmed by observers and researchers for many years. For example, McGraw, Skidmore, Lefevor, Docherty, and Mahone (2023, p. 303) conclude that "holding nonaffirming LDS beliefs may be related to and predict future depression, through internalized stigma among current and former LDS [sexual minorities]." However, to characterize religious beliefs in this singular manner fails to capture the considerable ambiguity of religious beliefs as they relate to personal problems. After all, research also confirms the importance of religious beliefs as major contributors to recovery from serious personal problems. For example, Jerome, Heath, Williams, Winters, and Cutrer-Pårraga (2023, p. 186) examined the role of religious/spiritual (R/S) beliefs in recovery from trauma and concluded that the process of successful coping "involves reframing one's situation to align with R/S beliefs, adapting oneself to accept the human condition while acknowledging divine communication and support, and increasing one's hope for a growth-oriented outcome."

Normative Developmental Issues

Very likely, many counselors and therapists have a good understanding of specifically religious issues that arise from developmental issues, not so much because they necessarily relate such issues to religion but because they understand human development. For example, pubescent adolescents question almost everything, including their religious views and, of course, the religious views of their parents. Their parents sometimes wonder whether their confrontational and probably annoying adolescent will ever grow beyond such thoughts and actions and become likeable again. Fortunately, such adolescents almost always grow beyond these things. Somewhat more seriously, counselors and therapists likely also understand the existential challenges that often accompany older adulthood, with Erikson's emphasis on integrity versus despair as a significant struggle. Counselors and therapists are unlikely to see integrity as a religious issue in therapy, but will often see despair in older adults who seek therapy. And, such despair may be expressed in specifically religious terms, but also understood in developmental terms.

Personal, Religion-Related Quirks

Mental health care professionals usually have experience in relating with clients who bring eccentricities to therapy. As many scholars have observed, when therapists encounter religion-related issues in therapy, they usually do not have good ways to think about how to provide treatment. When the religion-related issues pose visible eccentricity, providing treatment becomes even more difficult. For one thing, the eccentric character of an individual's religion-related issues may pose difficulty for therapists' ability to see them, due to the unusualness of the issue, if for no other reason. For another thing, therapists usually want to affirm the religious outlook/worldview of their clients. Such challenges may be seen in the following example. The client, a firefighter, commonly fights fires in residential neighborhoods.

> I see God everywhere—always have. When I was a kid, I remember thinking that the stains on the tablecloth were signs of God's presence. I don't believe that anymore. Nowadays, I'm different. I can't stand most of the ways people talk about God. Sometimes, I think to myself, "I hate love." When people speak of God's love, I feel a sneer coming on. But, it's not that I don't think about God. I do. A lot. My way of thinking about God means a lot to me. I still see God everywhere. But it's fire where I see God most. I know it sounds odd, but when I fight fires, I feel like I'm fighting God—sort of like Jacob fighting with an angel. I've never decided not to fight a fire when I have to. It's my job. So, I'm going to do all I can to put out the fire. When I'm on my own, though—like at home—it's different. I use fire for my worship. That's where God is. I go to church. Really. The thing that gets me there is that our church burns a lot of candles. Maybe, it's the flames as nature the way God made it that seems to connect me to God. ... You know, a lot of religions have a fire God. Well, me, too.

This client proceeds to describe his rich, meaningful spiritual life, strangely centered around his interest in "God" as "fire." Quite apart from a presentation such as this, religion-related eccentricities may be as much a cultural phenomenon as individual ones. Surely, this kind of eccentricity includes Christian snake handlers, speaking in tongues, and others.

To close this discussion of clients' presentation of religion-related issues, it should be said that clients bring to their counselors and therapists many more than this report can include and discuss. The list of these issues merely serves to bring them together for readers. Readers are encouraged to reflect on this list and to revise it, based on their clinical work, and, of course, to add to it.

Counselors and therapists can and will confront many, if not all, of these religion-related challenges in their clinical practices. Meeting these challenges, along with all of the others with which they are already well acquainted, such as depression, marital conflict, career frustrations, and so on, is the reason that they do what they do. Or, "This is what we live for." And, as caring, objective, and consummately professional as they are, they complete and enhance one another by welcoming these challenges, just as they welcome one another when they best relate with peers, with the highest integrity and competence of which they are capable.

References

Abernethy, A. D., & Lancia, J. J. (1998). Religion and the psychotherapeutic relationship: Transferential and countertransferential dimensions. *The Journal of Psychotherapy Practice and Research*, *7*(4), 281–289.

Adams, L. (2023, February 20). Firm named to create Southern Baptist Convention database of ministers accused of abuse. *The Tennessean*.

Barnett, J. E., & Johnson, W. B. (2011, March). Integrating spirituality and religion into psychotherapy: Persistent dilemmas, ethical Issues, and a proposed decision-making process. *Ethics and Behavior*, *21*(2), 147–164. 10.1080/10508422.2011.551471

Beit-Hallahmi, B. (1975). Encountering orthodox religion in psychotherapy. *Psychotherapy: Theory, Research & Practice*, *12*, 357–359.

Britannica. (2022). Peoples temple. https://www.britannica.com/topic/Peoples-Temple

Captari, L. E., Hook, J. N., Hoyt, W., Davis, D. E., McElroy-Heltzel, S. E., & Worthington, Jr., E. L. (2018). Integrating clients' religion and spirituality within psychotherapy: A comprehensive meta-analysis. *Journal of Clinical Psychology*, *74*, 1938–1951.

Coburn, K. O., & McGeorge, C. R. (2019). What do Christian clergy say?: Advice from Christian pastors to family therapists about working with LGB clients. *Contemporary Family Therapy*, *41*, 236–246.

Cotton, S., Grossoehme, D. H., & Tsevat, J. (2007). Religion/spirituality and health in adolescents. In T. G. Plante, & C. E. Thoresen (Eds.), *Spirit, science, and health: How the spiritual mind fuels physical wellness* (pp. 143–156). Westport, CT: Praeger.

Cragun, C. L., & Frielander, M. L. (2012). Experiences of Christian clients in secular psychotherapy: A mixed-methods investigation. *Journal of Counseling Psychology*, *59*(3), 379–391.

Friedson, M. L. (2015). Psychotherapy and the fundamentalist client: The aims and challenges of treating Jehovah's Witnesses. *Journal of Religion and Health*, *54*, 693–712. 10.1007/s10943-014-9946-8

Griffith, J. L., & Griffith, M. (2002). *Encountering the sacred in psychotherapy: How to talk with people about their spiritual lives*. New York, NY: Guilford.

Gross, T. (2022, June 2). How the Southern Baptist Convention covered up its widespread sexual abuse scandal. https://www.npr.org/2022/06/02/1102621352/how-the-southern-baptist-convention-covered-up-its-widespread-sexual-abuse-scand

Hathaway, W. L., & Ripley, J. S. (2009). Ethical concerns around spirituality and religion in clinical practice. In J. D. Aten, & M. M. Leach (Eds.), *Spirituality and the therapeutic process: A comprehensive resource from intake to termination* (pp. 25–52). Washington, DC: American Psychological Association.

Hill, P., & Pargament, K. (2003). Advances in the conceptualization and measurement of religion and spirituality: Implications for physical and mental health research. *American Psychologist*, *58*, 64–74.

Hall, T. W., & Edwards, K. J. (2002). The spiritual assessment inventory: A theistic model and measure for assessing spiritual development. *Journal for the Scientific Study of Religion*, *41*, 341–357.

Harris, N., Sisemore, T. A., Pargament, K. I., & Brown, G. S. (2014). The relationship of decline in spiritual struggles to psychotherapy outcomes: Evidence from a large scale survey of psychotherapy clients. *Christian Psychology*, *8*(2), 40–48.

Jerome, A., Heath, M. A., Williams, M. Winters, R., & Cutrer-Pårraga (2023). Traversing trauma: Resilient women's religious and spiritual stories of hope and strength. *Professional Psychology: Research and Practice*, *54*(2), 177–187. 10.1037/pro0000491

Kizilhan, J. I. (2014). Religious and cultural aspects of psychotherapy in Muslim patients from tradition-oriented societies. *International Review of Psychiatry*, *26*(3), 335–343.

Lauer, C., & Hoyer, M. (2019). Almost 1,700 priests and clergy accused of sex abuse are unsupervised. https://www.nbcnews.com/news/religion/nearly-1-700-priests-clergy-accused-sex-abuse-are-unsupervised-n1062396

Leighton, T. J. (2014). The therapeutics of counselling religious clients: Intake and assessment. *International Journal of Mental Health and Addiction*, *12*, 295–311. 10.1007/s11469-013-9454-1

Litjmaer, R., Moodley, R., & Sunderani, S. (2013). The therapist's self-disclosure in crosscultural treatment. *World Academy of Science, Engineering, and Technology*, *7*, 663–667.

McGraw, J. S., Skidmore, S. J., Lefevor, G. T., Docherty, M. & Mahone, A. (2023). Affirming and nonaffirming religious beliefs predicting depression and suicide risk among latter-day saint sexual minorities. *Journal of Counseling Psychology*, *70*(3), 293–306. 10.1037/cou0000659

McLemore, C. W., & Court, J. H. (1977). Religion and psychotherapy—Ethics, civil liberties, and clinical savvy: A critique. *Journal of Consulting and Clinical Psychology*, *45*, 1172–1175.

Murphy, C. (2015). Interfaith marriage is common in U.S., particularly among the recently wed. Pew Research Center. https://www.pewresearch.org/fact-tank/2015/06/02/interfaith-marriage/

Oxhandler, H. K., & Parrish, D. E. (2017). Integrating clients' religion/spirituality in clinical practice: A comparison among social workers, psychologists, counselors, marriage and family therapists, and nurses. *Journal of Clinical Psychology*, *74*, 680–694. 10.1002/jclp.22539

Paine, D. R., Sandage, S. J., Ruffing, E. G., & Hill, P. C. (2018). Religious and spiritual salience, well-being, and psychosocial functioning among psychotherapy clients: Moderator effects for humility. *Journal of Religion and Health*, *57*, 2398–2415. 10.1007/s10943-018-0612-4

Rosenfeld, G. W. (2011). Contributions from ethics and research that guide integrating religion into psychotherapy. *Professional Psychology: Research and Practice*, *42*(2), 192–199. 10.1037/a0022742

Shaler, L. (2019). Respecting the faith of clients and counselors. Counseling Today. https://ct.counseling.org/2019/05/respecting-the-faith-of-clients-and-counselors/

Shooter, S. (2016). *How survivors of abuse relate to God: The authentic spirituality of the annihilated soul.* Farnham, UK: Routledge.

Sunderania, S., & Moodley, R. (2020). Therapists' perceptions of their use of self-disclosure (and nondisclosure) during cross-cultural exchanges. *British Journal of Guidance and Counselling*, *48*(6), 741–756. 10.1080/03069885.2020.1754333

Tener, D., Katz, C., Marmor, A., & Lusky-Weisrose, F. (2020). "I was scared, like never in my life": Children's perspectives of nonfamilial sexual abuse within the Jewish ultraorthodox community in Israel. *Psychology of Violence*, *11*(1), 72–81.

Trusty W. T., Swift J. K., Black S. W., Dimmick A. A., & Penix E. A. (2021). Religious microaggressions in psychotherapy: A mixed methods examination of client perspectives. *Psychotherapy*, *59*(3), 351–362. 10.1037/pst0000408.

8 How to Improve Graduate Preparation for Clinical Practice

Francis A. Martin and Janet P. Turner

Because professional mental health care professionals completed graduate degrees, all of them have opinions about them. Typically, they place a high positive value on their respective programs and experiences as completers of graduate programs. The discussion here seeks to avoid either an easy conclusion that, without relevant evidence, preparation programs are failing or that their success is obvious, understood, and well-known. Instead, the necessary challenge is to first be honest about the real problems that beset preparation programs for mental health care providers. Then, of course, the necessary task of finding solutions to these problems ensues. This chapter aims to identify problems and to recommend solutions for them. Further, it is intended to contribute to the conversation and the consciousness raising that invites others to join the conversation, but also actively to join efforts toward improving preparation programs.

The next chapter is a necessary companion to this one. It presents recommendations that may be taken by individual counselors and therapists, professional associations, state legislatures, licensing boards, social service agencies, and businesses and corporations. Obviously, if reforms in counseling and therapy happen, all of these potential activists are needed in the effort.

A good beginning of this discussion is to be clear about the critically necessary role that graduate programs have in mental health care. The importance of preparation programs and the agencies that accredit them cannot be overestimated. These programs are the portal through which individuals enter the profession of counseling and therapy. An individual who completes a preparation program today may be providing clinical services for 40 years or more. Thus, what these programs do or fail to do imposes immense influence on mental health care for decades into the future.

"There's plenty of legitimate debate in clinical psychology and allied fields, such as psychiatry, social work, and counseling, but at least one proposition should not be particularly controversial: The state of mental

DOI: 10.4324/9781003472469-9

health care is in shambles" (Lilienfeld, 2014, *Evidence-Based Practice: The Misunderstandings Continue*). Concomitant to Lilienfeld's conclusion, professional education for counselors and therapists is "in shambles," too. It is failing. The data that indicate this are overwhelming. They are not new. The data have been published in various forms for many years. The evidence in this book joins, confirms, and adds to these data. No doubt, preparation programs have achieved remarkable success, while their graduates continue to demonstrate ongoing decline in competence and integrity. The accrued data capture the oft-cited quip, "The surgery was a success, but the patient died."

A General Assessment of Preparation Programs

Generally, preparation programs need to be clear about what they aspire to do. This is to ask, "What is their reason for being?" If they aim to produce minimally competent counselors and therapists, they should build their programs around this goal. The need for this emerges from the fact that most clinical preparation programs do not aim to prepare clinicians. While this may appear to be enigmatic, my review of the mission statements of randomly located 100 preparation programs indicates that a minority of presumed clinical preparation programs, including social work, mental health counseling, psychology, and marriage and family therapy, aim to prepare mental health care clinicians. Among the 100 programs, 33 indicated that preparing clinicians—expansively defined—is a feature of their aspirations. The aim or mission of such programs must include minimally competent clinicians. While academic success, including high standing through accreditation and research productivity, is important, it cannot and should not supplant clinical competence. Therefore, clinical preparation programs will be clear about gathering the best information about highly effective therapists and construct their mission, goals, courses, and other actions, accordingly.

Preparing practitioners provides the population of a profession's providers, whether they are physicians, attorneys, or others. If medical schools excluded preparation for practicing physicians or law schools excluded preparation of practicing attorneys, these schools would not likely continue to exist, let alone thrive. What may happen to counseling and therapy if their preparation programs fail to provide minimally competent practitioners?

Anticipating the obligation to prepare minimally competent mental health care clinicians, questions may help to frame the issues that need consideration, including these:

> Can faculty who populate preparation programs describe the characteristics of highly effective clinicians or refer to research that offers help with such a description?

Are faculty competent mental health care clinicians?

On what bases are faculty evaluated as being important to the institutions where they serve?

Are candidates for admission to the profession of mental health care assessed in such ways that indicate positive potential for becoming effective clinicians?

What are the criteria for determining that students are successful in their preparation programs?

What are the specific gatekeeping criteria that the program uses?

Although they are not an exhaustive list, these questions may help faculty and their leaders to consider their reasons for serving in such programs.

The multiple issues that characterize preparation programs cannot be adequately discussed in this chapter, simply due to the necessity of containing a vast amount of information in a relatively small space. Confirmed by numerous sources, as cited elsewhere in this book, suffice it to report that several deficiencies in preparation programs appear in the literature. Among these deficiencies,

Evidence-based teaching is rare.

Clinical efficacy rises only slightly because of graduate preparation programs.

Many programs severely lack emphases on preparing students to practice evidence-based interventions.

Old and non-relevant theories occupy too much space in the curricula of most preparation programs.

Candidates for careers in counseling and therapy are admitted to preparation programs when criteria for admission are weak.

Some programs focus on only one major treatment orientation, including Adlerian Therapy, Integral Therapy, Biblical Therapy, Contemplative Therapy, or others, denying their students the opportunity to gain needed, wide-ranging skills in research-validated therapies. Instead of professional education, according to Nuland (2001, p. 35), these approaches and many others are "indoctrinology," perpetuated by "indoctrinologists," politely but persuasively coercing large numbers of students and, later, practicing clinicians to provide incompetent mental health care. "I am an Adlerian therapist" or "I provide Christian Counseling" are the kinds of statements that indicate indifference, if not opposition to, counseling and therapy that is based on research-validated evidence.

Accreditation appears not to contribute to producing competent clinicians (Refer to information, below.)

Preparation programs vary extremely in size—from around 30 graduate semester hours to 120 graduate semester hours—although their graduates receive licenses that authorize them to practice very similar therapies, depending on state statutes and regulations. A license may be secured after only one year of preparation, on the low side, or after seven years, on the high side.

The level of clinical competence of faculty in preparation programs is generally low and likely does not improve over time.

Also, in anticipation of the recommendations for preparation programs, their leaders and faculty should assess their useful and positive professional assets and ask how they may best utilize them. They should not assume that their considerable assets are effectively utilized by their graduates. Many who study the performance of mental health care providers raise concerns about preparation programs. In short, many have described and attempted to explain the apparent, longstanding, and pervasive disconnection between preparation programs and clinical practice (e.g., Cummings & O'Donohue, 2011; Daniel et al., 2019; Even & Robinson, 2013; Goldberg et al., 2016; Gonsalvez & Crowe, 2014; Hill et al., 2015; Lane, 2023; Levy & Ellison, 2022; Lilienfeld, Ritschel, Lynn, Cautin, & Latzman, 2014; Lwin & Beltrano, 2022; O'Donnell, 2011; O'Donohue, Cummings, & Cummings, 2008; Society for the Advancement of Psychotherapy, no date; Spengler & Pilipis, 2015; Vannatta & Steen, 2019; Wike, Bledsoe, Bellamy, & Grady, 2013; and, Williams, Weinzatl, & Varga, 2021). Stated tersely, O'Donnell (2011, p. 258) calls for "radical reform" of preparation programs.

Specialized Accreditation: Betrayal or Betterment?

Does specialized accreditation improve outcomes for the programs that have it? As this discussion clarifies, the answer usually presupposes that an answer to this question is that specialized accreditation makes a preparation program a good one or, possibly, a superior one. Commonly, an assumption is that specialized accreditation, along with institutional accreditation, establishes a program as better than those that lack such accreditation. Usually, this assumption has a comfortable partner with the assumption that specialized accreditation also very likely produces competent clinicians. Are these assumptions correct?

Does accreditation by their respective agencies enhance the likelihood of preparation programs delivering minimally competent mental health care providers? Apparently, the answer is "no," although the answer depends on the criteria and methods that are used to determine this. Suffice it to report that a common conclusion about social work education is represented succinctly by Lane (2023, p. 27), "The research highlighted a gap between academic input and the realities and challenges of current social work practice, particularly in terms of depth and complexity of the knowledge and skills needed for frontline practice." Many others have examined social work education and reached similar conclusions. More broadly, also with regard to social work education, "the accreditation standards are rather lax" (Thyer & Pignotti, 2015, p. 264). These conclusions have real implications for the clinical work that social workers provide. As Lwin and Beltrano (2022) conclude, "While Evidence-based and Evidence-informed Practice (EBP; EIP) are woven throughout child welfare systems and discussed in social work education, they are rarely applied to everyday service" (p. 166). Advancing this idea to encompass accredited social work preparation programs and with caveats, Wike, Bledsoe, Bellamy and Grady conclude, "Our study found that websites of a random sample of schools of social work revealed little content related to EBP [Evidence-based Practices] or ESI [Evidence-supported Interventions] in general and even less evidence of partnerships between schools of social work and community agencies designed to advance the use of EBP or ESI in social work practice" (p. 445). So far, a research-validated connection between specialized accreditation and improved competence of graduates from social work preparation programs has not been established.

The references to social work education, above, appear to be echoes of data from research about psychology preparation programs and mental health counseling programs. With regard to preparation programs for psychologists, a narrowly gauged research conclusion by Levy and Ellison (2022, p. 376) is that "doctoral-level psychology programs are not sufficiently preparing their students with personality disorder training, which serves as a substantial disservice to both trainees and the public." As a real and unfortunate complement to this conclusion and slightly more specifically, Styck (2012, p. 11) asks whether accreditation of school psychology programs matters. With caveats, she concludes that there is no significant difference between accredited preparation programs and non-accredited programs. More broadly, Spengler and Pilipis (2015) prepared a comprehensive meta-analysis of clinical competence and concluded, "The results from the present meta-analysis establish that experience leads to some, but not much, improvement in clinical decision making—at least as currently and historically trained, practiced, and researched" (p. 372). Additionally, with several suggestions about the general inadequacy of clinical training in graduate programs, Spengler and Pilipis (2015, p. 372) also conclude, "With the glaring challenge these results pose to graduate training programs and practicing clinicians, they also raise important questions about how learning about clinical decision making occurs."

Extending the question about the relevance of accreditation for programs that prepare mental health care providers, Hill and her colleagues raise a simple question, "Is training effective?" The findings of Hill et al. (2015) partially moderate the conclusion that accredited professional education programs may not add significantly to the competence of trainees. Generally, they affirm that trainees in their externships "were able to form stronger working alliances [with their clients]" and "were better able to facilitate improvement in their clients' interpersonal relationships" among other findings (p. 198). However, they also conclude, "On the other hand, trainees did not change in terms of therapist- and client-rated session quality, therapist-rated real relationship, engagement of clients after intake or eighth session, or reductions in client's symptomatic distress" (p. 198). The carefully crafted research of Hill and her colleagues may be the feather in the storm, when compared with, say, the blunt assessment of psychology training programs by O'Donohue, Cummings, and Cummings (2008) who conclude that training programs have failed to prepare mental health care providers with clinical competencies. One of their colleagues, O'Donnell (2011), calls for "radical reform in educating and training" psychologists, with a needed emphasis on clinical competence.

Mental health counseling preparation—or professional counseling—programs show inconsistencies and deficiencies that are similar to those of accredited social work and psychology programs. An indicator of this comes from a study by Williams, Weinzatl, and Varga (2021). They report that "the results of this study suggest that CMHC students may not receive adequate training in couple and family counseling knowledge and skills within their programs." While training in couple and family counseling may be seriously lacking in preparation programs for mental health counselors, this kind of counseling is commonly practiced by mental health counselors. Further, they acknowledge, "CACREP-accredited CMHC programs offer limited preparation for students in couple and family counseling through required coursework."

Even and Robinson report convincing validation of certain outcome variables associated with accreditation by CACREP—the Council for the Accreditation of Counseling Related Educational Programs, by far the most common accreditor of mental health counseling programs. Specifically, the variables that CACREP accreditation supports are that graduates of these programs are more likely than graduates of non-accredited programs to pass standard examinations and less likely to receive ethical complaints against them (Even and Robinson, 2013, p. 30). Such a comparison may provide little reassurance for those who wish to promote program accreditation as a marker of competence of those who complete their programs. After all, to conclude that licensees who complete accredited programs are better—no matter what the specific measure is—than those who do not complete accredited programs may not make the case for how competent or incompetent such completers are. Significantly, according to a study by Martin (2020, pp. 54–72), licensees who complete either an accredited program or a non-accredited program are approximately equally likely—around 20%—to advertise aberrant, inappropriate approaches to counseling and therapy. In their examination of teaching group counseling skills in CACREP-accredited programs, Vannatta and Steen (2019, p. 146) acknowledge that "it is difficult to understand why there is not more of a balance between attending to the development of knowledge and the development of skills." Their observation refers to CACREP-accredited programs, but conclusions very similar to theirs commonly appear in the literature about programs that are accredited by other agencies and that ostensibly prepare mental health care professionals for clinical practice.

Clearly, this is not a thorough study of accreditation of preparation programs for mental health care providers. At least, this report serves to raise important questions about whether these programs prepare minimally competent clinicians. Inevitably, among the questions to be raised is whether accreditation may serve to enhance the academic prowess of preparation program completers far more than equipping them with clinical competencies. Before leaving the matter of accreditation, though, another largely unstudied feature of accreditation involves the accreditation of programs that conspicuously defy and reject the normative standards and values of the profession that presumably endorses these programs through accreditation. Issues related to this are discussed in the next topic.

Religion-Dominated Preparation Programs

For reasonably well-informed individuals, the idea of a Christian school of law likely seems like an odd combination of categories. By what conceivable rationale would anyone attempt to train aspiring attorneys to practice "Christian law," with little or no regard to law that has been duly established by local, state, and national jurisdictions? The combination of "Christian" and "law" would likely seem even more peculiar, if the Christian law school advertised—somewhat proudly—that it holds a view of the Bible as the inerrant Word of God, promotes the Gospel of a Christ-centered life, and roots its law curriculum in a Biblical worldview. Unlikely! Despite how peculiar such a law school would be, the fact is that numerous religion-based institutions and their professionally accredited programs hold such views and define their mental health care preparation in these terms.

Because we come from a CACREP-related history, we will use CACREP accreditation to illustrate certain phenomena, acknowledging that the other major types of accreditation (i.e., APA and NASW) could be presented here, too. Some CACREP-accredited programs and their institutions acknowledge that they hold professional, specialized accreditation by CACREP and simultaneously reject the accreditation. Others claim that they comply with the standards of accreditation, but that they are not accredited. They appear to pretend to be something that they are not—and apparently refuse to be. Thus, the three kinds of illustrations include those programs that are accredited by CACREP and that implicitly oppose the normative standards of the profession, those programs that are accredited but appear overtly to reject the accreditation, and those programs that claim to comply with accrediting standards but that are not accredited.

To be clear about the relevance of these illustrations, the specifically religious views of these programs and their institutions are not the topic of concern. Instead, the topic of concern is mental health care—the fundamentally important matters of meeting the clinically relevant needs of clients, with concern about client autonomy and well-being. Individuals associated with these programs and institutions may believe what they wish to believe. Their wishes should be protected, just as the wishes of those who have alternate religious beliefs or no religious beliefs should be protected. However, insofar as these individuals, programs, and institutions committedly suffuse their specifically religious beliefs with mental health care, the appearance is that they betray the integrity of every other mental health care provider, by defining mental health care in tightly constricted conceptualizations and practices. As such, they should be challenged by the larger mental health care community, if not filtered out of it. Here are the illustrations.

Asbury Seminary

The mission statement of Asbury Seminary says, "Asbury Seminary is a community called to prepare theologically educated, sanctified, Spirit-filled men and women to evangelize and to spread scriptural holiness throughout the world through the love of Jesus Christ, in the power of the Holy Spirit and to the glory of God the Father" (Asbury Seminary, 2023a, *About*). In the context of mental health care, the mission statement poses questions. Among them, if this is the mission of the Seminary, is it also the mission of the accredited mental health counseling program? Whether it is the mission of the accredited mission program or not, does the mission of the Seminary define the mission of the program as an ideological one and not necessarily a clinical one and/or an evidence-based one? In the presentation of its "defining values," the Seminary provides much of the answer to these questions.

> Asbury Seminary will be committed to graduate-level theological education which is faithful to God's Word. Serious biblical, theological, and pastoral reflection which is committed to historic orthodoxy is crucial for the long-term health and vitality of the Church. Asbury Seminary needs a well-trained, missionally alive, spiritually vibrant faculty

> and staff in order to "theologically educate" men and women. Although we are generously catholic with all those who are historically orthodox, we are called to highlight the distinctive contributions of the Wesleyan/Arminian tradition. We will resist attempts to downgrade our programs and scholarship and, instead, we will extend effective pastoral leadership and Wesleyan scholarship around the world. (Asbury Seminary, 2023a, *About*)

In the presentation of the mission of the CACREP-accredited mental health counseling program, Asbury Seminary provides explicit answers to these questions.

> Asbury Seminary's 75-hour Master of Arts in Mental Health Counseling allows you to pursue an understanding of wholeness, boundaries, ethics and diversity through theory and practice as you train to become a professional counselor. Within the degree, you'll understand and integrate a biblical and theological understanding with historical and contemporary theories in order to meet the professional standards of accrediting agencies.
>
> The mission of the Department of Counseling and Pastoral Care is to equip students to serve diverse communities by facilitating healing and growth through reflectively integrating Christian values, principles and resources with pastoral or professional counseling competencies and practices. (Asbury Seminary, 2023b, *Academics*)

Covenant Theological Seminary

The mission statement of Covenant Theological Seminary says, "Covenant Seminary exists to glorify the Triune God by training his servants to walk in God's grace, minister God's Word, and equip God's people—all for God's mission" (Covenant Theological Seminary, 2023, *About Us*). Extending the ideology of the Seminary's mission, the mission of the mental health counseling program says, "The Master of Arts in Counseling (MAC) program at Covenant Seminary is clinically focused and biblically grounded. Our MAC program will help you become a biblically faithful and clinically excellent counselor. We help you harmonize contemporary counseling theories and techniques with a Christian worldview, and when you graduate you are prepared for licensure, changed by a community of grace, and ready to help hurting people" (Covenant Theological Seminary, 2023a, *Master of Arts in Counseling*). The Seminary elaborates its commitment to a "biblically grounded" ideology, in its presentation of "The 5 Foundations" of the mental health counseling program. The most relevant and first one is "A BIBLICAL FRAMEWORK: Of the program's 75 credit hours, 15 provide a theological foundation for clinical practice. With this biblical understanding of God, human nature, and the process of change, our graduates evaluate and develop gospel-centered counseling theories and techniques" (Covenant Theological Seminary, 2023a, *Master of Arts in Counseling*). What is "gospel-centered counseling?" In the context of discussing a major health care service—counseling and therapy—how does gospel-centered therapy compare with, say, gospel-centered pharmacy, nursing, physical therapy, or proctology.

Trinity Evangelical Divinity School

Trinity Evangelical Divinity School presents more complexity, with several locations, and more breadth in its academic offerings than its name suggests. The School describes its mission, stating, "Trinity's mission is to educate men and women to engage in God's redemptive work in the world by cultivating academic excellence, Christian faithfulness, and lifelong learning. As an institution committed to inerrant Scripture, given by God as our final authority for faith and life, we hold ourselves accountable to it and to each other with regard to these values as we cultivate the mission mentioned above" (Trinity Evangelical Divinity School, 2023, *Mission and Values*). It adds, "We are here to model and to engender Christ centeredness in all that we do. The lordship of Christ should affect and be evident in every aspect of education, relationship, and endeavor at Trinity" (Trinity Evangelical Divinity School, 2023a). With regard to its CACREP-accredited mental health counseling program, Trinity Evangelical Divinity School says, "Our purpose as a divinity school is to know the Gospel, live the Gospel, and make the Gospel known. In today's ever-changing culture, Trinity immerses students in a community of biblical orthodoxy and practical living" (Trinity Evangelical Divinity School, 2023b, *Statement of Faith*). TEDS affirms these words, stating, "As the verbally inspired Word of God, the Bible is without error in the original writings, the complete revelation of His will for salvation, and the ultimate authority by which every realm of human knowledge and endeavor should be judged" (Trinity Evangelical Divinity School, 2023b, *Statement of Faith*).

Lincoln Christian University

Lincoln Christian University emphasizes that "It is a 60-hour, seminary based, clinical mental health counseling degree grounded in a Biblical worldview" (Lincoln Christian University, 2023, *MA in Counseling*). And, strangely, the Lincoln Christian University declares, "The addition of CACREP accreditation does not change the purpose of LCU's MA in Counseling program, which is to help students integrate a Biblical worldview with current and historical psychological theories and evidence-based, developmentally sound counseling methods in order to assist students to grow in counseling competencies, spiritual well-being, interpersonal relationships and personal awareness" (Lincoln Christian University, 2023a, *MA in Counseling Receives CACREP Accreditation*). Possibly, this conditional view of its accreditation comes from its view of The Bible. Lincoln Christian University states, "The Bible, the Old and New Testament Scriptures, is the uniquely inspired Word of God (2 Tim. 3:14–17; 2 Peter 1:16–21). The Bible is the rule of faith and practice for Christians. We affirm that Scripture is the authoritative revelation from God by which we know God's will and Christ's authority" (Lincoln Christian University, 2023b, *Statement of Faith*).

Erskine Theological Seminary

Erskine Theological Seminary advertises its Master of Arts in Christian Counseling (MACC), saying, "CACREP/Licensing: The MACC degree has been developed to CACREP standards" (Erskine Theological Seminary, 2023, *Accreditation*). With regard to the mission of the MACC, the Seminary says, "The MACC is a professional degree that prepares students to be effective, licensed counselors with a strong Christian worldview, eligible to work in any public or private institution providing psychological care. The 60-hour program is intended to provide a broad base of scriptural knowledge with an intensive, state-mandated core set of competencies" (Erskine Theological Seminary, 2023a, *Master of Arts in Mental Health Counseling*). These statements raise questions: If the MACC program has been developed to CACREP standards, why is the program not accredited? If the MACC program prepares "licensed counselors with a strong Christian worldview," what is a Christian worldview and how is this worldview related to "providing psychological care?" Is this the Seminary's way of opportunistically utilizing a mental health counseling preparation program that prepares mental health counselors to promote its strongly held religious beliefs, while evading the demands of being a part of the profession for which it ostensibly prepares licensees? Similarly, would the Seminary advertise that it complies with institutional accreditation without having it? Among its many statements that define its academic and clinical programs, a few of them may indicate reasons for the Seminary's avoidance of seeking accreditation of its mental health counselor preparation program and being a part of the profession for which it alleges to prepare its students. The Seminary says,

> OUR MISSION & OUR VISION: The mission of Erskine College is to glorify God as a Christian academic community where students integrate

> knowledge and faith, equipped to flourish as whole persons prepared for lives of service, leadership, and influence through the pursuit of undergraduate liberal arts, graduate, and seminary education.
>
> Erskine Theological Seminary (Theological Graduate Programs) Mission: Erskine Theological Seminary prepares men and women to fulfill the Great Commission of Jesus Christ through theological higher education that is ecclesial, missional, and confessional.
>
> Vision (How we lift the burden): Erskine Theological Seminary is a Biblical, Reformed, and Evangelical Seminary community of learning sustained in prayer, supported by a growing constituency, united in faith, and fueled by the power of the Holy Spirit for gospel transformation in every area of life. (Erskine Theological Seminary, 2023b, *Mission and Values*)

The Seminary emphasizes that it is "Biblical" and "Evangelical." Although it prepares its students for state-issued licenses, the Seminary declares that it is "committed to preparing students for ministry. Because we are committed to the Church, our primary focus is on preparing men and women to serve in Christ's Church." (Erskine Theological Seminary, 2023b, *Mission and Values*). Taken together, the Seminary's statements confirm that the Seminary utilizes its religion as therapy. As such, along with many similar institutions, it appears to immerse in an anti-intellectual, pre-scientific, highly conditioned, and arbitrary approach to therapy. Its place among mental health care preparation programs should be questioned and challenged.

Christian Theological Seminary

The Christian Theological Seminary defines its mission, stating, "To form disciples of Jesus Christ for church and community leadership to serve God's transforming of the world" (Christian Theological Seminary, 2023, *Mission*). To prepare its students for licensing as mental health counselors, Christian Theological Seminary offers a Master of Arts in Clinical Mental Health Counseling. The Seminary says that the "program provides professional counseling preparation and spiritual/theological integration for mental health counselors, pastoral psychotherapists and spiritual care specialists" (Christian Theological Seminary, 2023a, *Master of Arts in Mental Health Counseling*). This description may suffice, but the Seminary's description of the program also says, "The MACMHC degree prepares students for certified membership in the American Association of Pastoral Counselors. It is guided by the Council for Accreditation of Counseling & Related Educational Programs (CACREP) standards and the professional orientation of the American Counseling Association (ACA)"

(Christian Theological Seminary, 2023a, *Master of Arts in Mental Health Counseling*). This statement is truly lacking in reason, if not integrity. On the one side, it says that the Christian Theological Seminary will prepare its students for membership in AAPC and, on the other side, it follows the guidelines for training of the American Counseling Association. Along with similar institutions, is this another expression of an inauthentic, utilitarian, and opportunistic method through which the Seminary and its graduates can secure a license, without having to affiliate with the profession or association that enables them to secure a license? It prepares students and graduates for one thing, while presuming to practice another. It pretends to associate with CACREP and ACA, while preparing its students and graduates to practice outside the boundaries and accountability of CACREP and ACA. The Seminary asserts that its mental health counseling program is guided by CACREP standards, as if it may be accredited, but lacks accreditation by CACREP. As such, the Seminary appears to mislead prospective students.

Grand Rapids Theological Seminary

A unit of Cornerstone University, Grand Rapids Theological Seminary advertises a mental health counseling program. About the program, the Seminary asserts, "The Counseling Division faculty continue to review and assess the M.A. in Clinical Mental Health Counseling program to identify necessary changes to improve the program and its outcomes as well as to align with the standards of the Council for Accreditation of Counseling and Related Educational Programs (CACREP)" (Cornerstone University, 2023, *Master of Arts in Mental Health Counseling/Accreditation*). Further, it says, "The M.A. in clinical mental health counseling degree will prepare you clinically for a future career as a Licensed Professional Counselor" (Cornerstone University, 2023a, *Master of Arts in Mental Health Counseling*). This statement is misleading. The Seminary cannot assure its students and graduates that they can be licensed because some states require that prospective licensees must have completed a CACREP-accredited program.

Grand Rapids Theological Seminary is a unit of Cornerstone University. On the "About" page of Cornerstone University, the identity of both the Seminary and the University is clearly presented through these statements.

> At Cornerstone University, we are committed to the steadfast teachings of Christ. We teach, learn and live out God's word in all things. And we train and equip future leaders to do the same in whatever environment they are called to.

> Mission: Cornerstone University exists to empower men and women to excel as influencers in our world for Christ by offering a student-focused learning community where Jesus Christ is central. (Cornerstone University, 2023, *About*)

Grand Rapids Theological Seminary can "align with the standards of CACREP," but should they advertise that it aligns with such standards without normative external review? No doubt, Cornerstone University, of which the Seminary is a unit, would never dare to advertise that it aligns with academic, institutional accreditation, without actually having such accreditation. So, by what contorted rationale do Cornerstone University and Grand Rapids Theological Seminary advertise that they are something that they likely cannot be? Along with similar institutions, is this a way for Cornerstone University and Grand Rapids Theological Seminary to impound the opportunity for graduates of the mental health counseling program to receive a state-issued license to practice, without the inconvenience of minimal compliance with normative professional standards for such programs?

Missio Theological Seminary

Profiled elsewhere in this book, Missio Theological Seminary uses its refusal of accreditation as a selling point for its mental health counseling program. It says, "… you will not need to have graduated from a CACREP school to be eligible to apply for LPC in NJ." (Missio Theological Seminary, 2023b, *Counseling Licensure*). When the refusal of professional accreditation appears as a selling point for a clinical preparation program, it risks looking like ideological narrow-mindedness that withholds itself from professional accountability. It looks like out-of-control opportunism. Insofar as this may be a correct conclusion, does the Seminary betray the integrity of the faith by which it ostensibly lives?

The eight institutions and programs that are briefly presented here serve as illustrations. The number of such institutions is much larger than the small number presented here. To reiterate, the religious views of the institutions reviewed here should be protected. Nothing here is intended to malign these institutions and programs. They are using the current rules to their advantage. This means that the rules are much more the problem than these institutions and programs alone. As noted already in this book, at this time, the broadly defined profession of counseling and therapy has no way to filter treatment approaches into clinical practice nor to filter them out. Similarly, the profession cannot effectively filter out preparation programs that conspicuously dilute and compromise the profession.

Also, with regard to the many institutions and programs that opportunistically take inappropriate advantage of the rules, note must be taken of the profound and consequential failure of the major professional associations that worked for several decades to establish licensing for mental health care providers. In short, they failed to establish a secure connection between their programs and specialized accreditation (e.g., CACREP, APACOA, CSWE, or CAOMFTE) and licensing. As such, more than securing professionally accountable preparation programs and their profession, they became inadvertent collaborators with those who would harm them.

The mental health counseling programs briefly profiled here appear to reject the values of the profession that endorses it. The programs that are accredited promote their belief that The Bible is the inerrant Word of God. Regardless of longstanding and substantial scholarship that rejects this belief, individuals may believe in biblical inerrancy if they wish. However, insofar as they presume to regard their apparent absolutism as the guiding authority in mental health care, they harm counseling and therapy as a health care profession. To protect their beliefs, they appear to deny decades of valuable and necessary research about mental-emotional-relational problems. With certainty, none of these believers would restrict the dental care of their children to dentistry as it was practiced in or before the first century. Apart from mental health care, they would reject health care that boasted about its pre-scientific, anti-intellectual, and cultish rejection of good evidence for such health care.

If these institutions truly hold the beliefs that they conspicuously avow, why would they contaminate their beliefs with the approval of a largely secularist agency such as the American Counseling Association, American Psychological Association, or National Association of Social Workers? Why would they associate their "Biblical Worldview" with the inconveniently large and re-orienting views of professionally accountable mental health care? Is their entry into mental health care an acknowledgment of their assumption that their presumed stalwart beliefs are, in truth, inadequate and that, due to this inadequacy, they need an external agency and licensing to approve of them? Or, do they lack a believable foundation of self-approving authenticity and, lacking this, apply the makeup of mental health care to attempt to look better to themselves?

Surely, the leaders and faculty in these institutions and programs that promote biblical inerrancy, gospel-centered and Christ-centered therapy, along with closely related ideologies, understand that their views of The Bible lack internal consistency. Whether their point of reference is The Bible or derivatives of The Bible, such as *The Westminster Confession of Faith*, they select passages, mostly from The Bible, to accommodate views for which they need support and manifest obliviousness to many other views for which they do not want to be held accountable. For example, if they genuinely believe in inerrancy or similar things, how could they also pursue degrees in and practice medicine, pharmacy, psychotherapy, or any other approach to healing that may be pursued in the twenty-first century. After all, in James 5:15 ESV, The Bible says, "And the prayer of faith will save the one who is sick, and the Lord will raise him up." Usually, their rationalization for not accrediting the Lord as the direct instrument of healing is that the Lord works through those who heal sickness such as physicians or pharmacists. Still, the so-called inerrant view is that prayer, not trained physicians, heals.

However, the more carefully such biblical messages are studied, the less viable their rationalizations are. For example, more narrowly, with regard to trauma and distress, The Bible says, "Give strong drink to the one who is perishing, and wine to those in bitter distress" (Proverbs 31:6 ESV). This is "good news" for everyone who lives with compulsions to medicate their distress with alcohol. And, if taken seriously, those who practice counseling and therapy or almost any other form of health care should know that, if they comply with this biblical injunction, they should encourage others to take "strong drink" and "wine" as their medicine.

Apparently, training in counseling and therapy, particularly when it leads to a state-issued license, is not only unnecessary but also an act of disobedience of God. After all, as another reminder for those whose inerrancy views guide their healing-related behaviors, "Is anyone among you sick? Let him call for the elders of the church, and let them pray over him, anointing him with oil in the name of the Lord" (James 5:14 ESV). Those who practice counseling and therapy with an affirmation of the inerrancy view of The Bible obviously need, first, to ensure that they go to church leaders and pray for healing and, then, of course, have plenty of oil on hand. Probably, instead of re-assuring their hoped-for followers of the importance of personal beliefs and faith, they appear to suffer from their inhumanely manicured view of The Bible as the inerrant Word of God. This appears to be more an act of God-hoarding than a minimally honest commitment to mental health care.

Preparation Programs and Clients

With regard to specialized accreditation, as noted earlier, "The surgery was a success, but the patient died." The necessary question at the end of this brief discussion of the accreditation of professional education and training in mental health care is "When, if not now, will the major associations and honest colleges and universities begin to work toward establishing the credibility and durability of accreditation of mental health care preparation and licensing?"

In sum, when the value of accrediting professional preparation programs for prospective mental health care providers is examined, two things are clear. One, accredited programs can and do justifiably claim that they comply with the accreditation standards of their profession and that this refers almost exclusively to their minimal academic sufficiency. Two, accredited programs tacitly denounce the needs of those for whom such programs exist—the clients for whom their graduates will provide professional services. Or, regardless of the role of religion in accredited programs, as Vannatta and Steen (2019) describe their reaction to this disturbing imbalance, "it is difficult to understand why there is not more of a balance between attending to the development of knowledge and the development of skills" (p. 146). This imbalance is the condition of currently accredited programs.

Chapter 3 of this book includes a discussion of five organizations that sell licenses, with most of them having little or no basis for minimal credibility related to integrity or competence in counseling and therapy. Many of such organizations associate themselves with unaccredited colleges, seminaries, universities, or similar organizations. Commonly, these unsubstantial "academic" institutions are accredited by the Accrediting Commission International. The Accrediting Commission International is located in Beebe, Arkansas, after having suffered mandated closing and removal from other states (Academic.com, 2021). Wikipedia says,

> Accrediting Commission International (ACI), also known as Accrediting Commission International for Schools, Colleges, and Theological Seminaries, possibly associated with International Accrediting Commission (IAC), also known as International Accrediting Commission for Schools, Colleges and Theological Seminaries, is an unrecognized educational accreditation corporation in the United States. It primarily accredits religious schools, including seminaries and Bible colleges, and also offers accreditation to non-U.S. schools that offer business education programs. It is on a 2009 list of accreditation mills in College and University, the journal of the American Association of Collegiate Registrars and Admissions Officers. (Wikipedia, 2021)

Clients' views and understanding of mental health care preparation programs are largely unknown. On their behalf, though, note should be taken of their likely confusion that comes from multiple titles for degrees that their providers advertise. If they look for a therapist, what degree should appeal to them? In which degree, if any, should they believe? Without including titles of degrees, such as the PSC.D. or D.PSc., along with many others, which one(s) of these, if any, should clients identify with competent services?

M.A?	M.S.S.W.?	M.Ed.?
M.C.?	M.A.H.S.?	M.A.O.P.?
D.Min?	Ph.D.?	D.B.H.?

D.Div.?	M.D.?	PSYA.D.?
Th.D.?	M.S.W.?	M.S.N?
Ed.D.?	M.Div.?	M.S.?
Psy.D.?	DSW?	M.M.F.T?
M.H.D.L.?	D.O.?	M.A.M.H.C?

This list is not a complete one, but as limited as it is, it is likely a source of confusion, if not dismay, among prospective, conscientious clients who wish to understand the qualifications of therapists. However, the titles of degrees are a relatively small source of confusion, when it is compared with the number of titles for state-issued licenses. Martin (2020, pp. 254–257) reports a list of almost 200 titles for state-issued licenses. As such, this number does not include the many different licenses that are issued by non-state organizations. And, when the virtually limitless number of treatment models and orientation is added to the marketplace where prospective clients search for help, their confusion likely becomes even more intense and may prohibit them from seeking and receiving the help they need.

At least, clients should be able to expect a clearer picture of their providers than they can now see. Degree programs should be much more consistent in admission standards, graduation requirements, clinical competence, accreditation standards, and more. More broadly and necessarily, clients should be able to expect that their providers are competent clinicians. At this time, professional associations and preparation programs cannot give them this assurance. The burden of connecting academic acumen and clinical competence falls on the shoulders of preparation programs.

Strategic and Practical Recommendations

Many researchers have described the deficiencies of preparation programs. Merely counting or accounting for deficiencies is in itself deficient. Much more is needed. Actions are needed. Recognizing that a list of recommended actions is not likely to be complete nor readily utilized or necessarily utilizable by those who could be utilizing them, truly useful recommendations for preparation programs would likely include the following ones.

Assess and Affirm Faculty and Program Leaders' Assets

The importance of this may be simpler than it, at first, appears. In short, if faculty know what resources are available, including goodwill, positive expectations, academic talent, clinical talent, a network of supporters, positive relationships with administrative superiors, and so on, along with staff, funding, facilities, and so on, they will have established a foundation for developing strategies through which important constituents'—mainly, clients'—needs may be met.

Engage Constituent Representatives

Those who have important interests in a preparation program and its outcomes can assist in assessing the potential of a program. When the potential is directed toward equipping clinically competent counselors and therapists, all constituent groups and individuals can also assist with needed changes.

Emphasize Clinical Preparation

Preparation programs need to shift toward becoming clinical preparation programs, as a significant and necessary priority. Lacking this emphasis, the practice of counseling and therapy is likely to continue its slide toward definitional incompetence. When implemented, though, clinical preparation should include established standards for competent clinical performance, not only for students, to be sure, but also for the practicing, independent clinicians that they will become.

Move Beyond Theories

Preparation programs need to allow traditional theories of counseling and therapy to expire and to build on the substantial body of evidence for training clinicians. Evidence-based training including evidence-based teaching and clinical supervision is available. Preparation programs need to throw away the outdated belief that their students should choose their theory. Having to choose a theory has too much in common with choosing a personal, religious orientation. Such an expectation of students, graduates, and licensees perpetuates and exacerbates the seemingly inexorable decline of professional competence.

Build on Evidence That Clarifies What Highly Effective Therapists Do

Preparation programs need to carefully study and integrate into their basic functioning the evidence that facilitates the development of competent clinicians. The common expectation that professional preparation programs aspire to excellence is defied by the evidence to the contrary. Diligent, persistent program-saturated focus on developing competent counselors and therapists can draw from extensive literature that defines effective counselors and therapists (e.g., Blatt, Sanislow, Zuroff, & Pilkonis, 1996; Delgadillo et al., 2022; Eells, 1999; Fox, 2023; Goldfried, Raue, & Castonguay, 1998;

Huhra, Yamokoski-Maynhart, & Prieto, 2008; Lafferty, Beutler, & Crago, 1989; Liszewski, 2022; Martin & Turner, 2020; Owen et al., 2019; Skovholt & Jennings, 2004; Vaz & Sousa, 2021; Wampold & Owen, 2021).

Build an Evidence-Based Curriculum

No doubt, huge volumes of research confirm the effectiveness of counseling and therapy. However, typically the research is not utilized in preparation programs. Faculty should not assume that their knowledge of research-supported therapies is effectively utilized by their graduates. Such assumptions are challenged by many researchers, including Daniel et al. (2019). They raise caution about vaunted belief in evidence-based therapies, saying, "Despite continued emphasis on the dissemination of evidence-based therapies in the research literature, and increased access to information and resources via the Internet, many practitioners, clinical educators, and trainees note continued barriers to incorporating scientific evidence into the provision and supervision of clinical care" (p. 207). Faculty in preparation programs must explore the possibility that their programs may be one of the barriers to which Daniel et al refer.

Leaders and faculty in preparation programs need to examine the activities in their programs that may mitigate against the appropriate, clinical utilization of research-validated evidence. They may ask, "How do we ensure that students acquire awareness of and skills in supporting their clinical judgments with empirically validated evidence?" Or, "To what degree does our preparation program stand more firmly on various ideologies about counseling and therapy, teaching, clinical work, religion, and others, including conventional theories, than evidence-based approaches to counseling and therapy?" Generally, the appearance of preparation programs is that, instead of advancing and relying on valuable and agreed-upon evidence, ideologies reign. As a consequence of this ideological regality, practicing counselors and therapists enact their ideologies and, with no more than their clinical fantasies, merely invent orientations to their work. Instead of ideologies, as Whitney (2021, p. 18) wisely concludes, "With the establishment of evidence-based lists [of treatments], one could make the argument that there may not be a need to study PHTs [potentially harmful therapies] if every clinician practiced ESTs and EBP" [empirically supported treatments and evidence-based practices]. If clinicians practice ESTs and EBPs, they should begin their preparation programs.

An evidence-based curriculum should include evidence-based teaching. While this is a common deficiency in clinical preparation programs, several research reports about evidence-based teaching have emerged during the last two decades. Resources for understanding and implementing evidence-based teaching are available (e.g., Allan, 2019; Feinstein, Heiman, & Yager, 2015; Mackrill & Iwakabe, 2013; Malott, Hall, Sheely-Moore, Krell, & Cardaciotto, 2014; Martin & Turner, 2020; Osberg, 1997; Plakun, Sudak, & Goldberg, 2009; Wheeler & Delaney, 2008).

Carefully Assess Candidates for Admission to Clinical Preparation Programs

Because graduate programs are the portal through which individuals enter into the profession of counseling and therapy, the importance of the process, procedures, standards, and other reasons for admitting candidates for these programs cannot be overstated. The necessary question is whether the selection of candidates for admission to clinical preparation programs elevates the probability that graduates of these programs will become effective and competent clinicians.

Walfish and Moreira (2005) observe that the three most commonly cited variables for admission to graduate programs in marriage and family therapy are interview performance, grade point average, and personal statement (p. 400). Also, they observe that the criteria for interview performances and personal statements are highly ambiguous. This self-imposed ambiguity becomes more ambiguous, as highlighted by Ivey and Partington (2014) in their study of woundedness. They conclude, "One of the biggest challenges for those charged with selecting applicants for healing professions such as clinical psychology is to discriminate between facilitative and obstructive woundedness" (p. 174). Apparently, raters of candidates leaned toward suspicion of prospective students who reported that they overcame wounding experiences and similarly leaned toward doubt about prospective students who expressed current woundedness. The implication of this is that those who decide to admit students into their programs look for prospects who seem to be a lot like themselves. As another challenge to preparation program leaders and faculty, Hsueh et al. (2020, p. 118) advise, "Given the importance of programmatic commitments to diversity in students' decisions, there is a need for programs to critically evaluate existing policies, curricula, graduate training experiences, and the admissions process to strengthen their commitments to fostering inclusion."

More broadly and presumably, faculty in preparation programs generally understand that whom they admit to their programs not only shapes the outcomes of their respective programs but also influences the future of their profession. Allowing for this, a recent and not so surprising observation by Coogan and Homrich (2018) is that there is "a lack of supportive evidence for useful admissions procedures" (p. 282). Insightfully, Harwig adds, "[T]he emerging consensus from research participants regarding the counseling profession's graduate admissions screening processes is that these processes are an important responsibility entered into conscientiously and collaboratively while at risk of inconsistency, subjectivity, and need for improvement" (Harwig, 2021, *Counselor Educators' Perceptions of Their Gatekeeping Role in Assessing Personal Characteristics during Admissions Screening*).

Protect Students' Personal Beliefs, While Preparing Them for Competent Clinical Work

Successfully navigating the transition from being outside the profession of counseling and therapy to being on the inside as a competent therapist involves multiple levels of change. Indeed, the work and service of counselors and therapists call on them to pursue issues with their clients that they would not likely, in many cases, pursue with anyone else. This refers to such things as asking questions and expecting answers about hidden fears, marital betrayal, poor parenting, shame-saturated thinking and behavior, and so on. For most students and fresh graduates, the transition necessitates stressful experiences, particularly as they carry the demands that inhere in adapting toward competence in their clinical work.

The process of transitioning from outside to inside the profession includes professional accountability from those who train them. Such accountability requires that instructors, mentors, clinical supervisors, and others who oversee the development of students and early career counselors and therapists give attention to the well-being of their development. How well do the overseers maintain an honest and safe environment for them? How well do the overseers demonstrate respect for differences between themselves and those whom they oversee? How well do the overseers demonstrate fidelity to professional standards, including gatekeeping? How accurately do the overseers assess the impact of the power differential between themselves and the ones being overseen? Obviously, many other relevant questions about professional oversight could be raised. Suffice it to conclude, though, that faculty, their leaders, and clinical supervisors elsewhere must hold themselves to standards of healthy human relationships (e.g., honesty and respect for others) and professional accountability.

Develop Consistency among Preparation Programs

Currently, extreme inconsistency among preparation programs is conspicuous and pervasive. For example, a casual search of many major universities easily locates, say, a social work program in which 32 graduate semester hours are required and a counseling psychology program in which 110 graduate semester hours are required—programs within the same institution. If the aim of these programs is to equip their graduates to become competent clinicians, this inconsistency reeks of failure, either for the social workers or the psychologists. To achieve licensing, why should one licensure track program enable individuals to complete the process in one year, while another licensure track program and the residency that follows require seven years, recognizing that their clinical services are very much alike? And, by what conceivable rationale—particularly in looking at the fact of declining competence and the cacophonous world of preparation programs—should these extraordinary differences exist in one university, as they commonly do?

Deleterious inconsistency among preparation programs may be observed in relation to several other differences. Some will be comfortably connected with a major mental health care professional association, while others have no such connection. Some will display numerous indicators of tightly structured, anti-scientific, exclusionary, and ideological orientations, such as those that advocate for a Bible-based approach to therapy, while others display numerous indicators of their commitment to intellectual and clinical diversity, evidence-based clinical services, and more. Some vigorously promote gender equity, while others vigorously oppose it. Some are rigidly and permanently attached to an ideology—clinical or other—while others seek to be open and adaptable. And so on. Along with others, these inconsistencies have mired counseling and therapy in a swamp of massive uncertainty.

Utilize Technology

"Counselor educators [along with psychologist and social worker preparation trainers] need to increase the importance placed on technology in counselor education programs. The movement of technology into increasingly primary roles in health care is indicative of the need for it to become a primary focus during the education and training of counselors" (Wilkinson & Reinhardt, 2015, p. 416). The specific applications of technology that will enhance the development of competent mental health care providers are numerous. One of many good resources for this is *The Journal of Technology in Counselor Education and Supervision*. Another good one is Jewell, Anthony and Murphys's article, "Utilizing Technology in Social Work Education: Development of the Technology Effectiveness and Social Connectedness Scale" (2021).

To extend the emphasis on utilizing technology, preparation programs could provide valuable assistance to practicing mental health clinicians, particularly their respective graduates. Specifically, a need among practicing clinicians is access to research reports. A common and correct observation about these colleagues is that they do not utilize needed, relevant research. In response to this need, preparation programs and the institutions of which they are units could provide access to search platforms such as

EBSCO Host or other similar search platforms. Such access would not only help these colleagues; it would also likely bolster institutional loyalty.

Explore Innovative Methods for Improving Clinical Effectiveness

The examples of possibilities for innovative methods are numerous. Whatever the methodology may be, it should have good evidence to support it. An example of this may be quantifying therapeutic language (Miller, 2023), as an indicator of competence or potential competence. Another example, provided by Montan et al. (2022), demonstrates a careful examination of how to improve training within a commonly known model of psychotherapy—in their study, the model is psychodynamic psychotherapy. Other useful examples may be found in Hahn, Weck, Witthøft, and Kühne (2023); Kaslow et al. (2009); Kühne, Heinze, Maaß, and Weck (2022); and Teichman, Berant, Shenkman, and Ramot (2022).

Develop a Clinical Curriculum

No doubt, the development of a sufficient, clinical curriculum requires years, mainly because of ongoing change. Change may come in the form of new, evidence-based models of interventions, discoveries in neuroscience, revisions of the DSM, and so on. A clinical curriculum will require ongoing adaptation, just as the process of counseling and therapy with an individual client requires adaptation. With change as an ever-present reality, faculty and their leaders will make many decisions about what and how to deliver the program for their students and their profession. The critically important role of faculty leaders should be enhanced, through secure and appropriate salaries, to be sure, but also through clinical, academic, and intellectual freedom. However, given the chaotic and cacophonous condition of curricula among preparation programs, faculty and their leaders must also accommodate the necessity of preparing competent mental health care clinicians, regardless of their individual preferences. At least, this includes standards for the content of curricula and the size of the program, with demonstrable emphasis on developing competent clinicians. Without such an emphasis, a better option may be to terminate the program. While some clinically deficient programs need to end, others that place a relatively low priority on training students to become clinically competent may have other priorities that easily justify their important role in counseling and therapy. A commonly described alternative to training students for clinical competence are programs that place a high priority on faculty research and publishing. While such programs may not be directly oriented toward preparing clinicians, they often add some of the necessary evidence, insights, and techniques for those who prepare clinicians. Thus, such programs are necessary.

Another significant feature of developing a clinical curriculum is the need to seek a level of coherence among programs that supports credibility for all programs. While this should not involve uniformity, it should involve coherence and consensus about the characteristics of skilled clinicians and general agreements about how to train them. Among other difficult challenges, this involves urgently needed compromises from all of the major mental health types of organizations and licensing. Simply put, there is no future excuse for programs through which licensing may be achieved, with only 30 graduate semester hours required in one program and more than 100 in another program. When their respective graduates receive state-issued licenses and, subsequently, deliver very similar clinical services, the justification for this difference is no longer available.

The "right" curriculum will also be suffused with professional accountability, with a clear and necessary emphasis on the well-being of clients who receive or will receive mental health care from students and the eventual licensees they become. This means that clinically sophisticated programs will engage prospective therapists in achieving minimal standards of competence, as defined by research and the profession. In application, out of a clear commitment to clients, these programs will exclude those who cannot serve clients well. Or, as the Society for the Advancement of Psychotherapy (no date/online) says, in its article titled, "Graduate Programs Must Take Greater Responsibility for Students Who Are Not Achieving Appropriate Outcomes and May Not Be Suitable as Therapists,

> This can be a touchy subject. Yet, just like any other profession, students will vary in performance and some may not have the potential to be effective therapists. It is very difficult to accurately assess who will be inappropriate for clinical work during the graduate school application process. Therefore, once it is clear a student is not capable of providing appropriate clinical care, we should take it upon ourselves to ensure (with empathy and care) that they seek alternative career paths. Educators should ask themselves, "Would I want my partner/family member seeing this student?"

Unfortunately, faculty in clinical preparation programs generally believe that their students are profoundly precocial and will almost inevitably succeed, a delusion that may be fueled by students' admiration and idealization of faculty. The evidence clearly indicates that many of their students and the practicing clinicians that they become do not possess skills that may qualify them to be regarded as competent. The primary obligation of faculty is to ensure as best as they can that their graduates can provide competent professional care for their clients. This is the singularly most important marker of a successful clinical preparation program. Achieving this way of helping students to develop as clinicians should begin with admissions practices and by engaging students in clinical work from their earliest days in their graduate program. And, during their earliest days, students may, for example, be involved in clinical work as a client in "group therapy" that, among other things, is led by an advanced student and one of their clinical faculty. This or similar initiatives can help fulfill the program faculty's obligation to ensure that clients are likely to receive competent clinical services.

Institutionalize Practitioner-Scholars as Faculty

Those who prepare others to provide clinical services should be providing clinical services and include their supervisees in sessions that the teacher leads, as a way to provide an experiential model for how therapy is done—and hopefully, done well. In clinical preparation programs, skilled clinicians should have equal status, if not more status, with traditional scholars.

As curricula move toward increasing emphasis on developing competent counselors and therapists, they will be delivered by programs that recruit and hire faculty who have demonstrated effective clinical skills, including those who demonstrate effective clinical supervision. This evokes the question, "Who is qualified to serve as faculty in mental health care provider preparation programs?" Obviously, tradition dictates that those who hold relevant doctoral degrees and indicate potential for scholarly productivity usually have priority over others. Clinical competence is almost never a criterion for selecting faculty. This must change. Indeed, in many selection procedures, emphasis on degrees and the potential for scholarly productivity should be subordinated to the necessity of selecting individuals who can demonstrate high clinical competency. Program leaders should give at least equal standing for "professors of practice" as they give to faculty who are selected according to traditional criteria.

Established academic preparation programs in counseling and psychotherapy do not usually favor the effective training of competent counselors and therapists. Indeed, as several researchers, cited elsewhere in this book, consistently affirm, preparation programs are not generally effective. In their study of core clinical competencies in marriage and family training programs, D'Aniello and Hertlein (2017, p. 223) "propose that using the core competencies as a guide for quantifying and assessing student progress can assist MFT faculty in their gatekeeping responsibilities." Whether the core competencies are used for gatekeeping functions or not, an important question is "Why are the core competencies not already utilized for assessing students' progress toward becoming clinically competent?" When attention is turned toward faculty, another question is obviously important. "Why are the core clinical competencies not utilized to assess faculty effectiveness in their clinical work?"

The answer to this question involves (1) the fact that most faculty in counselor and therapist preparation programs are not practicing therapists (e.g., Perez-Rojaz, Bartheolomew, and Joy (2022), (2) faculty are generally prisoners of the mythology that, because they are training others to be therapists, they are necessarily competent therapists, and (3) their students often have widely different needs and expectations (e.g., Turns, Nalbone, Hertlein, & Wetchler, 2014), and, as almost inevitable outcomes, neutralizes the potential and necessary influence on students' development of clinical competence. These deficits have real, practical, and long-lasting consequences for graduates and licensees. For example, in their study of sexuality training in counseling psychology programs, Mollen, Burns, Lee, and Abbott (2020) conclude that sexuality training is largely outdated and that, among other proposals, faculty need training in this area of their teaching. At least, based on the ineffectiveness of training competent counselors and therapists, faculty who are not actively engaged in clinical practice or those who have not practiced for five—or, generously, ten—or more years should not presume to have the requisite understanding of clinical skills or ability to demonstrate these skills and, therefore, should not attempt to equip their students, including providing clinical supervision, with their needed clinical skills. Framed differently as a question, should clinical faculty be required periodically to record their clinical sessions with real clients and to have their clinical skills assessed?

Protect Scholarship and Research

Obviously, this book aims to make a case for integrity and competence in counseling and therapy and, in this chapter, to propose actions that will elevate collective integrity and competence. However, acknowledging that some individuals and their respective programs excel in scholarship and research, they should have a visible place in preparation programs, too. Nothing here should be construed to suggest that scholarship and research should be discounted, let alone eliminated.

Another aspect of protecting scholarship and research is that faculty and their leaders appear to protect themselves from scholarship and research when it comes to examining their respective programs. The research that supports counseling and therapy preparation curriculum may be somewhat easily located (e.g., Barrett, Gonsalvez, & Shires, 2020; Baynes, 2022; D'Aniello & Perkins, 2016; Hurley & Taiwo, 2016; Lonergan, Duchin, Fromson, & AhnAllen, 2020; Mennen et al., 2018; Tasca et al., 2019; Vannatta & Steen, 2019). The important question for faculty and their leaders is simple: As academic and clinical professionals, have you sought to implement relevant research that holds huge potential for informing your decisions about your program?

Like therapy itself, the immense positive potential of preparation programs can be actualized. To express and fulfill this potential, faculty and leaders of preparation programs need to do what we expect the best of therapists to do: engage themselves in the process of change, including welcoming the risks that inhere in such engagement. The profession and the clients who are served by it are well worth the effort.

References

Academic.com. (2021). *Accrediting Commission International.* Retrieved from https://en-academic.com/dic.nsf/enwiki/4736973

Allan, R. (2019). Teaching and learning evidence-based practices: Promoting dialogue for counsellors and psychotherapists. *Counselling and Psychotherapy Research, 19*, 206–213. 10.1002/capr.12223Citations: 3

Asbury Seminary. (2023a). *About.* https://asburyseminary.edu/about/theological-orientation/ten-core-values-of-strategic-vision/

Asbury Seminary. (2023b). *Master of Arts in Mental Health Counseling.* https://asburyseminary.edu/academics/degrees/master-of-arts/mental-health-counseling/

Barrett, J., Gonsalvez, C. J., & Shires, A. (2020). Evidence-based practice within supervision during psychology practitioner training: A systematic review. *Clinical Psychologist, 24*(1), 3–17. 10.1111/cp.12196

Baynes, K. (2022). Inspired supervision and mentorship: Creating a semi-structured curriculum for faculty development that enhances psychotherapy supervision and trainee teaching. *Journal of the American Academy of Child & Adolescent Psychiatry, 61*(10), S68–S68.

Blatt, S. J., Sanislow, C. A., Zuroff, D. C., & Pilkonis, P. A. (1996). Characteristics of effective therapists: Further analyses of data from the National Institute of Mental Health Treatment of Depression Collaborative Research Program. *Journal of Consulting and Clinical Psychology, 64*(6), 1276–1284.

Christian Theological Seminary. (2023). *Mission.* https://www.cts.edu/about/

Christian Theological Seminary. (2023a). *Master of Arts in Mental Health Counseling.* https://www.cts.edu/academics/degrees/master-of-arts-in-clinical-mental-health-counseling/

Christian Theological Seminary. (2023b, online). *Master of Arts in Mental Health Counseling.* https://www.cts.edu/academics/degrees/master-of-arts-in-clinical-mental-health-counseling/

Coogan, T. A., & Homrich, A. M. (2018). Preventing problematic behavior in trainees. In A. M. Homrich, & K. L. Henderson (Ed.). *Gatekeeping in the mental health professions.* Alexandria, VA: American Counseling Association.

Cornerstone University. (2023). *Master of Arts in Mental Health Counseling annual report.* https://www.cornerstone.edu/about/accreditation/clinical-mental-health-counseling-annual-report/

Cornerstone University. (2023a). *Master of Arts in Mental Health Counseling.* https://www.cornerstone.edu/programs/ma-clinical-mental-health-counseling/

Cornerstone University. (2023b). *About.* https://www.cornerstone.edu/about/

Covenant Theological Seminary. (2023). *About Us.* https://www.covenantseminary.edu/about-us

Covenant Theological Seminary. (2023a). *Master of Arts in Counseling.* https://www.covenantseminary.edu/mac

Cummings, N. A., & O'Donohue, W. T. (Eds.) (2011). *Understanding the behavioral healthcare crisis: The promise of integrated care and diagnostic reform.* New York: Routledge.

D'Aniello, C., & Hertlein, K. M. (2017). Integrating gatekeeping practices into core competencies in MFT training: Development of the core competency-based assessment measure. *Contemporary Family Therapy, 39,* 220–229. 10.1007/s10591-017-9416-z

D'Aniello, C., & Perkins, S. N. (2016). Common factors come alive: Practical strategies for implementing common factors in MFT Training. *Contemporary Family Therapy, 38,* 233–244. 10.1007/s10591-016-9377-7

Daniel, K. E., Jensen-Doss, A., Muroff, J., White, B. A., Reilly, E. E., Hollon, S. D., Mennin, D. S., Schuler, T. A., & Teachman, B. (2019). Characterizing evidence-based practice and training resource barriers: A needs Assessment. *Training and Education in Professional Psychology, 14*(3), 200–208.

Delgadillo, J., Deisenhofer, A-K. Probst, T., Shimokawa, K., Lambert, M. J., & Kleinstäuber, M. (2022). Progress feedback narrows the gap between more and less effective therapists: A therapist effects meta-analysis of clinical trials. *Journal of Consulting and Clinical Psychology, 90*(7), 559–567. 10.1037/ccp0000747

Eells, T. D. (1999). What do we know about master therapists? *Journal of Psychotherapy Practice Research, 8,* 414–317.

Erskine Theological Seminary. (2023). *Accreditation.* https://seminary.erskine.edu/erskine/accreditation/

Erskine Theological Seminary. (2023a). *Master of Arts in Mental Health Counseling.* https://seminary.erskine.edu/admissions/degrees/master-of-arts-christian-counseling/

Erskine Theological Seminary. (2023b). *Mission and values.* https://seminary.erskine.edu/erskine/mission/

Even, T. A., & Robinson, C. R. (2013). The impact of CACREP accreditation: A multiway frequency analysis of ethics violations and sanctions. *Journal of Counseling & Development, 91*(1), 26–34.

Feinstein, R., Heiman, N., & Yager, J. (2015). Common factors affecting psychotherapy outcomes: Some implications for teaching psychotherapy. *Journal of Psychiatric Practice, 21*(3), 180–189.

Fox, S. (2023). *Therapist perceptions on factors differentiating the most from least effective therapists.* [Doctoral dissertation]. Indiana University of Pennsylvania. http://gateway.proquest.com/openurl?url_ver=Z39.88-2004&rft_val_fmt=info:ofi/fmt:kev:mtx:dissertation&res_dat=xri:pqm&rft_dat=xri:pqdiss:29255578

Goldberg, S. B., Miller, S. D., Nielsen, S. L., Rousmaniere, T., Whipple, J., Hoyt, W. T., & Wampold, B. E. (2016). Do psychotherapists improve with time and experience? A longitudinal analysis of outcomes in a clinical setting. *Journal of Counseling Psychology, 63*(1), 1–11.

Goldfried, M. R., Raue, P. J., & Castonguay, L. G. (1998). The therapeutic focus in significant sessions of master therapists: A comparison of cognitive-behavioral and psychodynamic-interpersonal interventions. *Journal of Consulting and Clinical Psychology, 66,* 803–810.

Gonsalvez, C. J., & Crowe, T. P. (2014). Evaluation of psychology practitioner competence in clinical supervision. *American Journal of Psychotherapy, 68*(2), 177–193.

Hahn, D., Weck, F., Witthøft, M., & Kühne, F. (2023). What characterizes helpful personal practice in psychotherapy training? Results of an online survey. *Behavioural and Cognitive Psychotherapy, 51*(1), 74–86.

Harwig, B. J. (2021). *Counselor educators' perceptions of their gatekeeping role in assessing personal characteristics during admissions screening.* https://www.proquest.com/docview/2582988508

Hill, C. E., Bauman, E., Shafran, N., Morrison, A., Rojas, A. E., & Gelso, C. J. (2015). Is training effective? A study of counseling psychology doctoral trainees in a psychodynamic/interpersonal training clinic. *Journal of Counseling Psychology, 62*(2), 184–201. 10.1037/cou0000053

Hsueh, L., Hobaica, S., Lumley, M. A., Werntz, A., Owens, S. A., Jason, J. & Washburn, J. J. (2020). Clinical psychology PhD students' admission experiences: Implications for recruiting racial/ ethnic minority and LGBTQ students. *Journal of Clinical Psychology, 77*, 105–120.

Huhra, R. L., Yamokoski-Maynhart, C. A., & Prieto, L. R. (2008). Reviewing videotapes in supervision: A developmental approach. *Journal of Counseling and Development, 86*(4), 412–418.

Hurley, D., & Taiwo, A. (2016). Critical social work and competency practice: a proposal to bridge theory and practice in the classroom. *Journal of Social Work Education, 38*(2), 198–211. 10.1080/02615479.2018.1533544

Ivey, G., & Partington, T. (2014). Psychological woundedness and its evaluation in applications for clinical psychology training. *Clinical Psychology and Psychotherapy, 21*, 166–177. 10.1002/cpp.1816

Jewell, J. R., Anthony, B, & Murphy, A. (2021) Utilizing technology in social work education: Development of the technology effectiveness and social connectedness scale. *Journal of Social Work Education, 57*(2), 372–382.

Kaslow, N. J., Grus, C. L., Campbell, L. F., Fouad, N. A., Hatcher, R. L., & Rodolfa, E. R. (2009). Competency assessment toolkit for professional psychology. *Training and Education in Professional Psychology, 3*(4, Supplement), S27–S45. 10.1037/a0015833

Kühne, F., Heinze, P. E., Maaß, U., & Weck, F. (2022). Modeling in psychotherapy training: A randomized controlled proof-of-concept trial. *Journal of Consulting and Clinical Psychology, 90*(12), 950–956. 10.1037/ccp0000780

Lafferty, P., Beutler, L. E., & Crago, M. (1989). Differences between more and less effective psychotherapists: A study of select therapist variables. *Journal of Consulting and Clinical Psychology, 57*(1), 76–80.

Lane, D. (2023). Social work education and practice learning at a crossroads: Challenges. *Practice: Social Work in Action, 35*(1), 27–45.

Levy, K. N., & Ellison, W. D. (2022). The availability of training opportunities in personality disorders in American Psychological Association and Psychological Clinical Science Accreditation System-accredited clinical and counseling psychology doctoral programs. *Training and Education in Professional Psychology, 16*(4), 376–384. 10.1037/tep0000376

Lilienfeld, S. (2014). *Evidence-based practice: The misunderstandings continue.* https://www.psychologytoday.com/us/blog/the-skeptical-psychologist/201401/evidence-based-practice-the-misunderstandings-continue

Lilienfeld, S. O., Ritschel, L. A., Lynn, S. J., Cautin, R. L., & Latzman, R. D. (2014). Why ineffective psychotherapies appear to work: A taxonomy of causes of spurious therapeutic effectiveness. *Perspectives on Psychological Science, 9*, 355–387.

Lincoln Christian University. (2023). *MA in Counseling.* Retrieved from https://lincolnchristian.edu/academics/programs/masters/ma-counseling/

Lincoln Christian University. (2023a). *MA in Counseling receives CACREP accreditation.* Retrieved from https://lincolnchristian.edu/news/lcu-ma-in-counseling-receives-cacrep-accreditation/

Lincoln Christian University. (2023b). *Statement of faith.* Retrieved from https://lincolnchristian.edu/about-us/statement-of-faith/

Liszewski, K. (2022). *The qualities and characteristics that distinguish most effective therapists: A survey of clinical supervisors and directors.* [Doctoral dissertation, Indiana University of Pennsylvania]. http://gateway.proquest.com/openurl?url_ver=Z39.88-2004&rft_val_fmt=info:ofi/fmt:kev:mtx:dissertation&res_dat=xri:pqm&rft_dat=xri:pqdiss:28860875

Lonergan, B. B., Duchin, N. P., Fromson, J. A., & AhnAllen, C. G. (2020). Skills-based psychotherapy training for inpatient psychiatry residents: A needs assessment and evaluation of a pilot curriculum. *Academic Psychiatry, 44*(3), 320–323.

Lwin, K., & Beltrano, N. (2022). Rethinking evidence-based and evidence-informed practice: A call for evidence-informed decision making in social work education and child welfare practice. *Social Work Education, 41*(2), 166–174.

Mackrill, T., & Iwakabe, S. (2013). Making a case for case studies in psychotherapy training: A small step towards establishing an empirical basis for psychotherapy training. *Counselling Psychology Quarterly, 26*(3–4), 250–266. 10.1080/09515070.2013.832148

Malott, K. M., Hall, K. H., Sheely-Moore, A., Krell, M. M., & Cardaciotto, L. (2014). Evidence-based teaching in higher education: Application to counselor education. *Counselor Education and Supervision, 53*(4), 294–305. 10.1002/j.1556-6978.2014.00064.x

Martin, F. A. (2020). *Therapy thieves: How to save mental health care from its providers.* New York: Oxford University Press.

Martin, F. A., & Turner, J. P. (2020). *Clinical supervision in the real world: A practical guide to ethics, legal issues, and personal development.* New York: Routledge.

Mennen, F. E., Cederbsum, J., Chorpita, B. F., Becker, K., Lopez, O., & Sela-Amit, M. (2018). The large-scale implementation of evidence-informed practice into a specialized MSW curriculum. *Journal of Social Work Education, 54*(S1), S56–S64. 10.1080/10437797.2018.1434440

Miller, K. (2023). *Can we improve psychotherapy by quantifying therapists' language?* https://hai.stanford.edu/news/can-we-improve-psychotherapy-quantifying-therapists-language

Missio Seminary. (2022b). *Counseling licensure.* https://missio.edu/counseling-licensure/

Mollen, D., Burns, T., Lee, S., & Abbott, D. M. (2020). Sexuality training in counseling psychology. *Counseling Psychology Quarterly, 33*(3), 375–392. 10.1080/09515070.2018.1553146

Montan, I., Dinger, U., Dück, J., Ehrenthal, J. C., Storck, T., Taubner, S., Weintz, L. P. H., Thake, M., Friederich, H.-C., Schauenburg, H., Schultz, J.-H., & Nikendei, C. (2022). Psychotherapy trainees' perspective on a longitudinal curriculum for the training of psychodynamic intervention competencies. *Psychoanalytic Psychology, 39*(4), 321–329. 10.1037/pap0000418

Nuland, S. B. (2001). Indoctrinology: PC, M.D.: How political correctness is corrupting medicine. *The New Republic, 224*(8), 34–39.

O'Donnell, R. R. (2011). Reforms in professional education. In N. A. Cummings, & W. T. O'Donohue (Eds.), *Understanding the behavioral healthcare crisis: The promise of integrated care and diagnostic reform* (pp. 257–278). New York: Routledge.

O'Donohue, W. T., Cummings, N. A., & Cummings, J. L. (2008). The unmet educational agenda in integrated care. *Journal of Clinical Psychology in Medical Settings, 16*, 94–100.

Osberg, T. M. (1997). Teaching psychotherapy outcome research methodology using a research-based checklist. *Teaching of Psychology, 24*(4), 271–274. 10.1207/s15328023top2404_13

Owen, J., Kivlighan III, M., Kopta, M., Drinane, J. M., Miller, S., & Imel, Z. (2019). Are high-performing therapists both effective and consistent? A test of therapist expertise. *Journal of Consulting and Clinical Psychology, 87*(12), 1149–1156. 10.1037/ccp0000437

Perez-Rojaz, A., Bartheolomew, T. & Joy, E. (2022). Counseling psychology faculty's involvement in practice: A mixed methods study. *Counselling Psychology Quarterly, 35*(1), 61–88.

Plakun, E. M., Sudak, D. M., & Goldberg, D. (2009). The Y model: An integrated, evidence-based approach to teaching psychotherapy competencies. *Journal of Psychiatric Practice, 15*(1), 5–11. 10.1097/01.pra.0000344914.54082.eb

Skovholt, T. M., & Jennings, L. (2004). *Master therapists: Exploring expertise in therapy and counseling.* New York: Merrill Publishing.

Society for the Advancement of Psychotherapy. (n.d.). [no title] https://societyforpsychotherapy.org/10-ways-to-improve-psychotherapy-outcome/

Spengler, P. M., & Pilipis, L. A. (2015). A comprehensive meta-reanalysis of the robustness of the experience-accuracy effect in clinical judgment. *Journal of Counseling Psychology, 62*(3), 360–378. 10.1037/cou0000065

Styck, K. M. (2012). Preparing school psychologists for working with diverse students: Does program accreditation matter? *Current Issues in Education, 15*(2), 1–16. https://cie.asu.edu/ojs/index.php/cieatasu/article/view/964/340

Tasca, G. A., Rupal Bonli, R., Hunsley, J., Angus, L., Drapeau, M., Fitzpatrick, M., & Knoll, M. (2019). Outcome and progress monitoring in psychotherapy: Report of a Canadian Psychological Association Task Force. *Canadian Psychology/Psychologie canadienne, 60*(3), 165–177. 10.1037/cap0000181

Teichman, Y., Berant, E., Shenkman G., & Ramot, G. (2022). Supervisees' perspectives on the contribution of supervision to psychotherapy outcomes. *Counseling and Psychotherapy Research.* https://onlinelibrary.wiley.com/doi/pdf/10.1002/capr.12540

Thyer, B. A., & Pignotti, M. G. (2015). *Science and pseudoscience in social work practice.* New York: Springer.

Trinity Evangelical Divinity School. (2023a). *Mission and values.* https://www.tiu.edu/mission-core-values/

Trinity Evangelical Divinity School. (2023b). *Statement of faith.* https://www.tiu.edu/statement-of-faith/

Turns, B. A., Nalbone, D. P., Hertlein, K. M., & Wetchler, J. L. (2014). Perceptions of program enhancers and stressors by marriage and family therapy students and faculty. *Contemporary Family Therapy, 36*, 507–517. 10.1007/s10591-014-9313-7

Vannatta, R., & Steen, S. (2019) Pedagogical practices in CACREP accredited group counseling courses: A content analysis. *The Journal for Specialists in Group Work, 44*(2), 138–150. 10.1080/01933922.2019.1599477

Vaz, A., & Sousa, D. (2021). Persuasiveness: An underappreciated characteristic of effective therapists. *Psychology of Consciousness: Theory, Research, and Practice.* 1–16. 10.1037/cns0000309

Walfish, S., & Moreira, J. C. (2005). Relative weighting of admission variables in marriage and family therapy graduate programs. *The American Journal of Family Therapy, 33*, 395–402.

Wampold, B. E., & Owen, J. (2021). Therapist effects: History, methods, magnitude, and characteristics of effective therapists. In M. Barkham, W. Lutz, & L. G. Castonguay (Eds.), *Bergin and Garfield's handbook of psychotherapy and behavior change: 50th anniversary edition* (pp. 297–326). Hoboken, NJ: John Wiley & Sons.

Wheeler, K., & Delaney, K. (2008). Challenges and Realities of teaching psychotherapy: A survey of psychiatric-mental health nursing graduate programs. *Perspectives in Psychiatric Care, 44*(2): pp. 72–80.

Whitney, B. M. (2021). Ethical considerations for the study of potentially harmful or ineffective treatments. *Professional Psychology: Research and Practice, 52*(1), 12–20. 10.1037/pro0000341

Wike, T. L., Bledsoe, S. E., Bellamy, J. L., & Grady, M. D. (2013). Examining inclusion of evidence-based practice on social work training program websites. *Journal of Social Work Education, 49*, 439–450. 10.1080/10437797.2013.796791

Wikipedia. (2021). *Accrediting Commission International.* Retrieved from https://en.wikipedia.org/wiki/Accrediting_Commission_International

Wilkinson, T., & Reinhardt, R. (2015). Technology in counselor education: HIPAA and HITECH as best practice. *The Professional Counselor, 5*(3), 407–418. 10.15241/tw.5.3.407

Williams, A. E., Weinzatl, O. L., & Varga, B. L. (2021). Examination of family counseling coursework and scope of practice for professional mental health counselors. *The Family Journal, 29*(1), 10–16. https://journals.sagepub.com/doi/full/10.1177/1066480720978536

9 Advocacy among Therapists and Their Constituencies

Francis A. Martin and Janet P. Turner

The brief quote below is entirely fictional. However, it expresses a likely outcome from actions that are currently being considered by the legislature in South Carolina.

> Julie and Micah breathed uneasily, as if another breath could be delayed and, therefore, postpone the inevitability of life-changing, unwanted next steps. They felt the magnitude of change. Standing near the door for the last time, Micah reached for the light switch. There, in the doorway, they stood in the tomb-like silent darkness for a minute that seemed like an hour. Then, they quietly walked away from their fourteen-year-old office. Facing intense uncertainty, they left the career that had defined them for twenty-three years.
>
> Wistfully, with unusual nostalgia, Julie spoke, "It's hard. It's hard to think about all of this coming to an end. Who would have thought that when we met in grad school way back then that in mid-career everything would end? I never imagined in my wildest thoughts that the state would end my license—our license? It's really crazy. It doesn't make any sense. But here we are. We'll get by somehow. I think we can start by selling the house. I don't want to, but we need the money. We'll have to relocate. I don't know where, but we have to. Where would you like to go?"

"What are they talking about?"

In his book, *Therapy Thieves: How To Save Mental Health Care from Its Providers*, Martin (2020) described several external threats to mental health care providers. In this discussion, he referred to the actions by several states that would have led to the termination of professional licensing for mental health care providers (Martin, 2020, pp. 133–134). Now, in 2023, another state legislature is contemplating the termination of professional licensing for mental health care providers and others. Presented in all capital letters in the original, the summary of the bill, the *Entrepreneur Freedom Act*, that is moving through the South Carolina State legislature reads, as follows:

DOI: 10.4324/9781003472469-10

> Session 125 - (2023–2024)
> H 3515 General Bill, By Pace, Leber, Magnuson, S. Jones and White
> Summary: Entrepreneur Freedom Act
> A BILL TO AMEND THE SOUTH CAROLINA CODE OF LAWS BY ENACTING THE "ENTREPRENEUR FREEDOM ACT"; BY REPEALING SECTION 40-7-255 RELATING TO **HAIR BRAIDING PRACTITIONER** REGISTRATION; BY REPEALING CHAPTER 19 OF TITLE 40 RELATING TO **EMBALMERS** AND **FUNERAL DIRECTORS**; BY REPEALING CHAPTER 20 OF TITLE 40 RELATING TO LICENSED **DIETITIANS**; BY REPEALING CHAPTER 28 OF TITLE 40 RELATING TO **LANDSCAPE ARCHITECTS**; BY REPEALING CHAPTER 55 OF TITLE 40 RELATING TO **PSYCHOLOGISTS**; BY REPEALING CHAPTER 63 OF TITLE 40 RELATING TO **SOCIAL WORKERS**; BY REPEALING CHAPTER 67 OF TITLE 40 RELATING TO **SPEECH PATHOLOGISTS** AND **AUDIOLOGISTS**; BY REPEALING CHAPTER 75 OF TITLE 40 RELATING TO **PROFESSIONAL COUNSELORS, MARRIAGE AND FAMILY THERAPISTS**, AND LICENSED **PSYCHO-EDUCATIONAL SPECIALISTS**; BY REPEALING CHAPTER 77 OF TITLE 40 RELATING TO **GEOLOGISTS**; BY REPEALING CHAPTER 81 OF TITLE 40 RELATING TO THE STATE **ATHLETIC COMMISSION**; AND BY REPEALING SECTION 59-25-20 RELATING TO THE **QUALIFICATIONS OF TEACHERS**.
>
> [Bolding added.] (South Carolina Legislation, 2023)

If this bill succeeds, it will eliminate licensing for psychologists, social workers, professional counselors, and marriage and family therapists in the State of South Carolina. It may or may not succeed. However, as these bills become increasingly common, sooner or later, one of these expressions of political madness will pass through a legislature and be signed into law. The political push to accomplish this appears to be unrelenting among a minority of politicians.

So, what is this discussion about? Obviously, it is about the urgency of combatting the political madness in South Carolina. However, much more pervasively, it is about the intense urgency of trying to ensure that mental health care providers have a viable future. All conscientious counselors and therapists should give attention to real threats to their professional existence, including the threats that come within the "family." As this chapter and other sources make clear, numerous counselors and therapists have demonstrated their readiness to sabotage the future of counseling and therapy. To invent and sustain a viable future, many different actions must be taken. This chapter recommends many of these actions.

Before immersing in a discussion about actions that mental health care providers need to take, more should be said about the political madness in South Carolina. If counselors, psychologists, social workers, and marriage and family therapists dismiss the legislative initiative in South Carolina as wacky politicians who fail to understand mental health care, they have failed to understand the clinical mess that they have created. Whether counselors and therapists like it or not, they have overtly or tacitly contributed to the clinical madness with which counseling and therapy may now be characterized. The defense that says, "Well, the clinical madness isn't all of us. There are some of us who are truly professional," simply avoids the necessity of seeing the obvious realities before us. No doubt, there are truly professional clinicians among us, but for every one of them, there is at least one other who conspicuously lacks integrity and competence. This is what we have allowed to happen. This is what we must correct with numerous corrective actions, while we simultaneously seek to defeat legislative madness.

A Brief Orientation

Those of us who are counselors and therapists cannot achieve integrity and competence for ourselves or our profession unless we develop the strength to acknowledge our weaknesses and, therefore, to work toward overcoming them. At this time, no doubt, religion and other ideologies are weakening our profession. And, as a result, they weaken each of us. They require action toward claiming integrity for our profession. This chapter attempts to recommend some of the ways through which integrity can be claimed and maintained. However, no matter which ways may be pursued, they should not obviate the importance of the reason for the existence of counseling and therapy. In short, counseling and therapy exist to meet the clinically relevant needs of clients, within the broad range of mental-emotional-relational needs. This calls for clinically relevant actions that can establish and maintain the integrity and competence of the profession through which counselors and therapists seek to meet clients' needs.

The adage, "Nothing gets better, if nothing gets better," applies to the condition of counseling and therapy. If there is no improvement, no widespread refinement of professionalism, there is no improvement. And, without improvement, our profession continues to decline. Indeed, possibly, in concert with the legislators in South Carolina, the profession may be abetting their effort to terminate it.

Obviously, this book addresses the matter of the place of religion in counseling and therapy. It provides a huge volume of evidence to indicate that countless numbers of practicing counselors and therapists opportunistically, and typically without an evidentiary foundation, aim to utilize religion in their respective practices. Apparently, the common belief among many counselors and therapists is that their religion and their practice of counseling and therapy ought to be integrated. This belief expresses a misunderstanding of their role and the place of religion in it. And, they receive considerable support from some scholars. For example, Plante suggests that those who prefer not to integrate religion into clinical practice are biased against religion and that, instead of allowing this bias to skew their professional judgment, issues "a call for a more thoughtful, balanced, and evidence-based approach of integrating religious engagement within clinical and counseling psychological practice" (Plante, 2022, p. 1). Based on the profession's long and clear advocacy of diversity and inclusion, Plante's view represents numerous counselors and therapists.

However, along with numerous colleagues, Plante may be inviting others to practice their ideology as therapy and providing rationalizations for them to practice their ideologies. Inadvertently, those who advocate for diversity and inclusion may also be endorsing 99 Divine Principles, Abundant Life Christian Counseling, Adlerian Christian Therapy, Advanced DNA ThetaHealing, Agnostic Pastoral Counseling, Ancient Christian Wisdom, Animal Assisted Christian Counseling, Apostolic Counseling, Archangel Life Coaching, and Asana Buddhist Principles, to name only ten approaches from an accrued list of more than 5,000 specifically religious approaches to counseling and therapy, accompanied by approximately 10,000 religion-related approaches. What is the relation between these approaches and the evidence-based approach for which Plante calls? In short, there is none. As noted elsewhere in this book, large numbers of counselors and therapists not only fail to integrate evidence-based approaches in their therapy but also assertively oppose evidence-based approaches. On Plante's behalf, it should be said that many scholars have assumed for many years that religion could and should be integrated into clinical practice. They have thought about religion and therapy in very much the way that Plante thinks. As sincere as their assumption was, they must also acknowledge that we, including us, were wrong.

To acknowledge being wrong is obviously insufficient. Yes, many of us have been wrong. But the welfare of clients and the survival of mental health care services are issues that this acknowledgment does not address. "[P]erhaps it might be contended that our oft-claimed unique focus on caring for marginalized and other historically oppressed groups lays upon [us] a particular burden to ensure that the services provided to these individuals are not yet another way of exploiting their hopes and needs" (Thyer & Pignotti, 2015, p. 263). When counselors and therapists of good character and professionalism stand by while their colleagues and others exploit the hopes and needs of very large numbers of clients, they tacitly give permission to this exploitation. This chapter aims to encourage others to take actions that can elevate the integrity and competence among counselors and therapists. It recommends urgently needed actions. While the specific actions that we recommend will be—and should be—adjusted to accommodate the individuals and groups, taking action should not be optional. The issue is sometimes stated as "Not to decide is to decide." In the current situation, "Not to act is to act." The lack of action gives tacit approval to those who very publicly practice significantly below minimal professional standards of practice.

Toward accomplishing desperately needed reforms in counseling and therapy, *The Challenges of Integrating Religion and Spirituality into Psychotherapy* is not sufficient and cannot stand alone. It is an expression of a much larger dialogue. Much of the larger dialogue is reported by Martin (2020) in the chapter titled, "The Long Conversation about Counseling and Therapy." Many others have written sensitive, intellectually strong, insightful books and articles about the best expressions of counseling and therapy, including its many vulnerabilities. This book makes no attempt to capture all of this. Among the many books that take readers into the developing world of therapists, some almost always arise in discussions of important ones. They include Rogers' *A Way of Being* (1980), Yalom's *The Gift of Therapy* (2002), Cozolino's *The Making of a Therapist* (2004), and Ronnestad's and Skovholt's (2013) *The Developing Practitioner: Growth and Stagnation of Therapists and Counselors.* These luminaries in the profession of counseling and therapy have acknowledged the virtues of their understanding of counseling and therapy, along with their deficiencies. Following their enlightened leadership, this book offers a modest but sincere affirmation of their insights and inspiration, recognizing that we stand in awe of their contributions.

Needed Actions toward Integrity, Competence, and Inclusion

To create and sustain integrity and competence among counselors and therapists, many different actions are needed by many different individuals, groups, associations, legislatures, and others, possibly including decisions by juries and judges. The discussion here is not intended to address all possible courses of action. Instead, it is intended to offer a wide of array actions that almost inevitably arise from the evidence that this book and others have reported. The recommended actions fall into five categories, including those that should be taken by

Individual Counselors and Therapists
Professional Associations
Licensing Boards and State Legislators
Social Service Agencies
Businesses and Corporations

A brief statement about clients' perspective is added to some of the recommendations. This acknowledges that clients' views of what counselors and therapists do are critically important. At least, for the purpose of representing the profession with reasonable accuracy, the public image of the profession is important. If the public image is one that evokes doubt more than confidence, sneers more than smiles, or rejection more than welcome, needy individuals and family will not likely pursue and receive the professionally accountable services that they need.

Individual Counselors and Therapists

The current condition of counseling and therapy calls for change. All important, positive change begins in counseling and therapy begins with an individual, but individuals alone cannot achieve significant change in the large and complex clinical world. However, all individuals can improve their clinical work. Toward accomplishing such improvement, they can find valuable help. For example, they can, at least as a beginning, try to absorb the conclusion that "The accumulating evidence suggests that biases often adversely affect the accuracy of clinical judgments, even among the many clinicians and supervisors who are capable, knowledgeable, and intelligent" (Bowes, Ammirati, Lilienfeld, Costello, & Basterfield, 2020, p. 442). Quite beyond such an acknowledgment, these researchers offer the idea that such an acknowledgment is "a useful starting point" (p. 442) for significant change and improvement in clinical performance. As therapists seek to elevate their clinical effectiveness, they may move beyond a starting point, by utilizing the recommendations below and searching for additional actions.

With regard to the urgency and necessity of significant change in counseling and therapy, all of those who practice as counselors, therapists, teachers, administrators, or others within the profession are affected and influenced—whether they recognize this or not—by the massive proliferation of aberrant and often harmful religious and religion-related approaches to therapy. Thus, all counselors and therapists, regardless of their apparent professional security at this time, should get involved in efforts to save their profession and to ensure that it provides services that epitomize integrity, competence, and inclusion. Also, practicing clinicians need to recognize that they do not necessarily pursue improvement in their clinical performance alone.

As this book, along with other researchers, makes clear, professionally accountable counselors and therapists are swamped by those among them who are not professionally accountable. Including the information in this book and a substantial body of research from others, every practicing counselor and therapist is compromised by those who provide services that fall seriously below minimal professional standards. Instead of succumbing to helplessness in response to the compromisers, individual counselors and therapists can take actions that will neutralize the threat to their professional welfare and, more importantly, the welfare of their clients. In pursuing actions, they should keep in mind that they are not alone. They may join a large—hopefully, enlarging—body of mental health care providers who aspire to establish and maintain professional integrity and competence in the delivery of counseling and therapy services. Also, they should keep in mind that their best efforts may not produce immediate, positive results. Nevertheless, a collection of possible actions and initiatives appears below.

Ask and answer a simple question about your professional practice, regardless of your specific role: How may I improve my professional services? The answer may require you to acknowledge weaknesses or failures. In the process of such acknowledgments, though, you will also need to recognize your professional assets and clinical successes. Still, improving your clinical effectiveness also improves the profession.

Take actions to protect yourself from peers who are hurting/will hurt you. As you protect yourself, you will also be protecting your clients. Your actions may involve studying the websites of counselors and therapists whose practices are located near yours. Your actions may involve contact and conversation with some of those whose information appears to compromise, if not violate, normative professional standards. In situations where you identify clear violations of professional ethics and or state regulations and laws, you may wish to submit information to the appropriate, regulatory agency in your state.

Gather information. The data that call for reform of counseling and therapy are enormous. Maybe, a place to begin to gather information is to review the reference section of this book. If you are a social worker, you may want to get a copy of Thyer and Pignotti's book (2015), *Science and Pseudoscience in Social Work Practice*. Or, if you are a psychologist, a good source for beginning to gather information is Cummings and O'Donohue's book (2011), *Understanding the Behavioral Healthcare Crisis: The Promise of Integrated Care and Diagnostic Reform*. Or, you may wish to read Martin's book (2020), *Therapy Thieves: How To Save Mental Health Care from Its Providers*. These books provide a valuable, substantial, and stimulating foundation for considering the need for critically needed reforms in counseling and therapy and many recommendations about how to achieve these reforms.

Get involved with other counselors and therapists toward helping to elevate integrity and competence. Getting involved can be many different things. It may be conversations with and among your professional friends, maybe, along with having coffee and/or lunch. Or, it may be preparing presentations for professional meetings, with the emphasis on ways to improve our profession. Or, it may be seeking leadership positions through which needed improvements can be pursued. Or, it may be making contact with officers in the local, state, or national professional associations with which you are affiliated.

Share relevant information. Just as we discover when we help clients, we sometimes know and understand more than we anticipated. So, as you gather information about the needs of our profession, you may also give serious attention to all that you already know, as bases for helping to improve our profession.

Organize with others to seek changes in local and state counseling- and therapy-related professional groups. Analogous to helping clients with their treatment goals, you already have experience in creating useful goals and trying to achieve them. Consider how you may be able to use your skills to help our profession through your participation in professional groups.

Invite trusted peers to evaluate your clinical work and commit to them to evaluate their clinical work, too. This will help to not only improve clinical skills but also build honest confidence in your profession.

Contact professional association leaders, share information with them, and inquire about their efforts toward improving our profession. Sharing useful and relevant information may express needed interest in leaders with whom you share information, but also may help them to direct energy and resources toward making important changes.

Contact state legislators, share information with them, and inquire about their efforts toward helping our profession to protect itself. Generally, legislators depend on their constituents for information that can help guide legislation and public policy.

In states where either professional associations or licensing boards and procedures allow it, report counselors and therapists who advertise inappropriate approaches to counseling and therapy or those whom you know to be providing inappropriate and possibly harmful therapies.

Gather free and clinically useful materials from government agencies, foundations, and other sources that will enable you to share valuable resources with your peers and your clients.

When you see a professional peer who practices inappropriate therapies, contact your peer and inquire about the therapies that are practiced.

Explore affiliation with an advocacy group that shares your interests. For example, based in Kansas City, but with national outreach, The BMS Project advocates for the mental health of young athletes.

Create or help to create evaluation procedures for your individual practice, the group practice of which you are a member, or the agency where you are employed.

Within your practice group or practice, invent ways to advocate for our profession.

To secure your confidence in your clinical work, invite trusted peers to share mutual evaluations of your and their clinical work.

Nominate, campaign for, and vote for leaders of professional associations who have a clear and preferably demonstrated commitment to solve many of the problems addressed in this book and elsewhere.

As Robert Resnick advised in his APA presidential address in 1997, with regard to the need for ongoing reform of professional practice, "Psychologists must take an active role in shaping the next iteration of the health care delivery system, and the next, and the next. Psychologists and their patients must be players as well, not just providers!" (Resnick, 1997, p. 467). The message to psychologists stands as an entirely apt one for all mental health care providers, now, 20 some years later. Resnick's advice must be considered as a general and viable direction for practicing counselors and therapists. In the context of the concerns addressed in this book, his advice is more salient than ever. However, in a recent poll (Norcross, Pfund, and Cook, 2022) on the future of psychotherapy among 56 "psychotherapy experts," none identified the multiple threats, especially aberrant and inappropriate approaches to counseling and therapy that have become widely recognized. Among the more than 36 clinical orientations that the experts named in the poll, none referred to religion, spirituality, or religion-related orientations. This indicates that the work to be done is, indeed, huge.

Adding to the need for individual mental health care clinicians to initiate needed actions, clinical supervisors should be added to individuals who need to take actions, too. A discussion of needed actions by clinical supervisors could consume a great deal of space. Instead of this, readers are referred to our earlier book, *Clinical Supervision in the Real World: A Practical Guide to Ethics, Legal Issues and Personal Development* (Martin & Turner, 2020). The book contains several recommendations for ways clinical supervisors should prepare for their work and other actions that will improve their service to their supervisees and their profession.

Clients' perspective: Clients are not helped by "the profession," whether the profession is physical therapy or counseling and therapy. They are helped by an individual who is a therapist. Clients do not speak about "my profession" from which they get help, but speak of "my therapist" or "my counselor." In other words, counseling and therapy are almost always very personal and relational. Therefore, a client's perception of therapists will be shaped and colored by their peers who advertise "clinical" approaches such as Behavioral Christian Counseling, Bible Inspired Counseling, Bible Readings, Bible-Based Christian Approach, Bible-Believing Therapy, Biblical Discipleship Counseling, Biblical

Dream Analysis, Biblical Evangelical Counseling, Biblical Genetics, Biblical Insights Based Therapy, Biblical Nauthetic Principle, Biblical Transformational Healing, Biblical World View, Biblically Based Soul Care, and Bibliotherapeutic Christian Counseling, among thousands of others. All therapists should ask themselves, "Are these the approaches that I want to represent me and my professional services?" Or, "Do these approaches represent the profession in which I am a member?"

Similarly, among tens of thousands of examples of clinical madness, prospective clients may also see Buddhism and Indigenous Art Therapy, Buddhist and Sufi Integrated Therapy, Christa Energy Attunement, Dharmacharya—Buddhist, Dory Cote Shamanic Practices, or Divine Channeling. Do these so-called "therapies" represent you or the profession of which you are a member? If not, what would you like to do, in response to them?

Professional Associations

No matter which license for clinical practice an individual holds, it would not have been possible without professional associations. Psychologists would not have licensing in their individual or collective history without the American Psychological Association. Mental health counselors—also commonly called "Professional Counselors"—would not have licensing in their individual or collective history without the American Counseling Association. This simple acknowledgment refers also to licensing for social workers and marriage and family therapists, along with other smaller groups. However, at this time, none of these associations represent those who hold the licenses that the associations established through their considerable, lengthy efforts and expenses, mainly because the proportion of licensees who are members of these associations continues to decline. Therefore, all of the major associations must examine their reason for their respective existence and revise their activities so that they can re-claim their rightful and desperately needed influence. Otherwise, they tacitly agree with the proposition that the profession that they allege to lead is one that they no longer lead and, due to their apparent commitment to not leading, will continue to decline.

Such a conclusion may appear to be merely a sour one that lacks evidence or relevance. Many researchers and others have reported about the importance of professional mental health care associations and their complicity—usually, inadvertent—in contributing to the decline of counseling and therapy. For example, Thyer and Pignotti (2015, p. 226) refer to the "lax ethical standards that promote pseudoscience" in the clinical practice of social work. A feature of this laxity is that "most social workers do not belong" (p. 226) as members of the National Association of Social

Workers (NASW) and, therefore, are not exposed to appropriate accountability by their profession. The same lack of membership also characterizes the other major licensing categories, including mental health counselors, psychologists, and marriage and family therapists. Exacerbating this difficult environment for counseling and therapy, specifically religious associations have not only co-opted the prerogatives of professionally accountable counselors and therapists but also received tacit support from the major non-religious associations and have often adopted views of clients that the major non-religious associations reject such as misogyny. This sad phenomenon is described in detail elsewhere in this book. (Refer to the discussion of religion-based graduate programs in Chapter 8.)

Generally and minimally, professional associations must cooperate. "United we stand; divided we fall" comes as a relevant and urgent mantra. However, given the multiple and formidable challenges that currently beset counselors and therapists, much more than cooperation is needed. At least, cooperation must come. However, for the sake of the clients, no matter what kind of clients or the locations where they are served, professional associations should aim for more than cooperation. Anticipating the possibility of more than cooperation, they should consider an outcome beyond cooperation that is grander than cooperation, more substantial than cacophonous co-existence, more respectful of clients than the current and massive confusion permits, more clinically grounded and honest than the current environment generally allows, and much less corrupted by rampant and exaggerated individualism that characterizes the current situation. In short, they must unite. Yes, the major professional association should lower the currently high threshold of justifiable historic pride and, for the sake of having a viable profession in the future, pursue radical restructuring so that the major professional associations become one association.

While unifying is not likely to happen, despite the need for it, professional associations can take a number of needed actions. For now, the following actions are recommended. Professional associations should

Look for and eliminate aberrant therapies. This general recommendation emphasizes the need to expose aberrant and sometimes harmful therapies and to publicize such therapies. This could be a good beginning of urgently needed change.

Aggressively seek to enforce professional ethics, with regard to aberrant approaches to therapy and the issues related to these approaches such as potential harm to clients. Arguably, the most common violation of professional ethics is the intentional delivery of therapies that lack clinical credibility and that may cause harm. This form of violating professional ethics may be larger than all of the other forms of violating professional ethics.

Propose changes in licensing laws and regulations so that aberrant and often harmful therapies can be minimized, if not eliminated.

Work toward eliminating the several hundred titles of licenses issued to mental health care providers, with the idea that clients and prospective clients deserve a much better presentation of professional credentials than they currently see.

Aim to eliminate most of the titles for degrees that are earned by graduates who become licensees. (Refer to Chapter 8 for a list of degrees.)

Propose changes in licensing laws so that the vast array of fake licenses can be eliminated.

Propose increases in funding by state legislatures so that licensing boards or appropriate investigative, law enforcement procedures can not only discover and carefully monitor but also support the improvement of counseling and therapy within their respective jurisdictions.

Pursue legal actions against those who presume to practice "real" therapy but who lack relevant training and credentials for such practice.

Promote "practice formularies." These formularies would include (1) models of counseling and therapy that the association supports, (2) specific techniques that the association supports, recognizing that the techniques also have evidentiary support, and (3) the specific problems and/or disorders for which these models and techniques may be utilized. In addition, professional associations would emphasize that models and techniques that associations do not approve constitute a lapse(s) of professional ethics by those who practice them. This is a way to promote acceptable approaches to therapy and to eliminate unacceptable ones.

Prepare and distribute practice evaluation procedures and instruments.

Establish panels of reviewers who can examine the advertising of their peers. Currently, the only examination of advertising comes from those who receive income from the advertisers. Possibly, instead of reviewing the advertising of professional peers, a free evaluation of clinician's advertising would benefit the association and clinicians.

Define appropriate practice areas/specializations and inappropriate ones for practicing counselors and therapists, with emphasis on the necessity of appropriate preparation. They may all be MDs, but not all of them can opt to practice psychiatry or gynecology, merely because they want to. An example of this problem is that a small minority of those who advertise that they provide EMDR have either a related credential or training.

Establish mechanisms through which unethical approaches to counseling and therapy can be adjudicated. Currently, such mechanisms do not exist, except in the imagination of those who prefer the veneer of compliance with professional ethics. Also, currently, in the absence of monitoring and adjudication procedures, the only mechanism for enforcing professional ethics requires that clients who have been harmed or believe that they have been harmed file complaints against their providers.

Openly and energetically condemn and campaign against so-called "licenses" that have no basis in clinical reality. Several of these are presented in detail elsewhere in this book.

Deliver training events that give attention to clinical decision-making, with emphasis on treatments that lie securely within the boundaries of accountability and ethicality.

Carefully examine the recommendations, below, for state licensing boards and state legislatures and vigorously pursue the ones that they deem to be the most needed in their respective associations and states.

Licensing Boards and State Legislatures

Typically, licensing boards and state legislatures follow the leadership of professional associations and related groups, including colleges and universities. This is the way it should be. Thus, merely making recommendations for needed actions by licensing boards and state legislatures cannot omit the necessity of leadership from various professional groups.

Generally, the various professional groups and their leaders at a national and state level, including the American Counseling Association, American Psychological Association, National Association of Social Workers, American Association for Marriage and Family Therapy, and others, should coordinate their priorities so that they can ensure the collective well-being of all of their respective members and followers. Without such coordination, mental health care will continue to suffer from the massive fragmentation among mental health care provider groups and, therefore, the inevitable weakness that accompanies it.

Anticipating their efforts to influence licensing boards and legislatures, to what should these various groups give priority? Surely, one thing is minimal coherence in requirements for preparation programs. Another is minimal coherence in licensing requirements. Similar to training for physicians, mental health care providers need to assure clients and prospective clients that they have minimally relevant training and a relevant license. Another is that professional groups should develop mutually agreed upon titles for licenses and related references so that clients can more likely understand the potential capabilities of their providers. At this time, these things are not possible. Until these things are achieved, other recommendations to licensing boards and state legislatures should be considered.

Pursue periodic licensee evaluation, including evidence for ongoing training and, more importantly, clinical competence. The clinical practice of therapists should be carefully examined by other therapists. The preferred outcome of such an evaluation is the steady and assured improvement of clinical practice, not a means of merely punishing licensees.

Initiate reviews of counselor's records and feedback from clients or, alternately, work with professional associations toward ensuring that such reviews are regularly completed. At least, this ensures that a provider of mental health care services does not practice alone with no feedback for long periods of time. More than this, though, such reviews ensure that clients are receiving appropriate services.

Institute procedures through which practicing clinicians can refine their clinical competence through periodic peer reviews. This, too, may involve coordination with professional associations.

Initiate open reporting systems that encourage practicing clinicians to report inadequate clinical performance by a peer, with the goal of improving client services, not with the goal of exposing poor therapists or of punishing them.

Establish a secure "court" through which compromised and/or poorly performing therapists can be monitored, again, not only for the purpose of improving service to their clients but also for the purpose of providing support for these therapists.

Require preparation programs in their jurisdiction to demonstrate that they are truly preparing providers with real clinical competence.

Likely, in coordination with professional associations and academic leaders and their programs, licensing boards should collect and distribute practice-related guidance and relevant information. Among other things, the information could/would include research related to clinical practice (e.g., What may be some of the better ways to work with personality disordered individuals?"), therapies and clinical procedures that are not useful, directories of resources for specific clinical needs, and more.

Establish "practice formularies." These formularies would indicate which approaches to therapy are acceptable and which ones are not acceptable. Further, the formularies would also specify requirements for training and indicate sources of training for those who need to acquire training in acceptable approaches.

Consider the possibility of providing research-related tools, such as EBSCO Host, for their licensees.

Likely, in coordination with professional associations and university programs, licensing boards should prepare and distribute practice evaluation procedures and instruments.

Seek to include a broad array of its licensees in formulating its policies, procedures, and regulations.

As some currently do, should require practicing clinicians to maintain a public file in which they include

A philosophy of treatment
Clinical areas of confirmed specializations
Aggregated data from client feedback
Indications of clients who are not treated
Training and certifications completed
Certifications of relevant specializations
Material used in advertising clinical services

Establish panels of reviewers who can examine the advertising of their peers and serve as sources of guidance for practicing clinicians.

Likely, in coordination with professional associations and university programs, licensing boards should define appropriate practice areas/ specializations and inappropriate ones.

Work with other licensing boards, both within their respective states and among states, to establish as much coherence as they can, with respect to the titles of degrees, the titles of licenses, and minimal requirements among all kinds of licenses.

Invite responses to any licensee or preparation program to assess rules and regulations that influence either the clinical work of practicing clinicians or the work of preparation programs.

Communicate their deliberations with all practicing clinicians under their jurisdictions.

Consider comprehensive reviews of licensing for mental health care providers, with the aim of establishing minimal coherence in such licensing, to end the current chaos.

Consider how they can mandate standards of competence for mental health care providers and ways to confirm competence.

Consider ways to eliminate fake licenses.

Consider ways to eliminate from clinical practice those who practice without a license.

Consider the immense volume of evidence that indicates what works in mental health care and the evidence that assesses the numerous approaches to treatment that have no basis in clinical reality and effectiveness.

Consider how to establish priorities of commonly recognized, clinically appropriate mental health associations that have recognized authority among licensed providers so as to assign designated regulatory authority to them. Specifically, just as they do with medical practice or engineering practice, state legislatures should consider how professional associations can enforce appropriate professional standards of clinical practice.

Along with experts among mental health care providers, should develop standards for all mental health care licensees that are reflected in every statute and regulation and that, specifically and with enforcement procedures and resources, ensure that clients receive appropriate professional mental health care. This is to place priority on the needs of clients, not their providers.

Develop statutes and regulations that protect clients from predator "providers" who lack training, appropriate credentials, and/or competence to deliver what they provide to their clients or assign the task to licensing boards.

Develop ways to regulate the advertising of mental health care providers, to ensure that members of the public are not mislead, defrauded, or otherwise harmed or potentially harmed.

Examine all corporate entities that operate as purveyors of clinical practice, when they exist, first, as non-clinical entities. These entities may include social service agencies, online corporations (e.g, BetterHelp and Calmerry), or church-sponsored services.

Examine the marketing of mental health care services, to ensure that the consuming public within their respective jurisdictions receive accurate, professionally accountable information.

Create procedures for clients to report about the quality of the mental health care services that they receive. This calls for careful examination of current, laws, rules and regulations related to such reporting. Clearly, in some states, clients—the consuming public—have little or no voice in the determining the quality of services that they receive.

Clients' perspective. Licensing boards and state legislatures seldom become the focus of attention for clients who seek and/or receive mental health care. Probably, they do not usually comprehend the critical importance that these entities of their respective state have in the care that they receive. This situation is not likely to change, at least, in the near future.

Among the likely unknown deficiencies in the services that licensing boards and state legislatures provide is that they do not protect clients from incompetent and otherwise unethical therapists, including those who practice with no license, fake licenses, harmful approaches to therapy, and more. Insofar as they become aware of these deficiencies, clients need to request and demand that their legally designated servants protect them from these deficiencies.

Social Service Agencies

More likely than not, when a social service agency provides food services for its constituency, its delivery of services is carefully regulated by the state. On behalf of the citizens of the state, the safety and nutritional value of these services for those who are served must be monitored and approved. In contrast, in most jurisdictions, there is no such assurance for those who need mental health care and receive such care from social service agencies. This lack of assurance diminishes the importance of mental health care and those elsewhere who are well-trained and qualified to provide such care.

Typically, social service agencies are very rightly mission-driven, but too often lack an evidentiary basis for what they do. In their advocacy for research in social service agencies, Tyler, Mason, Vollmer, and Trout (2021, p. 162), conclude, 'Increased practitioner and consumer involvement from the start could improve the identification and use of evidence-based solutions in practice.' Because of the extraordinary variety of social service agencies—missions, sizes, locations, funding, leadership, and so on—the advice from Tyler et al. may cover much of what needs to be recommended, with regard to those agencies that provide mental health care. Generally, if their services include mental health care, these agencies should seek consultation with duly credentialed mental health professionals, professional associations, and others, or contract with qualified providers to deliver mental health care services to their clients.

Also, individual, licensed mental health care providers who deliver counseling and therapy in the context of social service agencies should be ever mindful of their duty to their clients. This may involve not only the delivery of counseling and therapy but also advocacy within the agency for their clients and high-quality caring environments.

Businesses and Corporations

Together, counseling and therapy are a major health care service. Their providers have approached one million in number in the United States. As such, mental health care involves huge sums of money. To no one's surprise, at this time, businesses have discovered that they can own and operate counseling and therapy services for profit-making. Among them,

Talkspace	Alma	Hurdle	ReGain
Faithful Counseling	Teencounseling	Brightside	Talkiatry
BetterHelp	Pride Counseling	Calmerry,	Psychology Today
Cerebral	Core	WellVia	Telemynd,

and many others, offer online services, but some make onsite services available, too. Possibly, due to the necessity of competing successfully with other corporations, each of the corporate mental health care businesses will be driven by their obligation to ensure that services come from counselors and therapists who demonstrate integrity and competence—maybe.

For decades, the move toward the corporatization of health care generally and mental health care in particular has been an inexorable one. The reality of an individual counselor or therapist thriving in a solo practice has faded during the past few decades. Instead of this somewhat quaint view of counseling and therapy, profit-driven corporations have not only moved into the consulting room; they have also determined whether there is a consulting room, which therapists will occupy the room, and how much they can earn (e.g., Pingitore, 1999; Yenney, 1994). Rudden (2022) concludes that the ongoing expansion of corporate control of mental health care holds negative outcomes for many of the providers who deliver their professional services in and through corporations. The history of the corporatization of medical care has seen physicians lament their loss of autonomy, as autonomy has been supplanted by corporate regulations (Casalino, 2004). Whether the health care service is medical or mental health care, the challenge for all professionals who are involved is to try to achieve a workable, client-oriented, and client-serving balance between corporate control and clinician autonomy.

Given how exploitive corporations often can be, mental health care providers who demonstrate integrity and competence should be wary of excessive corporate control of their professional services. Simply put, the more money goes into the pockets of investors, the less money goes to counselors and therapists and, therefore, to serving clients. The long-term benefits or negative outcomes for the clinical practice of counseling and therapy cannot be known at this time. Given how very much is unknown, mental health care providers should not only be wary of corporate interests, but should also aim to establish cohesion among their leaders and followers so as to protect the interests of their clients and, of course, themselves. For now, some of the needed recommendations include the following ones. Corporations should

With diligence comply with the highest standards of clinical service and professional ethics, with clear priority placed on the clinically relevant needs of clients.

Take a bottom-line view of their work, of course, they should also refuse to ignore the fundamental priority of client welfare.

Examine the work of their associated counselors and therapists, with an emphasis on ensuring that clinical work stands firmly on good evidence.

Examine the work of their associated counselors and therapists, with the aim of eliminating aberrant, inappropriate procedures and orientations to counseling and therapy.

Invent or contract with those who have already invented reliable methods of evaluating clinical services, including securing feedback from clients.

Evaluate their mental health care services, with an emphasis on the outcomes of their services.

Collaborate with professional associations, with the aims of ensuring that preparation programs produce competent clinicians, seeking ways to enhance the work of the corporation and mental health providers, refining professional ethics so that they maintain currency, and sharing the pursuit of needed research that leads to support for mental health care services.

Insurance companies that issue payments to duly credentialed counselors and therapists should examine the professional advertising of their payees, to ensure that aberrant, inappropriate, and possibly harmful approaches to clinical practice are not utilized and paid for.

Insurance companies should heavily invest in their long-term welfare and profitability by intensifying its auditing of the outcomes of their mental health care providers.

Clients' perspective. The belief that counselors and therapists are good-willed and competent providers who operate an office alone or with another person or two is fantasy. The easiest, but not necessarily the most lucrative, way to develop a practice is to cooperate with a corporation. The long-term impact of these corporations is unknown. For now, professionally accountable counselors and therapists must demonstrate their rightful clinical autonomy, so long as such autonomy delivers professional services within the boundaries of the highest standards of clinical practice. Whether clients know about the dynamics of doing business as mental health care providers, they should expect that their providers can and will deliver services that express the highest standards of their profession.

A Report from the Front Lines

The urgent need for changes in clinical mental health care may seem, at times, to be a largely abstract or even an irrelevant matter. Among others, including many researchers whose work is referenced in this book, Angela Parham, Licensed Professional Counselor-Mental Health Service Provider, along with the authors of this chapter, led an effort to understand what the picture of mental health clinical practice looks like "on the front lines" and gathered information about licensed mental health care providers in Tennessee. The information that she gathered led to important observations and conclusions about the current condition of counseling and therapy in Tennessee, with added implications for counseling and therapy everywhere. Her findings have been confirmed by many others, including Cuijpers, van Straten, Bohlmeijer, Hollon, and Andersson (2010); Daniel et al. (2019); Goldberg et al. (2016); Lilienfeld, Ritschel, Lynn, Cautin, and Latzman (2014); Martin (2020); Martin and Cannon (2010); Singer and Lalich (1996); Spengler and Pilipis (2015); and Thyer and Pignotti (2015). Parham randomly selected information from the websites of 200 mental health care providers in Tennessee. The providers include

Licensed Professional Counselors	80
Licensed Clinical Social Workers	44
Licensed Marriage and Family Therapists	32
Licensed Psychologists	17
No clear identification	18
Licensed Addiction Counselor	4
Other*	4
Certified Behavior Analyst	1

*These individuals report that they have licenses in other states.

Although many different features of these providers could be analyzed and reported, only two are analyzed here: licensing status and treatment orientations. With regard to the licensing status of the providers whose information was taken from their websites, licensing may not be what it appears to be. A surprising number of individuals indicated that they held a current license, but did not. Among the 200 individuals whose advertising appeared on Psychology Today's platform, an examination of their licensing status produced the following results:

No license*	15
Confusing information**	5
Licensed in another state, but not Tennessee	3
Licensed in another state, but license expired	3
Fake licenses***	3
Tennessee licensee on probation	1
Tennessee license expired	1

* These individuals did not report that they had a license in any jurisdiction. Nothing in the records of the State of Tennessee indicated that they held a license.

** The licensing status of these individuals could be neither confirmed nor disconfirmed.

*** These are licenses that are verifiably purchased from vendors who require only payment of fees for the license. This book profiles some of these vendors elsewhere.

If no other information is reported here, the information about the licensing status among the counselors and therapists in this sample should raise concerns about licensing or the lack of licensing.

In addition, though, this report includes information about treatment orientation. The term, "treatment orientation" refers to many common approaches, such as Cognitive Behavior Therapy or Person-Centered Therapy, along with many that are not so commonly recognized. Among the 200 counselors and psychotherapists in this sample who advertise their services in Tennessee, a total of 639 treatment orientations were identified. Of these, only two—Cognitive Behavioral Therapy (172) and Trauma Focused Therapy (126)—are advertised by a majority of counselors and therapists. A more revealing number is that 535 treatment orientations are "solo" approaches. Each of these approaches is advertised by only one individual, with each of these approaches being one that none of the other 199 advertise. Forty-four treatment orientations are advertised by only two individuals.

In the context of this book, treatment orientations from this sample indicate that religion and religion-related therapies are commonly advertised, including those that are advertised by those who appear to have no training for the approaches to therapy that they advertise. Also, the likelihood is that for many of these therapies, no professionally accountable training is available.

By far, the largest identified, specifically religious approach in this sample is "Christian Counseling." Like other samples, a small minority of the individuals—only 9 of 50—who report this as a treatment orientation indicate that they have training, membership, certification, or anything else that would validate such an approach. Otherwise, the disaggregated number of religious or religion-related approaches is 294. To be clear, for example, when 50 "Christian Counseling" approaches are added to two "Christian Worldview" approaches, the total number of disaggregated approaches is 52. In contrast, an aggregated number of "Christian Counseling" approaches and "Christian Worldview" approaches is two. Thus, in contrast with the disaggregated number of 294 religious and religion-related approaches, the aggregated number is 159. Thus, among 200 counselors and therapists, 159 different religious and religion-related approaches were advertised.

Among the approaches found in the sample of 200 therapists, some were found that were truly unusual, but with some appearing to be new to the investigators and others to be truly strange, if not inappropriate. Some of those that may be new to many readers appeared to be quite broadly acceptable, if they were well-known, including AIR Network Therapy, SOMEX, BAUD Therapy, and Living-Systems Approach. Some of those that may be new to readers and likely inappropriate include Access Bars, After Death Communications, Aromatherapy, Blue Health Therapy, Herbal Medicine, Horticulture Therapy, and Sincere Approach.

A selection from the 159 different religious and religion-related approaches depends on the judgment of the reporters. Quite apart from their judgment, the necessary questions are "Are these therapies appropriate?" "Are the advertising counselors and therapists qualified to provide these therapies?" And, "What are the implications of their advertisements for the much larger body of counselors and therapists?" These questions are important, but answering them is not necessary in this discussion. Only 30 are selected, as a means of encouraging reflection on possible answers to these questions. Here are the selected approaches.

Christian Worldview	Judaeo-Christian Counseling
Past Life Regression Therapy	Ancient Hebraic Dream Interpretation
Arno Profile System	Biblical Solutions
Biblical Worldview	Christ-Centered Framework
Christian Counseling Ministry	Christian Integrative Therapy
Christian Outreach	Christian Sex Therapy
Creation Therapy	Enneagram Typing and Consultation
Honor God Therapeutic Work	Judaism Integrative Faith Counseling
Kundalini Arousal	Metaphysical Teaching and Healing
Past Life Soul Retrieval Therapy	Prayer Focused
Reiki Energy Healing	Shamanic Healing
Shamanic Journeying	Soul Collage
Spiritual Root System	Spiritual Technology
Splankna	The Art of Hearing God
Transpersonal Theology	Wisdom of the Mystics

Obviously, the future of counseling and therapy is mostly unknown. However, based on the evidence gathered for this brief report, several observations about the current condition of counseling and therapy provide important clues about possible directions of such a future. While many more observations could be made, the following ones appear to be necessary.

Understanding what counseling and therapy are is lacking. There is no broadly acceptable agreement about what counseling and therapy are and how counseling and therapy work. There is no broadly acceptable agreement about individual discretion in clinical decision-making, including the individual's options to provide explicitly religious approaches, claim expertise that is clearly lacking, or virtually every other feature of functioning as a therapist.

There is no way to eliminate incompetent therapists from practice. If they could be or had been eliminated, this report would not exist.

There is no way to eliminate from clinical practice those who hold fake licenses and pose harm to clients. This report confirms that such "licensees" are "out there" in large numbers.

Counselors and therapists, including licensing boards and professional associations, have no way to filter approaches into or out of counseling and therapy.

Clinical competence continues to decline, when this and similar reports are taken seriously.

Counselors and therapists do not like research- and evidence-based treatments. Instead, they appear to oppose evidence.

Exaggerated individualism among counselors and therapists expresses itself in wildly inappropriate ways, including numerous specifically religious ways.

Licensing boards appear to make little difference, with regard to ensuring competent mental health care.

The attributions of integrity and competence cannot now be assigned to counseling and therapy. And, until the groups named in this chapter take actions, including many of the actions recommended in this chapter, the future of counseling and therapy will see indefinite chaos, cacophony, declining integrity and competence, and dubious and declining relevance. Each conscientious, professionally accountable therapist needs to ask, "So, what can I do?"

The Right Beginning Is the End: It's All about the Client

Why do we—counselors and therapists—exist? We know the answer to this. We exist as professional mental health caregivers to provide professional services to clients. Practicing only within the boundaries of our individual areas of expertise, we diligently pursue what is best for our clients. Indeed, client welfare transcends all other considerations. This is what we believe, practice, and embody. And, when we do this, we fulfill the incredible promise of counseling and therapy. We help clients to move toward ways of living that exhibit their improved lives. When we do this, we embody hope.

References

Bowes, S. M., Ammirati, R. J., Lilienfeld, S. O., Costello, T. H., & Basterfield, C. (2020). Cognitive biases, heuristics, and logical fallacies in clinical practice: A brief field guide for practicing clinicians and supervisors. *Professional Psychology: Research and Practice*, *51*(5), 435–445. 10.1037/pro0000309

Casalino, L. P. (2004). Physicians and corporations: A corporate transformation of American medicine? *Journal of Health Politics, Policy, and Law*. *29*(4–5), 869–883.

Cozolino, L. (2004). *The making of a therapist: A practical guide for the inner journey*. New York: W. W. Norton & Company.

Cuijpers, P., van Straten, A., Bohlmeijer, E., Hollon, S. D., & Andersson, G. (2010). The effects of psychotherapy for adult depression are over-estimated: A meta-analysis of study quality and effect size. *Psychological Medicine*, *40*, 211–223.

Cummings, N. A., & O'Donohue, W. T. (Eds.) (2011). *Understanding the behavioral healthcare crisis: The promise of integrated care and diagnostic reform*. New York: Routledge.

Daniel, K. E., Jensen-Doss, A., Muroff, J., White, B. A., Reilly, E. E., Hollon, S. D., Mennin, D. S., Schuler, T. A., & Teachman, B. (2019). Characterizing evidence-based practice and training resource barriers: A needs Assessment. *Training and Education in Professional Psychology, 14*(3), 200–208.

Goldberg, S. B., Miller, S. D., Nielsen, S. L., Rousmaniere, T., Whipple, J., Hoyt, W. T., & Wampold, B. E. (2016). Do psychotherapists improve with time and experience? A longitudinal analysis of outcomes in a clinical setting. *Journal of Counseling Psychology, 63*(1), 1–11.

Lilienfeld, S. O., Ritschel, L. A., Lynn, S. J., Cautin, R. L., & Latzman, R. D. (2014). Why ineffective psychotherapies appear to work: A taxonomy of causes of spurious therapeutic effectiveness. *Perspectives on Psychological Science, 9*, 355–387.

Martin, F. A. (2020). *Therapy thieves: How to save mental health care from its providers.* New York: Oxford University Press.

Martin, F. A., & Cannon, W. C. (2010, May). A profession in peril. Counseling Today. 50–53.

Martin, F. A., & Turner, J. P. (2020). *Clinical supervision in the real world: A practical guide to ethics, legal issues, and personal development.* New York: Routledge.

Norcross, J. C., Pfund, R. A., & Cook, D. M. (2022). The predicted future of psychotherapy: A Decennial e-Delphi poll. *Professional Psychology: Research and Practice, 53*(2), 109–115.

Pingitore, D. (1999). The corporatization of psychotherapy: A study in professional transformation. In Weisgerber, K. (Ed.). (1999). *The traumatic bond between the psychotherapist and managed care.* Lanham, Maryland: Jason Aronson. pp. 217–235.

Plante, T. G. (2022). Religion has a public relations problem: Integrating evidence-based thinking into clinical practice. *Spirituality in Clinical Practice.* Advance online publication. 10.1037/scp0000292

Resnick, R. (1997). A brief history of practice expanded. *American Psychologist, 52*(4). 463–468.

Rogers, C. (1980). *A way of being.* Boston, MA: Houghton Mifflin.

Ronnestad, M. H., & Skovholt. (2013). *The developing practitioner: Growth and stagnation of therapists and counselors.* New York: Routledge.

Rudden, M. G. (2022). "A weird culture of coercion": The impact of health care corporatization on clinicians. *International Journal of Applied Psychoanalytic Studies, 19*(3), 270–290.

Singer, M. T., & Lalich, J. (1996). *Crazy therapies: What they are, do they work?* Hoboken, NJ: Jossey-Bass.

South Carolina Legislation. (2023). Entrepreneur Freedom Act. https://www.scstatehouse.gov/billsearch.php?billnumbers=3515&session=125&summary=B

Spengler, P. M., & Pilipis, L. A. (2015). A comprehensive meta-reanalysis of the robustness of the experience-accuracy effect in clinical judgment. *Journal of Counseling Psychology, 62*(3), 360–378. 10.1037/cou0000065

Thyer, B. A., & Pignotti, M. G. (2015). *Science and pseudoscience in social work practice.* New York: Springer.

Tyler, P. M., Mason, W. A., Barb Vollmer, B., & Trout, A. L. (2021). Practice to research and back in a social service agency: Trying to DO BETTER. *Child & Youth Care Forum*, *50*, 149–165. 10.1007/s10566-020-09548-3

Yalom, I. D. (2002). *The gift of therapy: An open letter to a new generation of therapists and their patients.* New York: HarperCollins.

Yenney, S. L. (1994). Trends in mental health care delivery: The corporatization of a caring profession. In S. L. Yenney (Ed.). *Business strategies for a caring profession: A practitioner's guidebook.* Washington, D.C.: American Psychological Association. pp. 17–22 10.1037/10506-003.

10 Integrity

Aspirations and Encouragement

Integrity, competence, and pluralism matter. Indeed, as individuals and a profession, we cannot thrive without demonstrated commitment to these values as operative principles and significant assets. Clearly, this book is an attempt to advocate for these principles and assets, believing that, if they are compromised and neutralized, those who need the professional assistance of counselors and therapists may not seek help and, if they seek help, will not likely find competent therapists to provide it. The large volume of empirically supported evidence that confirms the importance of these assets is undeniable. Nevertheless, doubt about the evidence may prompt others to locate their own evidence. They can locate it easily. They can visit readily available online websites of licensed and practicing therapists who may remove their doubt. For example, within a minute of beginning a search, I located a licensed therapist who blends her faith with her clinical service, saying, "I have christian [sic] prinicipals [sic] that I incorporate in therapy. (2 Timothy 1:7 KJV For God hath not given us the spirit of fear; but of power, and of love, and a sound Mind.) 'God Bless and Don't be stressed'" (Licensed Professional Counselor, 2023). I can affirm her faith and I can also feel doubt about her clinical judgment.

The urgent need for major changes in clinical practice is clear. This is a cause for action, not anxiety or panic. To gather some of the emphases in this book and add encouragement, this brief chapter comes in three parts. The first part is a brief, integrative statement about several of the challenges that this book presents. The second part is a professional's working definition of integrity. The third part is an attempt to define the work of counselors and therapists in terms of its incredibly large potential, as a heartfelt statement of encouragement.

A Brief, Integrative Statement

No doubt, numerous individuals find life-sustaining and life-affirming meaning in their religion. Nothing in this book should be construed as

DOI: 10.4324/9781003472469-11

an attack on or an affront to religion or to those who are committed to their religion. After all, I am an individual who has found significance in my religion.

Instead of an assessment of religion, this book is an assessment of the place of religion in the practice of counseling and therapy. In short, with chagrin and identifiable personal angst, I conclude that, in its tens of thousands of iterations in the practice of counseling and therapy, religion compromises and sometimes harms clients and, more broadly, the practice of counseling and therapy, while simultaneously both holding the hope that life can be better because of religion and the reality of helping clients to achieve better lives. This tormenting enigma will not disappear because it is discussed here. Instead, if this book engages counselors and therapists with their duty to maintain professional integrity and competence, they will improve their profession. Without actions toward improving it, they may lose their profession.

The most important duty of counselors and therapists is to meet the clinically relevant needs of their clients. The implementation of therapists' religion in the process of conducting therapy demonstrably and frequently mitigates against the effective fulfillment of this duty.

Counselors and therapists have a duty to continue their personal and professional development, through relevant and ongoing training, avoiding the comforting trap of resting securely in their personal experience of religion or their approach to counseling and therapy.

Counselors' and therapists' personal experiences and points of view should be honored, only because of their unique, personal, and likely positive meaning for them as individuals. However, all counselors and therapists must neutralize their preferred, personal interests and personality proclivities so that they protect the profession of which they are members and, moreover, protect the interests of their clients.

By now, the desperate need for integrity and competence in counseling and therapy has been largely made. While such a case will always be incomplete, the commitment to and the active pursuit of integrity and competence should be welcomed and pursued. Similar to the need for regular nourishment for their bodies, counselors and therapists should demonstrate their commitment to growing and sustaining their integrity and competence, perpetually replenishing them. For counselors and therapists who seek to become competent and to maintain competence with integrity, acknowledging their weaknesses becomes a duty. The process of professional development challenges all practicing therapists to actively pursue competence.

Such a pursuit likely includes active involvement in developing healthy pluralism, too. To maintain itself or thrive, the professional mental health care community must invite many differences among its members, while refusing to endorse differences that menace, threaten, and harm professional accountability within the community. Through its expanding cognizance of diversity, the community also maintains its ability to welcome differences among clients, too.

Counselors and therapists have a duty to contribute to the health and maintenance of their profession. Maximizing personal and shared accountability, this involves protecting the image and integrity of their profession and commensurately suppressing their individual desires to promote their individual interests, at the expense of their clients and/or their profession.

Counselors and therapists have a duty to express interest in, advocate for, and confidently believe in their profession and the positive potential of treatment that clients receive from it.

An individual's belief in professional accountability may be an empty belief if such a belief fails to lead to accountable actions. When expressed with integrity, though, this belief encompasses actions that demonstrate support for the duty to the welfare of clients and the profession, reliance on the best evidence for clinical practice, and, at the heart of such accountability, an ever-expanding determination to live well.

Effective provision of mental health care, including mental health care, does not and should not depend on the religious ideology of the counselors and therapists. Sooner or later, the professionally accountable mental health care community will take urgently and immediately needed actions toward eliminating the practices of those who lack minimal qualifications for practicing or suffer the consequences of their failure to do so and reckon with the possible demise of their profession. The community is bound by duty to take such actions, but not because it wishes merely to expose those with whom it seriously disagrees. Toward them, the community should demonstrate acceptance and grace, while also advocating for their improvement as professional caregivers. Ultimately, though, as this book has stated many times, the reason for the existence of mental health care professions is that they serve the clinically relevant needs of their clients. And, when individual counselors and therapist cannot or will not validate this reason for their existence, they must be excluded from the profession.

So, Now, Integrity?

Throughout this book, the concept of integrity has been a common reference. As counselors and therapists embody and enact integrity, though, it is no longer a concept, as if seeing it in print and approving it are sufficient. Indeed, if it rightly exists, integrity is embodied and enacted, because it is personal. As such, integrity is living secretly and privately the way we live openly and publicly fulfilling the highest standards of promises that we make to ourselves and our clients. In the practice of counseling and therapy, this means that living "privately" in the consulting room—or whatever the specific physical place is—closely matches the ideals that we publicly claim to be the services we deliver.

Integrity comes when *individual counselors and therapists* embody and enact the highest standards during their private consultations with their clients and vigorously uphold these standards in their public associations and relationships.

Integrity comes when the *leaders of professional associations* embody and enact the highest standards of our profession, practicing servanthood, transparency, honesty, and generosity in their leadership, and energetically investing in the ongoing improvement of our profession.

Integrity comes when faculty in *preparation programs* embody and enact the highest standards of teaching, assessing, and training effective mental health clinicians and modeling for them persons of conscience and compassion whose academic achievements are suffused with service to our profession.

Integrity comes when all of us diligently and persistently work to maintain it. This is the way it is. However, even when an individual's level of integrity is high, it may also be disappointingly low. Because the level of integrity among mental health care providers continues to sink, those who possess the highest level of integrity have seen theirs compromised, if not rejected.

Although the current condition of therapy is not what it should be, religion can be integrated into clinical practice, if it is competently and inclusively integrated with the highest integrity. This is the theme of this book. More than a mere theme for a book, though, the challenges of such integration are a sad and growing reality. In this book and elsewhere, the evidence is clear. Professional accountability among mental health care providers is being wrecked. Nevertheless, instead of lamenting the compromised condition of counseling and therapy, this book is a call to all of us to vigorously pursue integrity, competence, and inclusion. The pursuit must involve all of us—individuals, association leaders, preparation program faculty and their leaders, and others. The recommendations for action in Chapter 8 partially show us the way.

Counselors and Therapists Persist

In matters of faith, an attitude of elitism or superiority seldom serves anyone very well. Among counselors and therapists, this kind of attitude about conducting therapy, likewise, seldom serves anyone very well. In contrast with elitism and its expression in an overconfidence bias, when counselors and therapists diligently seek to prioritize the experience of their clients as the necessary focus of attention, an attitude of humility likely arises and serves the interests and needs of both clients and their professional caregivers. For counselors and therapists, this involves thoughtful, reflective honesty with one's self and, when feasible, with trusted peers. It necessarily involves growth and change. It elevates the possibility that counselors and therapists who conscientiously pursue excellence, along with the risks that inhere in such a pursuit, may acquire the characteristics of highly effective counselors and therapists and enjoy the active engagement in risking more, to achieve more, recognizing that this recursive process is a virtually endless one.

The significance of the pursuit of excellence in this discussion is that, when done well, it acknowledges, affirms, and enhances the clinical skills of counselors and therapists. More specifically, it releases them from easy comfort with familiar clinical habits and, therefore, permits them to serve the interests of their clients, including the religious interests of their clients, with elevated effectiveness. In practice, they can welcome the diverse and complex religious needs and issues that their clients bring to counseling and therapy and enjoy providing professional care for their clients. They can enact the guidelines that were discussed earlier in this book.

Religion in the practice of counseling and therapy is inevitable. After all, those who are religious are more fundamentally human than religious. And, like parenting, careers, marriages, or other human pursuits, the widest range of human concerns find their expression in religion, including everything from despair and suicide to ecstatic pleasure. This is the nature of being human, no matter what the particular pursuit may be. Likewise, counseling and therapy, as human pursuits, exhibit a very similar range of expression. Whether the population is clients or their professional caregivers, the reality of their humanity will express itself. In the end, it is this reality, along with whatever connection with transcendent beings they may discover, that holds immeasurably large potential for hope, personal meaning, positive identity, and life-affirming community. All of this is possible because we are human. Clearly, our discomfort and occasional disillusionment that come from being human confirm more than it denies. To be sure, our humanity is what alienates us from one another, particularly when we succumb to fear-based thinking, with special and specific reference to "the other," but ultimately provides the source of our unity, meaning, and purposefulness. Our humanity.

Indeed, humanity holds us captive to all things human, including the need for food, the irresistible drive to belong, and much more, but that also stimulates within us the need to feel the adventure of living, to find comfort, if not joy, in living. Those who live well persist in the adventure, discovering both the inexplicable delights and the crushing disappointments that come with it, but persistently look for ways to select and elevate the delight, while knowingly risking the reality of threatening change and disturbing losses. With all of its attendant uncertainties, the adventure of living well is worth all of the risks that inhere in it. Along with clients whom we serve, this is what we—counselors and therapists—do and who we are, when we live well.

And, even when we are beset with painful challenges—cancer, a parent with dementia, diabetes, an anguished child, an "empty nest," divorce, and many other possibilities—we persist. We persist because this is what we expect of ourselves, in our personal and relational attempts to live well, recognizing that we are indefinitely unfinished. At least, we have discovered, sometimes over and over again, that persistence meets our expectations that we can, indeed, live well. Further, our example of living well assures our clients that, during their bleakest moments, they may live well, too. Also, as ones who live well, we are far better able to help our clients. Again, this is what we do and who we are. Each of us is captive of our individual humanity, a life that comes with unspeakable potential for good. And, when we live well, almost inevitably we release this potential and invite others to find it for themselves. This is the lived ideal of freedom. We are truly free when we fulfill this potential. We soar! We persist!

As a young professional, Carl Rogers, along with his wife, Helen, determined that they would raise their children by the dictates of Watsonian behaviorism (Martin, 1973, p. 5). If they had done this, very few of us would have heard of Carl Rogers. Obviously, Rogers grew well beyond Watsonian behaviorism and, because of his growth, influenced and enriched our profession. This is to say that, within our profession, we have influencers, individuals who will forever have an impact on our profession. For me, some of them have become heroes, as I immersed in their biographies. Knowing that I cannot acknowledge all of them, I count Sigmund Freud, Carl Rogers, Aaron Beck, and George Kelly as necessary figures on my list of professional heroes. As I contemplate these figures from our history, I ask, "Why? Why are these figures important to me?" Almost inevitably, my answer is that they grew. They dared to challenge their own ideas. By risking failure, they gained success, when they opened their ideas to the scrutiny of their professional community. Instead of beginning their unknown professional trajectory with certainty about their inevitable rise to prominence, they risked going nowhere. Because they dared to be challenged, though, they became stronger and increasingly prominent in our profession. More than growing or becoming prominent, they contributed—almost immeasurably—to our professional well-being. We should emulate them, knowing that we may never achieve prominence, but also knowing that we will have made a positive difference because, like them, we dared to grow. Each of us can make a positive difference.

Finally, as we attempt to make a positive difference in our profession, our personal place in it should be recognized for what it is. Our place—my place—is not one of ownership. I can no more own my profession than I can own democracy. Like democracy, our profession must be shared. Instead of an owner's place, it is a custodian's place, a shared place. For a short time and with my peers, I have custody of this wonderful adventure called counseling and therapy. Sooner or later, no matter how strong or positive your and my custodial management of it is, you and I must pass it to others. Thus, each activity, whether it's with my peers or with clients or students, the compelling obligation is to try to ensure that their inheritance warrants their investment in sharing their custodial duty with the next generation of counselors and therapists.

References

Licensed Professional Counselor. (2023). [no title]. https://www.psychologytoday.com/us/therapists/vondolyn-lane-buffalo-ny/1061895

Martin, F. A. (1973). *A study of Carl Rogers' philosophy of persons. [Doctoral Dissertation].* Southern Baptist Theological Seminary.

Appendix

Partial List of Religion-Oriented Approaches to Counseling and Therapy

The 400 religion-related approaches to counseling and therapy in the list below is, indeed, a partial list. It is representative of the much larger, mostly not widely recognized, number of such approaches. The much larger number is not precisely known, but a gathering of religion-related approaches to counseling and therapy for this book indicates that the known number rises to approximately 11,000. Readers are encouraged to review the list, with the question about whether the items in this list represent them as individual therapists and the profession in which they are members.

99 Divine Principles
Abundant Life Christian Counseling
Adlerian Christian Counseling
Advanced Spirit Releasement Therapy
Agnostic Pastoral Counseling
Alien Abduction Therapy
Ancestral Regression Therapy
Ancient Shamanic Drum Journeys
Animal-Assisted Christian Counseling
Apostolic Counseling
Archangel Life Coaching
Asana Buddhist Principles
Authentic Christian Compassion (ACC)
A Course in Miracles
Actualized Christian Truth
Advanced DNA ThetaHealing
After-Life Christian Affirmative
Alchemical Hypnotherapy Approaches
Analytic Christian Spiritual Therapy
Ancient Christian Wisdom
Angelic Massage
Animal Spirits Guidance
Applied Christian Theology
Art-Based Christian Counseling
Attachment-Based Christian Counseling
Ayahuasca Ceremonies

Behavioral Christian Counseling
Bible Readings
Bible-Based Christian Principles
Bible-Based Theological Counseling
Bible-Centered Eclectic Approach
Biblical Christian Sex Therapy
Biblical Dream Analysis
Biblical Genetics
Biblical Life Coaching
Biblical Recasting Therapy
Biblical World View
Bible Inspired Counseling
Bible-Based Christian Approach
Bible-Based Process-Oriented Therapy
Bible-Believing Therapy
Biblical Christian Counseling and Prayer
Biblical Discipleship Counseling
Biblical Evangelical Counseling
Biblical Insights-Based Therapy
Biblical Nauthetic Principle
Biblical Transformational Healing
Biblically Based Soul Care

Biblically Based Marital Coaching
Bibliotherapeutic Christian Counseling
Brain Health Assessments—Christian
Brain-Based Christian Counseling
Buddhism and Christian Spirituality
Buddhism and Diamond Heart
Buddhism and Indigenous Art Therapy
Buddhism-Cognitive Behavioral Therapy
Buddhism/Hinduism/A Course in Miracles
Buddhism/The Chakra System/The Christ Path
Buddhist and Daoist (Taoist) Philosophies
Buddhist and Earth-Based Beliefs
Buddhist and First Nation Traditions
Buddhist and Law of Attraction Teachings
Buddhist and Shamanic Practices
Buddhist and Sufi Integrated
Buddhist Energy Psychologies
Buddhist Meditation/Soto Zen Tradition
Buddhist Psychology/Hakomi Method
Buddhist Recovery Models
Buddhist Theravada & Vajrayana Traditions
Buddhist Transpersonal & Positive Psychology
Calvary Care—Christian
Buddhist, Christian, Earth-Based et al. Therapies
Caring Christian Model
Catholic Christian Faith Oriented
Celtic Christian Orientation
Centering Christian Prayer and Meditation
Ceremonial Magic
Chakra Healing and Chakra Dance
Charismatic Christian Psychology
Chassidic Spirituality
Child-Centered Christian Play Therapy
Christa Energy Attunement
Christian Adlerian Therapy
Christian Acceptance & Commitment Therapy
Christian Archetypical Psychology
Christian Art Therapy
Christian Auditory Meditation Therapy
Christian-Based Belief Therapy
Christian-Based Existential Therapy
Christian-Based Treatment (CBT)
Christian Behavior Analysis
Christian Bible-Based Morality Orientation
Christian Body-Based Modalities
Christian Buddhism
Christian Buddhist Therapy
Christian Client-Centered Techniques
Christian Coaching
Christian Cognitive Behavior Therapy
Christian Cognitive Processing Therapy
Christian Cognitive Behavioral Play Therapy
Christian Control Mastery Therapy
Christian Counseling—Holy Spirit Guided
Christian Counseling—Shamanic Processes
Christian Couples Therapy
Christian Creationist Approach
Christian Dialectical Behavior Therapy
Christian Diamond Approach
Christian Domestic Violence Counseling
Christian Dream Interpretation
Christian Eclecticism
Christian EMDR
Christian Energy Healing
Christian Experiential Therapy
Christian Family Solutions
Christian Feminist Therapy
Christian Gestalt
Christian Gestalt Therapy
Christian God-Focused Counseling
Christian Gospel-Based Therapy
Christian Healing Process
Christian Humanistic Psychology
Christian Hypnotherapy
Christian Identity Therapy
Christian Imago Therapy
Christian Integrated Approach
Christian Integration with Depth Psychology
Christian Jungian Therapy
Christian LDS Counseling
Christian Life Coaching
Christian Marriage Sex Therapy
Christian Meditation
Christian Mysticism
Christian Narrative Therapy
Christian Natal Charts
Christian Person-Centered Therapy
Christian Philosophy
Christian Psychoanalysis
Christian Psychodrama

Christian Psychodynamic Therapy
Christian Recovery Model
Christian Sex Addiction Therapy
Christian Sex Therapy
Christian Soul Attachment
Christian Spirituality
Christian Wisdom-Based Counseling
Clearing Past Life Relationship
Dharmacharya
Distinctive Christian Point of View
Divine Nurture
Earth-Based Beliefs
Eastern Esotericism
Energy-Quantum and Spiritual Healing
Family Systems Theory-Buddhist Thought
Gnosticism
Herbalism/Buddhist Meditation/Shamanism
Indian Buddhist Tantra
Indo-Tibetan Buddhism/Christianity
Integration of Secular Buddhist Psychology
Islamic Integrated Psychotherapy
John of God Crystal Healing
Kabbalistic and Buddhist Psychology
Kabbalistic Ideology
Metaphysical Healing
Missionary Worldview
Mother Earth/Elements of Spirit
Muslim Psychotherapy
Nature-Based Buddhist-Agnostic
Nondual Kabbalistic Healing
Nouthetic Counseling
Past Life Soul Retrieval
Principles of Soul Healing Love
Quantum Angel Healing
Sacred Acoustics
Sacred Card Readings
Sacred Geometry
Sacred Plants and Nature
Salt (or Halo) Therapy
Salve Regina Expressive Arts for Healing
Samatha Samadhi (Buddhism)
Sankhya and the Upanishadic Traditions
Sat Nam Rasayan Healing
Scientology
Seichem Egyptian Energy Healing

Christian Psychology
Christian Reiki
Christian Romantic Compatibility Counseling
Christian Solution Focused
Christian Soul Coaching
Christian Systemic Therapy
Christian Yoga
Daoist (Taoist) Philosophies
Dharmacharya—Buddhist
Divine Channeling
Dory Cote Shamanic Practices
Earth-Based Religious
Eastern Mystical Traditions
Entheogenic Shamanism
Frum Therapy
Golden Angel Healing Work
Hinduism
Indo-Tibetan Buddhism
Integrated Sufism
Islam
Japanese Soto Zen Buddhism Style
Jung and Mahayana Buddhism
Kabbalistic Healing
Mary Queen of Angels Cards Readings
Buddhist Jungian Philosophy
Modern Soul Therapy
Muslim Healing
Mystery School Teachings
Nature-Based Mysticism
Neurobiology/Neuroscience/Buddhist Practices
Past Life Regression and Spirit Release
Prayer Therapy
Qabalistic Pathworking
Sacral Bars
Sacred Activations Practice
Sacred Dance
Sacred Heart Alchemy
Sai Shakti Healing
Salvation Divine Therapy
Samadhi Therapy
Samatha Samadhi Practices
Santosha Psychotherapy
Satvic Living
Scripturally Rooted Therapy
Shadow Alchemy

Shake Your Soul
Shalem Spiritual Formation
Shamanic Astrology & Meditation
Shamanic Practices
Shamanic Practices
Shambhala Buddhist Approach
Shambhala/Tibetan Vajrayana Buddhist
Shifaa Soul Counseling
Shiva Samhita
Slender Stoic Behavioral Coaching
Soto Zen Tradition
Soul and Life Purpose-Oriented
Soul Beauty Recovery
Soul Card Creation
Soul-Centered Authenticity
Soul Coaching w/Oracle Cards
Soul Coaching/Spirit Release
Soul Collage/Dreamwork
Soul Crossing
Soul Detective Protocols
Soul Discovery Counseling
Soul Encounters
Soul Evolution Processing
Soul Full Counseling
Soul Healing Love
Soul Illumination Focusing-Transformation
Soul Intentions
Soul Level Positive Psychology
Soul Life/Sacred Feminine
Soul Navigation
Soul Parenting
Soul Re-Contracting
Soul Regression Therapies
Soul Restorative Treatment
Soul Retrieval After Loss or Trauma
Soul Retrieval Hypnotherapy
Soul Sacred Journey
Soul Searching and Eclectic Techniques
Soul Sport
Soul Synergy and Coherence Therapy
Soul Therapy and Heart Relief
Soul to Soul Readings
Soul Tracking
Soul Travel & Dreamwork
Soul Work and Biblical Affirmation
Soul Work-Christ-Centered

Shakti Rising Model
Shamanic and Ancestral Journeying
Shamanic Drumming Circle
Shamanic Healing (Mesa Carrier, Peruvian Inkan)
Shamanism
Shambhala & Tibetan Vajrayana Buddhist Traditions
Shaolin Temple Energy Healing
Shiome Therapy
Skydancing Tantra
Soteriological Counseling
Soul Alignment
Soul Attachment Work
Soul Biofield Tuning
Soul Care Christian Counseling
Soul Circle
Soul Coaching—Scripture/Prayer/Worship
Soul Collage (Split Eye Reading/Lineage Work)
Soul Communion
Soul Cultivation
Soul Directed Advanced Energy Healing
Soul Drama
Soul Entrainment Therapy
Soul Expansion Shamanic Mentorship
Soul Growth Methods
Soul Healing Love and Imago Therapy
Soul Integration Therapy
Soul Journeys for Akashic Studies
Soul Life
Soul Loss/Soul Retrieval
Soul Oriented Empathic Counseling
Soul Play
Soul Reading
Soul Repair
Soul Retrieval & Past Life Regression
Soul Retrieval & Spiritual Emergency Therapy
Soul Retrieval/Functional Nutrition Coaching
Soul Schooling
Soul Spa
Soul Surfing
Soul Therapy and Generational Healing
Soul Ties
Soul Ties-Trust and Love-Based Connections
Soul Travel
Soul Wisdom Therapy
Soul Work Interventions
Soul Work/Regression Therapy

Soul Wounds Therapy
Soul-Based Ceremonies
Soul-Centered BreathWork
Soul-Centered Depth Psychology-informed
Soul-Centered Embodied Experiencing
Soul-Centered Psychoshamanic Approaches
Soul-Centered Work/Contemplative
Soul-Focused Feng Shui
Soul-Level Experiential Therapy
Soul-Life Integration/Crystals-Essential Oils
Soul-Satisfying Attachments Orientation
SoulCollage the Divine Spirit
SoulCycle Barre or Pilates
Soulshine Astrology
SoulTalk/SoulCare
SOULution-Focused Therapy
Sound Foundation in the Word of God
South American Toltec Shamanic Traditions
Spinal Release Technique
Spirit Junkie Masterclass
Spiritual Ascension Therapy (SAT)
Spiritual Herbalism
Spiritual Mentoring (Order of Melchizedek)
Spiritual Sex Therapy
Spiritual Treatment/Theophostic Prayer
Spiritual Warriorship Therapy
Splankna: EMDR TFT NET ACT RRCMT
Star Astronumerology
Sufi Mysticism
Swami Omkarananda Model
Sychronizes Soul
Tarot and Mediumship Readings
Theravada and Vajrayana Traditions
Tibetan Buddhist Chod Ritual
Torah-Based Therapy
Transpersonal & Positive Psychology
Trauma-Informed Buddhism
Whole Christian Life Integration
Wicca
Women's Christian Therapy

Soul Writing
Soul-Body-Mind Therapy
Soul-Centered Counseling/Sacred
Soul-Centered Dream Work
Soul-Centered Jungian Depth Psychotherapy
Soul-Centered Regression Hypnosis
Soul-Directed Energy Healing
Soul-Heart-Mind-Body Perspective
Soul-Life Integration Healing
Soul-Life Integration/Shamanic Healing
Soul/Spirit/Imaginal/Abstract Levels
SoulCollage Transpersonal Therapy
SoULL
SoulSpace
Soulumination
Sound Alchemy-Crystal/Tibetan singing bowls
Sound Mnemonics and Crystal Healing
Spartan SGX Coaching/Sports Contexted
Spirit 2 Spirit-CTT
Spirit Releasement and UFO/ET encounters
Spiritual Golden Angel Healing Support
Spiritual Medium/Clairvoyant
Spiritual Root System
Spiritual Stargates
Spiritual Warfare Preparation
Spiritually Fluent Psychotherapy
Sri Kaleshwar Follower/Approach
Stardreaming
Stoic Philosophical Orientation Therapy (STOP)
Sweatlodge Ceremonies
Tao of Self-Realization
The Christ Path
Throne Room Therapy
Tibetan Mongolian Buddhism
Transformational Christian Therapy
Transpersonal Therapy
Twelve-Step Christian Approach
Whole Person Christian Approach
Wise Christian Counseling
Word of God Christian Counseling

Index

Note: **Bold** page numbers refer to charts.